Cardiac Biomarkers

Alan S. Maisel • Allan S. Jaffe

Editors

Cardiac Biomarkers

Case Studies and Clinical Correlations

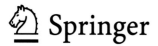 Springer

Editors
Alan S. Maisel
Division of Cardiovascular Medicine
University of California San Diego
La Jolla, CA
USA

Allan S. Jaffe
Cardiology Department
Mayo Clinic
Rochester, MN
USA

ISBN 978-3-319-42980-9   ISBN 978-3-319-42982-3   (eBook)
DOI 10.1007/978-3-319-42982-3

Library of Congress Control Number: 2016955804

Printed on acid-free paper

This Springer imprint is published by Springer Nature
The registered company is Springer International Publishing AG Switzerland

Dedicated to Dr. Burton E. Sobel, whose pioneering work on creatine kinase and tireless mentoring were instrumental in helping us understand the importance of biomarkers, and my partner in crime at Washington University where we validated the initial assay for cTnI, Dr. Jack Ladenson.

Allan S. Jaffe, MD

Preface

Biomarkers now play an integral role in the treatment and management of patients with congestive heart failure and acute ischemic heart disease because of the important information the values provide. All of us in the field are terribly interested in how to optimally use these biomarkers and particularly to understand when values provide actionable information. However, extrapolating a large compendium of information to the average clinician is difficult because many do not have the underlying basic science, laboratory, and/or clinical expertise about the use of these markers.

Accordingly, it seemed to us that there was a need to develop a case-based compendium of learning. For that reason, we asked our most knowledgeable colleagues to help us generate a book that hopefully comprehensively informs clinicians about how to optimally deploy the major clinically utilized biomarkers in a case-based manner. From scrutinizing the chapters, it appears we have succeeded. We hope you will enjoy and learn from the case studies as much as we have.

La Jolla, CA, USA   Alan S. Maisel, MD
Rochester, MN, USA   Allan S. Jaffe, MD

Acknowledgments

I would first like to acknowledge the now deceased Dr. Ralph Shabetai, who, as my first cardiology section chief, taught me the fine balance with the art and science of medicine. Never have I met a more selfless and giving man than Ralph. Second, I would like to thank my laboratory personnel, without whose help and support over these many years I would never have been half as productive as I have been. A special thanks to my lab director, Stever Carter, for 30 years of unwavering loyalty. I would be remiss if I did not thank my five children, who remind me on a daily basis why I inhabit the earth. Finally, my wife, Fran, thank you for putting up with long hours, extensive travel, and a crazy sense of humor.

Alan S. Maisel, MD

Contents

Contributors

Joseph S. Alpert, MD Department of Medicine, Sarver Heart Center, University of Arizona College of Medicine, Tucson, AZ, USA

Mayo Clinic, Rochester, MN, USA

Fred S. Apple, PhD Clinical Laboratories, Hennepin County Medical Center, Minneapolis, MN, USA

Department of Laboratory Medicine and Pathology, University of Minnesota, Minneapolis, MN, USA

Boris Arbit, MD Division of Cardiovascular Medicine, Department of Medicine, University of California, San Diego, La Jolla, CA, USA

Antoni Bayes-Genis, MD, PhD Department of Cardiology, Heart Failure Unit, Heart Institute, Hospital Universitari Germans Trias i Pujol, Badalona, Barcelona, Spain

Hospital Universitari Germans Trias i Pujol, Badalona, Spain

Daniel Chan, BMedSci, BMBS Department of Cardiovascular Sciences, University of Leicester, Leicester, UK

NIHR Leicester Cardiovascular Biomedical Research Unit, Glenfield Hospital, Leicester, UK

Horng H. Chen, MB, BCh Division of Cardiovascular Diseases, Department of Internal Medicine, Mayo Clinic and Foundation, Rochester, MN, USA

Robert Colbert, BS University of Minnesota Medical School, Minneapolis, MN, USA

Paul Ormandy Collinson, MA, MB, BChir, FRCPath, MD Clinical Blood Sciences and Cardiology, St George's Hospital and Medical School, London, UK

Louise Cullen, MB, BS Department of Emergency Medicine, Royal Brisbane and Women's Hospital, Herston, QLD, Australia

Lori B. Daniels, MD, MAS Division of Cardiovascular Medicine, University of California, San Diego, CA, USA

Christopher R. deFilippi, MD Department of Medicine, University of Maryland School of Medicine, Maryland Heart Center University of Maryland Medical Center, Baltimore, MD, USA

Salvator DiSomma, MD, PhD Department of Internal Medicine, Emergency Medicine, San Andrea Hospital, San Andrea, CA, USA

Department of Medical-Surgery Sciences and Translational Medicine, University Rome Sapienza, Rome, Italy

Kai M. Eggers, MD, PhD Departments of Medical Sciences, Cardiology, Uppsala University Hospital and Uppsala University, Uppsala, Sweden

Ugochukwu O. Egolum, MD Division of Cardiovascular Medicine, Vanderbilt University Medical Center, Nashville, TN, USA

Roxana Ghashghaei, MD Department of Internal Medicine, University of California San Diego Health System, San Diego, CA, USA

Evangelos Giannitsis, MD Department of Internal Medicine III, Cardiology, University Hospital Heidelberg, Medizinische Klinik III, Heidelberg, Germany

Trenton M. Gluck, BS Division of Cardiovascular Medicine, Department of Medicine, Veterans Affairs San Diego Healthcare System, San Diego, CA, USA

James Iwaz, MD Department of Internal Medicine, UCSD Medical Center, San Diego, CA, USA

Allan S. Jaffe, MD Cardiology Department and Department of Laboratory Medicine and Pathology, Mayo Clinic, Rochester, MN, USA

Steven R. Jones, MD Division of Cardiology, Johns Hopkins Hospital, The Johns Hopkins Ciccarone Center for the Prevention of Heart Disease, Baltimore, MD, USA

Hugo A. Katus, MD Department of Internal Medicine III, Cardiology, University Hospital Heidelberg, Medizinische Klinik III, Heidelberg, Germany

David E. Krummen, MD Division of Cardiovascular Medicine, University of California San Diego, San Diego, CA, USA

Division of Cardiovascular Medicine, VA San Diego Healthcare System, San Diego, CA, USA

Elizabeth Lee Division of Cardiovascular Medicine, Department of Medicine, University of California, San Diego, La Jolla, CA, USA

Noel S. Lee, MD Division of Cardiovascular Medicine, Department of Medicine, Sulpizio Cardiovascular Center, University of California, San Diego, La Jolla, CA, USA

Daniel J. Lenihan, MD Division of Cardiovascular Medicine, Vanderbilt University Medical Center, Nashville, TN, USA

Bertil Lindahl, MD, PhD Uppsala Clinical Research Center and Department of Medical Sciences, Uppsala University Hospital, Uppsala, Sweden

Josep Lupón, MD, PhD Heart Failure Unit, Heart Institute, Hospital Universitari Germans Trias i Pujol, Badalona, Spain

Department of Medicine, Universitat Autònoma de Barcelona, Barcelona, Spain

Johannes Mair, MD Department of Internal Medicine III – Cardiology and Angiology, Innsbruck Medical University, Innsbruck, Austria

Alan S. Maisel, MD, FACC Division of Cardiovascular Medicine, Department of Medicine, University of California San Diego, La Jolla, CA, USA

Department of Medicine, Coronary Care Unit and Heart Failure Program, Veterans Affairs San Diego Healthcare System, San Diego, CA, USA

Nicholas Marston, MD Department of Internal Medicine, UCSD Medical Center, San Diego, CA, USA

Seth S. Martin, MD, MHS The Johns Hopkins Ciccarone Center for the Prevention of Heart Disease, Baltimore, MD, USA

Wayne L. Miller, MD, PhD Department of Cardiovascular Diseases, Mayo Clinic, Rochester, MN, USA

Rohit Mital, MD Department of Internal Medicine, University of California, San Diego, Medical Center, San Diego, CA, USA

M. Möckel, MD, PhD Division of Emergency Medicine and Department of Cardiology, Campus Virchow Klinikum and Campus Charité Mitte, Charité – Universitätsmedizin, Berlin, Germany

Leong Ng, MD Department of Cardiovascular Sciences, University of Leicester, Leicester, UK

NIHR Leicester Cardiovascular Biomedical Research Unit, Glenfield Hospital, Leicester, UK

Ravi H. Parikh, MD Department of Medicine, University of Maryland School of Medicine, Baltimore, MD, USA

W. Frank Peacock, MD, FACEP Department of Emergency Medicine, Baylor College of Medicine, Houston, TX, USA

Ben Taub General Hospital, Houston, TX, USA

Alex Pearce, BA Department of Internal Medicine, University of California, San Diego, San Diego, CA, USA

Matthew N. Peters, MD Department of Cardiovascular Medicine, University of Maryland Medical Center, Baltimore, MD, USA

Nicholas Phreaner, MD Department of Internal Medicine, University of California, San Diego, San Diego, CA, USA

Renato Quispe, MD The Johns Hopkins Ciccarone Center for the Prevention of Heart Disease, Baltimore, MD, USA

Amy K. Saenger, PhD, DABCC Department of Laboratory Medicine and Pathology, University of Minnesota, Minneapolis, MN, USA

Yader Sandoval, MD Division of Cardiology, Hennepin County Medical Center/Abbott Northwestern Hospital, Minneapolis, MN, USA

J. Searle, MD, MPH Division of Emergency Medicine and Department of Cardiology, Campus Virchow Klinikum and Campus Charité Mitte, Charité – Universitätsmedizin, Berlin, Germany

Kevin Shah, MD Department of Internal Medicine, University of California San Diego, San Diego, CA, USA

Pam R. Taub, MD, FACC Division of Cardiovascular Medicine, Department of Medicine, University of California, San Diego, La Jolla, CA, USA

Martin Paul Than, MB, BS Emergency Department, Chirstchurch Hospital, Christchurch, New Zealand

Kristian Thygesen, MD, DSc, FACC Department of Cardiology, Aarhus University Hospital, Aarhus, Denmark

Per Venge, MD, PhD Departments of Medical Sciences, Cardiology and Clinical Chemistry, Uppsala University Hospital and Uppsala University, Uppsala, Sweden

Siu-Hin Wan, MD Department of Internal Medicine, Division of Cardiovascular Diseases, Mayo Clinic and Foundation, Rochester, MN, USA

Alan H.B. Wu, PhD Department of Laboratory Medicine, University of California, San Francisco, San Francisco General Hospital, San Francisco, CA, USA

Part I
Ischemic Heart Disease

Chapter 1
Pre-analytical Factors and Analytical Issues Affecting Interpretation of Cardiovascular Biomarkers

Amy K. Saenger

Abstract The Universal Definition of Myocardial Infarction globally endorses cardiac troponin (T and I; cTnT, cTnI) as the biomarker of choice for the diagnosis and assessment of acute coronary syndrome (ACS) and should be utilized routinely in patients with symptoms suggestive of acute myocardial infarction (AMI) [1]. Despite the widespread use of troponin in clinical practice there remain a number of pre-analytical, analytical and interpretive issues which can confound clinical interpretation and will likely be magnified with high-sensitivity troponin assays. The following case studies and discussion highlight some of these issues and nuances associated with troponin assays.

Keywords Troponin • High-sensitivity troponin • Myocardial infarction • Acute coronary syndrome • Chest pain • Biomarker • Hemolysis • Interferences • Heterophile • Antibody

The Universal Definition of Myocardial Infarction globally endorses cardiac troponin (T and I; cTnT, cTnI) as the biomarker of choice for the diagnosis and assessment of acute coronary syndrome (ACS) and should be utilized routinely in patients with symptoms suggestive of acute myocardial infarction (AMI) [1]. Despite the widespread use of troponin in clinical practice there remain a number of pre-analytical, analytical and interpretive issues which can confound clinical interpretation and are likely magnified with high-sensitivity troponin assays. The following case studies and discussion highlight some of these issues and nuances associated with troponin assays.

A.K. Saenger, PhD, DABCC
Department of Laboratory Medicine and Pathology, University of Minnesota,
Minneapolis, MN, USA
e-mail: saen0006@umn.edu

© Springer International Publishing Switzerland 2016
A.S. Maisel, A.S. Jaffe (eds.), *Cardiac Biomarkers*,
DOI 10.1007/978-3-319-42982-3_1

Case 1

A 68-year-old African-American male presents to the emergency room with complaints of indigestion, mild chest pain and shortness of breath. The onset of pain began approximately 4 h prior and would last intermittently for 15 min. He has no previous history of overt coronary heart disease but was overweight with a body mass index of 28 and new onset of mild hypertension. His initial electrocardiogram (ECG) shows mild T-wave flattening in the lateral leads along with other non-specific changes. A cardiac chest pain protocol was ordered which included serial cardiac troponin testing. The baseline plasma cTnT was 0.04 ng/mL (99th percentile: <0.01 ng/mL) and the patient was placed in the chest pain observation area where he was given nitroglycerin to assist with his chest and abdominal discomfort. Three hours later nursing staff in the emergency department drew another sample for cTnT testing. The laboratory called approximately 30 min later to inform ED staff that the 3-h sample was hemolyzed and recommended the patient be redrawn. There was insistence that the result be released and the technologist reported the 3-h cTnT result of 0.02 ng/mL. The patient's pain appeared to be resolving, his TIMI score was 1 and he was deemed low-risk and discharged. Ten hours post-discharge his wife found him unconscious and called 911. She was able to rouse him and he was transported to the same emergency department via ambulance. Upon arrival it was noted that his ECG remained non-diagnostic but cTnT was now 0.12 ng/mL. He was admitted for coronary catheterization and ultimately diagnosed with NSTEMI. Further investigation into the laboratory results reveal the patient's first cTnT specimen was deemed "mildly hemolyzed but acceptable" and the second cTnT specimen was "grossly hemolyzed" but released per physician request.

Discussion of Case 1

This scenario illustrates how pre-analytical variables such as hemolysis can drastically affect the analytical results and potentially result in serious patient safety risks. Reliability of the cTn measurement depends on the quality and integrity of the blood specimen collected, as with all analytes measured using central laboratory or point-of-care (POC) assays. Pre-analytical variables have significant potential to confound cTn measurement and can produce falsely elevated or falsely decreased results. Serious risk exists if a rise and/or fall in cTn values is masked or falsely detected by the presence of interfering substances in patient specimens and can adversely impact medical decision-making and patient care. Understanding about the pre-analytical factors and interferences that can influence cTn measurements is critical in order to establish strategies to assure collection of quality specimens, prevent reporting erroneous results, and identify scenarios when cautious interpretation of cTn results is warranted.

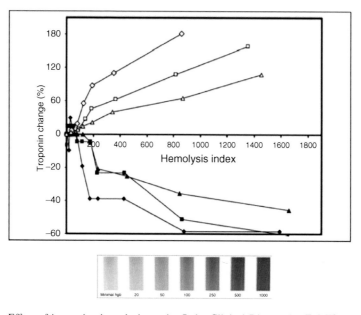

Fig. 1.1 Effect of increasing hemolysis on the Ortho Clinical Diagnostics TnI ES assay (*open symbols*) and the Roche hs-cTnT assay (*closed symbols*). *Note that the negative and positive scales are not equal (From Bais [4], reproduced with permission from the American Association for Clinical Chemistry)

Hemolysis is defined as the breakdown of erythrocytes with subsequent release of intracellular contents and is a known interference of a majority of cTnI and cTnT immunoassays [2–4]. Specimens collected from patients in the Emergency Department have high rates (up to 20%) of contamination due to hemolysis [5]. Hemolyzed specimens can cause either a positive or negative bias in troponin measurements, and although the bias is assay-specific in general hemolysis causes false-negative results in cTnT assays and false-positives in cTnI assays (Fig. 1.1) [4]. Florkowski *et al.* illustrated that specimens with cTnT concentrations near the 99th percentile reference interval (<14 ng/L) exhibited up to a 50% negative interference with increasing hemolysis in the Roche high-sensitivity cTnT (hs-cTnT) assay, whereas the Vitros ECi cTnI assay demonstrated a positive interference up to 576% with increasing hemolysis [2]. The mechanism of hemolysis interference remains unclear; it has been suggested that the release of hemoglobin and proteases from erythrocytes upon lysis may cause interference with the detection method or anti-cTn antibody recognition of degraded cTn fragments [3, 6, 7]. Plasma specimens are also more sensitive to hemolysis compared to serum which is unfortunate since plasma is the primary specimen type used in the emergency room and critical care patient areas [8].

The presence of hemolysis can be visually detected as a pink to red color when hemoglobin concentrations are >0.2 g/dL [9]. However, visual examination of specimen color is extremely subjective. Central laboratory analyzers are typically capable of performing automated spectrophotometric detection of hemoglobin to reliably detect hemolysis and aid in defining acceptable specimen rejection criteria. Unfortunately, there is no way to detect hemolysis in whole blood samples which is the primary specimen type used for POC cTn testing. Laboratories must implement acceptance/rejection criteria for hemolyzed specimens to assure accurate troponin results are reported, as well as monitor hemolysis rates originating from areas such as the emergency department where specimens are often not collected by phlebotomy staff.

Case 2

A 58-year-old Caucasian male with type 2 diabetes has been on hemodialysis for approximately a year and currently being evaluated for renal transplantation. He abruptly develops acute dyspnea and is unable to remain ambulatory without mild chest pain, therefore he is transported to the local emergency room. He denies a history of prior cardiovascular events or known coronary disease. His ECG is notable for an ST-segment depression and T waves. A baseline cTnI was measured using a point-of-care (POC) assay which was within normal limits (99th percentile: <0.08 ng/mL). A second POC cTnI result obtained 4 h later was also <0.08 ng/mL. The biomarker protocol at this institution required confirmation of all POC cTnI results with the central laboratory cTnI automated assay. The emergency medicine physician treating the patient received a call from the laboratory that the central lab cTnI results were 0.06 ng/mL for the baseline sample and 0.11 ng/mL for the 4-h sample, which was greater than the automated cTnI assay's 99th percentile (<0.04 ng/mL) and indicated a significant delta (change) over this acute time period. Based on this information, the patient is immediately taken to cardiac catheterization and a diagnosis of NSTEMI is made. The physician was puzzled regarding the lack of concordance between the two cTnI methods and also inquired if the reason was due to the automated "high-sensitivity" cTnI assay.

Discussion of Case 2

This case demonstrates the critical importance of understanding the limitations of the troponin assay used, regardless if the assay is POC or performed in the central laboratory. In addition, it highlights issues related to the lack of standardization between cTnI assays and the heterogeneous nomenclature used to describe assays.

Contemporary POC troponin methods are analytically and clinically less sensitive compared to central lab assays and there are currently no high-sensitivity POC assays available [10, 11]. Therefore, current guidelines recommend use of central laboratory troponin testing as opposed to POC. In a study reported by Apple et al., the ratio of measured 99th percentile to the limit of detection (LoD) across five different POC cTn test systems demonstrated considerable variability and substantially lower than automated hs-cTn and contemporary cTn assays [12]. Consequently, POC assays often produce undetectable cTn concentrations with lower clinical sensitivity to rule-in AMI or to use for predicting future adverse events in patients presenting to the emergency department with symptoms suggestive of cardiac ischemia [13–17]. This is a major concern in clinical practice as the limited analytical sensitivity of POC assays can lead to missed or delayed diagnosis of patients at-risk for ACS who may benefit from medical intervention. Further improvement in the analytical sensitivity of POC cTn test systems by manufacturers is needed in order to complement the growing utilization and superior diagnostic performance of high-sensitivity assays.

If the central laboratory is unable to meet a 60-min turnaround time (TAT; defined here as time from collection to reporting in the electronic medical record) a majority (>90 % of the time) for cTn testing, then POC testing should be considered although frequently an optimal TAT can be achieved after resolving operational issues and/or inefficiencies. Although use of POC cTn assays clearly improves TAT and availability of results [18, 19], having a more rapid test does not guarantee improved patient outcomes, operational efficiency, or cost effectiveness. Results vary regarding the effect of POC testing in reducing patient length of stay (LOS), patient charges and overall cost effectiveness [18, 20–22]. Whether POC cTn testing improves triage, treatment, and/or discharge of NST-ACS patients largely depends on the effectiveness of integration into the operational workflows and clinical protocols for each hospital or healthcare system.

Standardization and harmonization efforts have focused on cTnI assays, which are available from a wide variety of manufacturers and analytical platforms. Standardization is generally not an issue for cTnT because only one diagnostic company (Roche Diagnostics) holds the patent and antibodies for cTnT, with the caveat that there are known cTnT analytical differences evident between small and large platforms [23]. There are several cTnI diagnostic assays commercially available with variable analytical and clinical performance characteristics and different target antibodies (Table 1.1). The International Federation of Clinical Chemistry (IFCC) website (http://www.ifcc.org/) maintains a collated and updated list of these assays. Anti-cTnI antibody cross-reactivity with cTnI is dependent upon epitope recognition; however, the cTnI complex can also undergo substantial modifications after release into circulation including oxidation, reduction, phosphorylation and proteolytic degradation which can change its interaction with other troponins and anti-cTnI antibodies.

Despite some success with harmonization efforts for cTnI, significant inter-assay differences remain with up to a ten-fold difference in absolute cTnI concentrations [24]. The discordance in numeric cTnI values between assays and methods can largely be attributed to the diversity of different materials utilized for calibrators, as well as the variety of detection and capture antibodies used which have differing antigen epitope specificities (Table 1.1). Current cTnI calibration materials are only traceable to different calibrators selected by each manufacturer; consequently, cTnI results are not interchangeable between different assays and testing platforms.

Table 1.1 Analytical characteristics of selected contemporary troponin assays

Company/platform/assay	Cardiac troponin concentrations at:			Amino acid residues of epitopes recognized by capture (C) and detection (D) mAbs
	LoD[a], ng/mL	99th percentile, ng/mL (CV)[b]	10 % CV concentration, ng/mL	
Laboratory test systems				
Abbott AxSYM ADV	0.02	0.04 (14 %)	0.16	C: 87–91, 41–49; D: 24–40
Abbott ARCHITECT	0.009	0.028 (14 %)	0.032	C: 87–91, 24–40; D: 41–49
Beckman Access AccuTnI	0.01	0.04 (14 %)	0.06	C: 41–49; D: 24–40
bioMerieux Vidas Ultra	0.01	0.01 (27.7 %)	0.11	C: 41–49, 22–29; D: 87–91, MAb 7B9
Ortho Vitros ECi ES	0.12	0.034 (10 %)	0.034	C: 24–40, 41–49; D: 87–91
Roche Elecsys TnT Gen 4	0.01	<0.01	0.03	C: 136–147; D 125–131
Roche Elecsys TnI	0.16	0.16 (10 %)	0.3	C: 87–91, 190–196; D: 23–29, 27–43
Siemens Centaur Ultra	0.006	0.04 (8.8 %)	0.03	C: 41–49, 87–91; D: 27–40
Siemens Dimension RxL	0.04	0.07 (20 %)	0.14	C: 27–32; D: 41–56
Siemens Vista	0.015	0.045 (10 %)	0.04	C: 27–32; D: 41–56
Tosoh AIA	0.06	<0.06 (NA)	0.09	C: 41–49; D:87–91
Point of care test systems				
Abbott i-STAT	20	0.08 (16.5 %)	0.1	C: 41–49, 88–91; D: 28–39, 62–78
Alere Triage	50	<0.05 (NA)	NA	C: NA; D: 27–40
Alere Triage Cardio3[c]	10	0.02 (17 %)	NA	C: 27–39; D: 83–93, 190–196
Mitsubishi Pathfast	8	0.029 (5.0 %)	0.014	C: 41–49; D: 71–116, 163–209
Radiometer AQT90 cTnI	9	0.023 (17.7 %)	0.039	C: 41–49, 190–196; D: 137–149
Radiometer AQT90 cTnT	8	0.017 (15.2 %)	0.026	C: 125–131; D: 136–147
Response RAMP	30	<0.01 (18.5 % at 50)	0.21	C: 85–92; D: 26–38
Roche cobas h232 Cardiac T[c,d]	50	NA	NA	C: 125–131; D: 136–147
Roche Cardiac Reader cTnT[c]	0.03	NA	NA	C: 125–131; D: 136–147
Siemens Stratus CS	0.03	0.07 (10 %)	0.06	C: 27–32; D: 41–56

Table 1.1 (continued)

Adapted from Apple et al. [10], reproduced with permission from the American Association for Clinical Chemistry

[a]*LoD* limit of detection, *mAbs* monoclonal antibodies, *NA* not available, *Gen 4* fourth-generation

[b]*CV* coefficient of variation at 99th percentile

[c]Not cleared by the US Food and Drug Administration

[d]Standardized against hs-cTnT assay

[e]Standardized against Gen 4 cTnT assay

Although release of cTnT and cTnI from damaged cardiomyocytes should theoretically occur in equimolar amounts, absolute values for cTnT and cTnI between different assays are vastly different and poorly correlate. Some differences can be attributed to different clearance rates, ratio of free cTnI and cTnT pools and stability of circulating cTnI and cTnT.

In the absence of standardized cTnI assays, assay-specific cTnI decision thresholds (99th percentiles and acute change criteria) must be validated or verified for each assay and laboratory which a majority of facilities are underpowered to carry out, in terms of resources and expertise. It is important not to extrapolate cTnI reference values, results and decision thresholds between cTnI assays until cTnI assay standardization is successfully achieved, although in the author's opinion this is unlikely to happen anytime soon. Accordingly, healthcare systems reporting cTnI results across multiple manufacturer assays or testing platforms and merging results into a single electronic patient medical record must effectively differentiate the cTnI results by assay in order to minimize patient safety risks associated with misinterpretation of results.

While there are some analytical differences in cTnT assays dependent upon platform, the major differences are between the fourth-generation cTnT assays used in the United States and the fifth-generation TnT (also referred to as "high-sensitivity cTnT" or hs-cTnT) assays available everywhere except for the United States. The fourth-generation cTnT assay uses the M11.7 capture antibody and M7 detection antibody to recognize residues 136–147 and 125–131, respectively [23, 25]. The hs-cTnT assays utilize the M7 detection antibody and a chimeric derivative of the M11.7 detection antibody to generate the 5D8 detection antibody that similarly recognizes residues 136–147. Analytical evaluation between 4th and 5th generation cTnT assays demonstrate substantial positive bias (76 %) in measured cTnT values at the low end of the measuring range (<50 ng/L; <0.05 ng/mL) using the hs-cTnT assay compared with a fourth-generation cTnT assay [23]. The discordance between designated contemporary assays and high-sensitivity assays for both cTnT and cTnI could generate significant clinical confusion and potentially impact future standardization efforts of cTnI assays.

The lack of standardization in automated and POC troponin assays necessitates the need for assay-specific reference limits. Diverse 99th percentile reference intervals and systematic biases between POC and automated assays exist, even in methods which use the same antibodies designed to recognize the same antigen epitopes.

Table 1.2 Analytical characteristics of high-sensitivity troponin assays

| Company/ platform/assay | Cardiac troponin concentrations at: | | | Measureable values in reference participants > LOD (%) | Amino acid residues of epitopes recognized by capture (C) and detection (D) mAbs[b] |
	LoD[a], ng/L	10 % CV concentration, ng/L	99th percentile, ng/L		
hs-cTnI test systems					
Abbott ARCHITECT[c,d]	1.2	3.0	F: 16 M: 34	96	C: 24–40; D 41–49
Beckman Access[d]	2.1	8.6	F: 9 M: 11	80	C: 41–49; D: 24–40
Ortho-Clinical Diagnostics Vitros[d]	1.0	6.5	F: 16 M: 19	75	C: 24–40, 41–49; D: 87–91
Singulex Erenna MTP[e]	0.1	0.9	F: 15 M: 27	100	C: 41–49; D: 27–41
Siemens Vista[d]	0.8	3.0	F: 33 M: 55	86	C: 30–35; D: 41–56, 171–190
hs-cTnT test system					
Roche E601[c,d]	2.0	13	F: 14 M: 22	25	C: 136–147; D: 125–131

[a]*LOD* limit of detection
[b]*mAbs* monoclonal antibodies
[c]Not cleared by the US Food and Drug Administration
[d]For research use
[e]Available as commercial test through Singulex

Dupuy *et al.* identified discrepant results in a comparison of a POC cTnT assay versus a central laboratory hs-cTnT, with 41 % of samples presenting with cTnT values above the central laboratory hs-cTnT 99th percentile reference limit (<14 ng/L) but below the POC cTnT 99th percentile reference limit (<17 ng/L) [15]. Noteworthy, poor clinical concordance was observed despite the use of assay-specific cutoffs [15, 17], which is likely attributed to varying analytical sensitivities of the assays. Discordance in cTn results obtained between POC and lab cTn assays can confound appropriate interpretation of the clinical situation [14]; therefore, dual utilization of POC and central lab cTn testing within a hospital or healthcare system should be avoided.

Finally, review of peer-reviewed literature reveals descriptive verbiage and terminology regarding troponin assays (e.g., ultrasensitive, high performance, highly sensitive, high-sensitivity) which leads to a common misperception that one may be using a high-sensitivity assay when indeed they are not. The analytical characteristics of current high-sensitivity troponin assays are shown in Table 1.2; no hs-cTn assays are approved by the Food and Drug Administration for use in the United States. An analytical troponin scorecard has been developed and endorsed by the International Federation of Clinical Chemistry (IFCC) (Fig. 1.2) [26]. The first tier

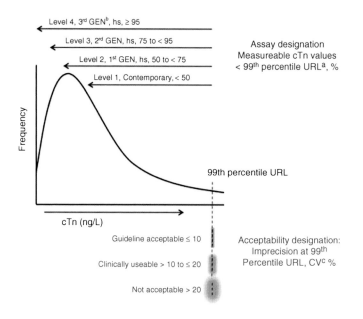

Fig. 1.2 IFCC scorecard classification of troponin assays. [a]*URL* upper reference limit, [b]*GEN* generation; hs, high-sensitivity, [c]*CV* coefficient of variation at 99th percentile URL (Adapted from Apple et al. [26], with permission)

criteria are based upon analytical sensitivity and designated based on the percentage of normal subjects who have measureable values above the limit of detection (LoD) but below the 99th percentile reference limit. The second tier criteria evaluate assay imprecision at the 99th percentile and classify as "guideline acceptable," "clinically useable" or "not acceptable". Accordingly, the definition of a high-sensitivity troponin assay requires having a detectable concentration above the LoD in a minimum of 50 % of normal subjects and a CV ≤ 10 % at the 99th percentile using sex-specific cut-points. The scorecard approach provides objective criteria for evaluating cTn assays and can be used to assess potential strengths and weaknesses of each assay used in clinical practice or the research setting. Notably, one way to distinguish high-sensitivity from contemporary troponin assays in literature or when in use clinically is that hs-cTn results should be reported in whole numbers (ng/L) to distinguish them from contemporary assays and avoid potential patient safety issues associated with rounding errors or decimal misplacement.

Case 3

An 80-year-old female with a chronic history of aortic stenosis presents with chest discomfort. Her baseline cTnI was markedly elevated at 1.43 ng/mL (99th percentile: <0.04 ng/mL) and she was admitted for observation. Additional sequential samples drawn 6, 12 and 24 h later confirmed the baseline results with a range between 1.22 and 1.55 ng/mL, all performed using the same cTnI assay. Her ECG was non-diagnostic with no changes over time. The physician consulted the laboratory director for additional discussion about these potential false-positive results. The specimens were analyzed using a different cTnI method and all results were below the 99th percentile for that assay (<0.03 ng/mL). The samples were then incubated with heterophile blocking reagent (Scantibodies, Inc., Saentee, CA) due to a suspected heterophile antibody interference and post-incubation cTnI results were all within the original assays reference interval (<0.04 ng/mL).

Discussion of Case 3

This case illustrates a case of false-positive troponin results due to heterophile antibody analytical interference. Assessment of troponin is the biochemical gold standard for the diagnosis of myocardial infarction and false-positive results carry a very high-risk of jeopardizing accurate clinical decision making. Heterophile antibodies are human antibodies with the capacity to bind to animal immunoglobulins, thereby potentially interfering with the interaction between animal-derived antibodies and analyte, which are components of all immunoassays. The mechanism of interference generally involves a bridging effect between the capture and detection antibody (Fig. 1.3).

The frequency of heterophile antibodies in the general population is estimated between 0.1 and 3.1% but can be significantly increased up to 50% in specific populations who have been therapeutic interventions with monoclonal antibody drugs such as chemotherapy or autoimmune diseases [27]. Heterophile antibodies can be classified into three broad groups:

- Polyspecific antibodies have mild to modest affinity to many different antigens, including animal antigens, but also autoantigens. A majority of the time the titer and affinity are low enough such that they will not cause interference in immunoassays but may be transiently increased in situations such as viral infections whereby their concentrations and affinity increases.
- Anti-immunoglobulin antibodies with cross-reactivity to animal immunoglobulins. Examples include rheumatoid factor and related antibodies; generally problematic in a sub-group of patients.
- High-specificity, high-affinity antibodies against antigens from one or several animal species. This class of antibodies arise from specific immunization and sensititization of individuals to an animal species. Examples include human anti-mouse antibodies (HAMA) and human anti-goat antibodies (HAGA).

Clinically, analytical interferences in troponin assays are particularly troublesome due to the critical nature of its involvement in acute diagnostic decisions. Clinical laboratories have mechanisms in place to investigate suspected interferences including confirmation of results by a different method, assessing linearity

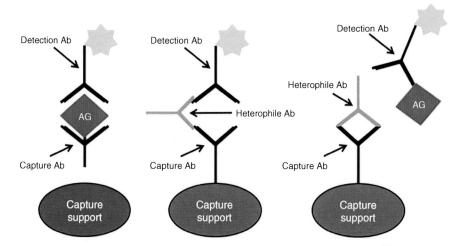

Fig. 1.3 Mechanism of immunoassay interference from heterophile antibodies. (**a**) illustrates how immunoassays are designed to work. The analyte/antigen (*AG*) is trapped between the capture and detection antibodies (*Ab*) and detected. (**b**) illustrates the most common form of heterophile antibody interaction in immunoassays. The heterophile antibody binds to both the detection and the capture antibody, simulating the presence of analyte in its absence and resulting in a false-positive result, or, if analyte is also present, a falsely elevated result. (**c**) illustrates a rare type of heterophile interaction that leads to a false-negative result. The heterophile antibody binds to the capture (or detection) antibody and prevents antigen-antibody interaction. (**a**) No interference. (**b**) False high/positive. (**c**) False low/negative. *AG* analyte/antigen, *Ab* antibodies

and recovery, utilizing heterophile blocking tubes, polyethylene glycol precipitation and/or immunoadsorption methods to remove non-specific assay interferences. It is important to note that the pre-analytical and analytical issues appear to be magnified in high-sensitivity cTn assays compared to contemporary assays, examples including skeletal muscle interference with the hs-cTnT assay [28], plasma versus serum differences [29] and disparate centrifugation practices [30]. Small changes or elevated troponin concentrations are highly clinically relevant, and remaining cognizant about the pre-analytical and analytical assay issues which can affect interpretation of results is critical.

References

1. Thygesen K, Alpert JS, Jaffe AS, et al. Third universal definition of myocardial infarction. Circulation. 2012;126:2020–35.
2. Florkowski C, Wallace J, Walmsley T, George P. The effect of hemolysis on current troponin assays–a confounding preanalytical variable? Clin Chem. 2010;56:1195–7.
3. Lyon ME, Ball CL, Krause RD, Slotsve GA, Lyon AW. Effect of hemolysis on cardiac troponin T determination by the Elecsys 2010 immunoanalyzer. Clin Biochem. 2004;37:698–701.
4. Bais R. The effect of sample hemolysis on cardiac troponin I and T assays. Clin Chem. 2010;56:1357–9.

5. Ong ME, Chan YH, Lim CS. Observational study to determine factors associated with blood sample haemolysis in the emergency department. Ann Acad Med Singapore. 2008;37:745–8.
6. Sodi R, Darn SM, Davison AS, Stott A, Shenkin A. Mechanism of interference by haemolysis in the cardiac troponin T immunoassay. Ann Clin Biochem. 2006;43:49–56.
7. Katrukha AG, Bereznikova AV, Filatov VL, et al. Degradation of cardiac troponin I: implication for reliable immunodetection. Clin Chem. 1998;44:2433–40.
8. Koch CD, Wockenfus AF, Saenger AK, Jaffe AS, Karon BS. BD rapid serum tubes reduce false positive plasma troponin T results on the Roche Cobas e411 analyzer. Clin Biochem. 2012;45:842–4.
9. Sonntag O. Haemolysis as an interference factor in clinical chemistry. J Clin Chem Clin Biochem. 1986;24:127–39.
10. Apple FS, Collinson PO, Biomarkers ITFoCAoC. Analytical characteristics of high-sensitivity cardiac troponin assays. Clin Chem. 2012;58:54–61.
11. Amundson BE, Apple FS. Cardiac troponin assays: a review of quantitative point-of-care devices and their efficacy in the diagnosis of myocardial infarction. Clin Chem Lab Med. 2015;53:665–76.
12. Apple FS, Ler R, Murakami MM. Determination of 19 cardiac troponin I and T assay 99th percentile values from a common presumably healthy population. Clin Chem. 2012;58:1574–81.
13. Aldous S, Mark Richards A, George PM, et al. Comparison of new point-of-care troponin assay with high sensitivity troponin in diagnosing myocardial infarction. Int J Cardiol. 2014;177:182–6.
14. Palamalai V, Murakami MM, Apple FS. Diagnostic performance of four point of care cardiac troponin I assays to rule in and rule out acute myocardial infarction. Clin Biochem. 2013;46:1631–5.
15. Dupuy AM, Sebbane M, Roubille F, et al. Analytical evaluation of point of care cTnT and clinical performances in an unselected population as compared with central laboratory highly sensitive cTnT. Clin Biochem. 2015;48:334–9.
16. Singh J, Akbar MS, Adabag S. Discordance of cardiac troponin I assays on the point-of-care i-STAT and Architect assays from Abbott diagnostics. Clin Chim Acta. 2009;403:259–60.
17. Venge P, Ohberg C, Flodin M, Lindahl B. Early and late outcome prediction of death in the emergency room setting by point-of-care and laboratory assays of cardiac troponin I. Am Heart J. 2010;160:835–41.
18. Loten C, Attia J, Hullick C, Marley J, McElduff P. Point of care troponin decreases time in the emergency department for patients with possible acute coronary syndrome: a randomised controlled trial. Emerg Med J. 2010;27:194–8.
19. Di Serio F, Antonelli G, Trerotoli P, Tampoia M, Matarrese A, Pansini N. Appropriateness of point-of-care testing (POCT) in an emergency department. Clin Chim Acta. 2003;333:185–9.
20. Apple FS, Ler R, Chung AY, Berger MJ, Murakami MM. Point-of-care i-STAT cardiac troponin I for assessment of patients with symptoms suggestive of acute coronary syndrome. Clin Chem. 2006;52:322–5.
21. Blick KE. The benefits of a rapid, point-of-care "TnI-Only" zero and 2-hour protocol for the evaluation of chest pain patients in the Emergency Department. Clin Lab Med. 2014;34:75–85, vi.
22. Collinson PO, John C, Lynch S, et al. A prospective randomized controlled trial of point-of-care testing on the coronary care unit. Ann Clin Biochem. 2004;41:397–404.
23. Saenger AK, Beyrau R, Braun S, et al. Multicenter analytical evaluation of a high-sensitivity troponin T assay. Clin Chim Acta. 2011;412:748–54.
24. Tate JR, Bunk DM, Christenson RH, et al. Evaluation of standardization capability of current cardiac troponin I assays by a correlation study: results of an IFCC pilot project. Clin Chem Lab Med. 2015;53:677–90.
25. Giannitsis E, Kurz K, Hallermayer K, Jarausch J, Jaffe AS, Katus HA. Analytical validation of a high-sensitivity cardiac troponin T assay. Clin Chem. 2010;56:254–61.

26. Apple FS, Jaffe AS, Collinson P, et al. IFCC educational materials on selected analytical and clinical applications of high sensitivity cardiac troponin assays. Clin Biochem. 2015;48:201–3.
27. García-Mancebo ML, Agulló-Ortuño MT, Gimeno JR. Heterophile antibodies produce spuriously elevated concentrations of cardiac Troponin I in patients with Legionella pneumophila. Clin Biochem. 2005;38(6):584–7.
28. Jaffe AS, Vasile VC, Milone M, Saenger AK, Olson KN, Apple FS. Diseased skeletal muscle: a noncardiac source of increased circulating concentrations of cardiac troponin T. J Am Coll Cardiol. 2011;58:1819–24.
29. Kavsak PA, MacRae AR, Yerna MJ, Jaffe AS. Analytic and clinical utility of a next-generation, highly sensitive cardiac troponin I assay for early detection of myocardial injury. Clin Chem. 2009;55:573–7.
30. Kavsak PA, Caruso N, Beattie J, Clark L. Centrifugation - an important pre-analytical factor for the Abbott Architect high-sensitivity cardiac troponin I assay. Clin Chim Acta. 2014;436:273–5.

Chapter 2
Troponin Basics for Clinicians

Yader Sandoval and Fred S. Apple

Abstract Cardiac troponin (cTn) is the preferred biomarker for the diagnosis of acute myocardial infarction (AMI), including each specific MI subtype (i.e., type 1–5 acute myocardial infarction), due to cTn's high myocardial tissue specificity and high clinical sensitivity [1]. cTn are regulatory proteins with both cytosolic (predominant) and structural pools (minor) [2]. Clinical implementation of cTnT and cTnI assays in the late 1980s revolutionized the diagnostic approach of patients with symptoms suspicious for AMI [3, 4]. Global utilization of high-sensitivity (hs) cTnI and cTnT assays has brought upon clinicians another transformational stage in the diagnostic approach of patients presenting with symptoms suspicious for AMI. It is essential for clinicians, in particular emergency physicians and cardiologists, to understand the nuances of cTn testing, as proper understanding of the analytical characteristics of assays will lead to sound clinical implementation and improved research observations.

Keywords Cardiac troponin • Troponin assays • Biomarkers in cardiac disease • cTn assays

Background

Cardiac troponin (cTn) is the preferred biomarker for the diagnosis of acute myocardial infarction (AMI), including each specific MI subtype (i.e., type 1–5 acute myocardial infarction), due to cTn's high myocardial tissue specificity and high clinical sensitivity [1]. cTn are regulatory proteins with both cytosolic (predominant) and structural pools (minor) [2]. Clinical implementation of cTnT and cTnI

Y. Sandoval, MD
Division of Cardiology, Hennepin County Medical Center/Abbott Northwestern Hospital, Minneapolis, MN, USA

F.S. Apple, PhD (✉)
Clinical Laboratories, Hennepin County Medical Center, Minneapolis, MN, USA

Department of Laboratory Medicine and Pathology, University of Minnesota in Minneapolis, Minneapolis, MN, USA
e-mail: apple004@umn.edu

© Springer International Publishing Switzerland 2016
A.S. Maisel, A.S. Jaffe (eds.), *Cardiac Biomarkers*,
DOI 10.1007/978-3-319-42982-3_2

assays in the late 1980s revolutionized the diagnostic approach of patients with symptoms suspicious for AMI [3, 4]. Global utilization of high-sensitivity (hs) cTnI and cTnT assays has brought upon clinicians another transformational stage in the diagnostic approach of patients presenting with symptoms suspicious for AMI. It is essential for clinicians, in particular emergency physicians and cardiologists, to understand the nuances of cTn testing, as proper understanding of the analytical characteristics of assays will lead to sound clinical implementation and improved research observations.

Fundamental Analytical Characteristics

In order to properly use cTn assays, in particular hs-cTn assays, clinicians must understand several test parameters that have important implications, including: limit of blank (LoB), limit of detection (LoD), limit of quantitation (LoQ), coefficient of variation (%CV) and the 99th percentile upper-reference limit (URL).

LoB, LoD and LoQ are terms used to describe the smallest concentration of cTn that can be reliably measured by an analytical procedure [5]. LoB is defined as the highest apparent cTn concentration measurement expected when replicates of a sample containing no cTn is tested [5, 6]. LoD is a concentration greater than the LoB; defined as the lowest detectable cTn concentrations reliably distinguished from the LoB in a sample containing a low cTn concentration [5, 6]. The clinical relevance of LoB and LoD relates to the emerging potential value of using very low cTn concentrations to exclude acute myocardial infarction sooner and/or risk-stratify patients [7–9]. These analytical parameters are of no clinical value with contemporary cTn assays, as these assays are unable to reliably measure cTn concentrations at these low levels. Conversely, hs-cTn assays are able to provide measurable values in >50 % of normal patients at these low concentrations with an acceptable total imprecision of <20 % [10].

LoD, LoB and LoQ are reported in the manufacturer's insert package and often described in peer-reviewed literature. For example, the hs-cTnT has been reported to have a LoB of 3 ng/L and a LoD of 5 ng/L [9, 10]. The clinical correlation of these concentrations corresponds to the potential value of ruling-out AMI faster with a high negative predictive (NPV) value. Body and colleagues examined the sensitivity and NPV of presentation hs-cTnT concentrations using both the LoB and LoD cutoffs for AMI [9]. Using the LoB the sensitivity and NPV for AMI were both 100 %; in contrast to 98.7 % and 99.0 % respectively for the LoD. Using the same hs-cTnT assay, Bandstein et al. hypothesized a similar concept using the LoD cutoff and concluded that among patients with chest pain who had an initial hs-cTnT <5 ng/L and no signs of ischemic electrocardiographic changes, there was minimal risk of myocardial infarction or death within 30-days [8]. These studies underscore the importance of understanding analytical parameters below the 99th percentile upper-reference limit (URL) and their potential clinical use in ruling out AMI earlier, as well as reducing serial cTn testing and hospital admissions.

From an analytical perspective, it is important to understand what is the total imprecision (analytical variation) at these very low concentrations and whether results obtained at these levels have a satisfactory precision to support clinical decision-making. This is highly relevant in the United States, where the Food and Drug Administration (FDA) will not allow cTn concentrations to be reported if values are below the LoQ (20% imprecision) [6, 11]. For example, the most recent FDA cleared cTn assay, the contemporary Beckman Coulter cTnI assay, has been reported to have a 99th percentile of <0.03 ng/mL. Notably, the 20% LoQ corresponds to 0.03 ng/mL. Hence, values under the LoQ (which in this case equates the 99th percentile) are unable to be reported in the United States, and therefore neither the LoB nor LoD would be of clinical relevance in such context.

An observed limitation of using either the LoB or LoD to exclude AMI using hs-cTn assays is that such strategy applies only to a modest proportion of patients [6]. In the same study by Body and colleagues, only 5.2% of patients had values under the LoB, whereas only 21% had values under the LoD [9]. While in some studies these rule-out strategies appear to have a potentially acceptable sensitivity and NPV, they are not applicable to most patients being evaluated for possible AMI. Based on these concepts that examined analytical parameters (LoB and LoD), Shah et al. examined a similar approach, but rather than using an analytical cutoffs, these investigators selected a threshold on the basis of a clinical need [12]. This was a testable concept based on the improved analytical precision at very low concentrations with the studied hs-cTnI (Abbott ARCHITECT) assay. In this study, inter-laboratory coefficient of variation was examined across 33 instruments and reported to be 12.6% at 3.5 ng/L. Therefore, based on the improved total imprecision at low levels, Shah et al. were able to examine a range of concentrations at these low levels and determined that in patients without AMI at presentation, hs-cTnI concentrations <5 ng/L were present in 61% of patients (2311 of 3799 with values under the 99th percentile), with a negative predictive value of 99.6% (95% confidence interval: 99.3–99.8%) for the primary outcome of composite index type 1 MI, or type 1 MI or cardiac death at 30-days.

Total Imprecision: Coefficient of Variation (%CV)

The coefficient of variation (CV) is a useful measure of relative spread in data and is used frequently in laboratory testing and quality control procedures [13]. Each laboratory result is associated with analytical variation, which can be calculated by repeatedly measuring one sample and calculating the analytical %CV from the mean and standard deviation (CV = (standard deviation/mean) * 100%) [13, 14]. Total imprecision (CV) at the 99th percentile URL for each assay should ideally be ≤ 10%, as improved precision facilitates the detection of serial changes in cTn (delta [δ]) [1]. Even though a CV ≤10% is preferred and deemed guideline acceptable, cTn assays with a CV ≤20% at the 99th percentile are clinically usable [1, 15]. Assays with a CV >20% at the 99th percentile URL should not be used clinically [1].

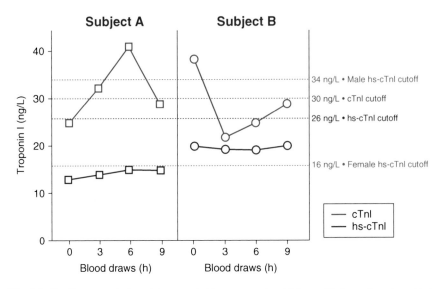

Fig. 2.1 Cardiac troponin I serial concentrations comparing high-sensitivity and contemporary assays in two suspected acute coronary syndrome patients presenting with 30 min of symptom onset

Notably, most contemporary cTn assays don't have an optimal imprecision ($\leq 10\%$ CV) at the 99th percentile, whereas high-sensitivity assays by definition have a $CV\% \leq 10\%$ [6]. This is clinically relevant as better imprecision facilitates detection of changing values, particularly at low cTn concentrations [1, 6, 10].

In a study comparing a contemporary cTnI assay with a %CV at the 99th percentile of 14% to a hs- cTnI assay with a %CV at the 99th percentile of 5.6%, the use of the hs-cTnI assay with higher precision was associated with fewer AMI diagnoses, a finding related to the improved total imprecision (less analytical noise), as using hs-cTn assays, only cTn increases indicative of true myocardial injury should be observed [10, 16]. The clinical impact of the relationship between the 99th percentile URL as the decision cutoff for acute MI and the %CV is illustrated in Fig. 2.1. Total imprecision has an important value not only at the 99th percentile, but also at lower concentrations such as the LoB and LoD as mentioned before, when considering whether rapid rule-out strategies using hs-cTn assays have satisfactory imprecision at these low levels.

cTn concentrations are also commonly reported by clinical laboratories at the 10% CV. For example, the contemporary Abbott Architect cTnI assay has a 99th percentile of 0.028 µg/L with a corresponding CV of 14% at this concentration. Against guideline-recommendations using the 99th percentile, some laboratories and/or clinicians may opt to use a concentration threshold at which the CV is 10%. Hence, based on this example, some may use the 10% CV concentration of 0.032 µg/L as the URL, rather than the 99th percentile concentration of 0.028 µg/L. Similarly, some laboratories may still use the World Health Organization (WHO) cutoffs based on receiver-operator-characteristic (ROC) curve analysis for the diagnosis of AMI. For example, the hs-cTnT assay has a reported 99th percentile of 14 ng/L and a ROC-derived concentration of 100 ng/L. Based on the old WHO recommendation, some laboratories may use the ROC derived concentration. It is important to emphasize that all major guidelines and societies in contemporary practice currently recommend the 99th percentile URL, ideally with a total imprecision of ≤10%, rather than any other concentration such as the 10% CV or ROC-derived concentrations.

The 99th Percentile Upper-Reference Limit

The detection of a rising and/or falling pattern of cTn with at least one value above the 99th percentile URL of a normal reference population is an essential component of the current definition of acute MI according to the Third Universal Definition of Myocardial Infarction consensus document [1]. Consequently, it is imperative to understand why the 99th percentile URL cutoff value is endorsed and how it is determined. The 99th percentile URL has been endorsed as the operative threshold on the basis that an acceptable false-positive rate would be approximately 1% [17, 18]. The 99th percentile URL is derived from a normal reference population using nonparametric statistical analysis to establish reference intervals [19]. However, the methodology used to define normal reference populations is heterogeneous and no uniform guideline exists to guide how researchers or manufacturers should define normality [19]. It has been recommended that as minimum studies screening for normal individuals should perform a clinical history to exclude history of cardiovascular disease and medication usage, surrogate biomarker for diabetes mellitus (hemoglobin A_{1C}), myocardial dysfunction (NT-proBNP) and renal dysfunction (creatinine, eGFR calculation), a minimum of 300 men and 300 women and inclusion of an imaging modality if financially feasible [19]. From a clinical standpoint it is important to understand that currently with contemporary cTn assays one single cutoff value is utilized. However, hs-cTn assays studies have shown differences in 99th percentile URLs among men and women and therefore sex-specific 99th percentiles will need to determined and reported for clinical use [19–21]. This concept is of relevance to clinicians as it has been studied that the use of a single diagnostic threshold with contemporary assays has contributed to the under-diagnosis of AMI in women [21]. Using a hs-cTnI assay with gender-specific cutoffs, Shah and colleagues demonstrated an increase in the diagnosis of MI in women and a minimal effect in men (Table 2.1) [21].

Using hs-cTn assays, age has been recognized as an important factor influencing the 99th percentile. In a large study including three well-characterized population studies: the Dallas Heart Study (DHS), the Atherosclerosis Risk in Communities (ARIC) Study, and the Cardiovascular Health Study (CHS); the 99th percentile URLs calculated on each cohort were significantly above the standard general cutoff specified by the manufacturer in all strata of men ≥50 years and women ≥65 years [22]. For example, in sub-cohort of the DHS that included individuals

Table 2.1 Diagnostic accuracy of type 1 myocardial infarctions comparing contemporary and high-sensitivity troponin assays in men and women using sex-specific vs. a single 99th percentile URL

Proportion of men and women with type 1 MI	Contemporary cTnI: single URL (50 ng/L)	High sensitivity cTnI: single threshold (26 ng/L)	High sensitivity cTnI: sex-specific URLs
Men	19 % (n = 117)	23 % (n = 142)	21 % (n = 131)
Female	11 % (n = 55)	16 % (n = 80)	22 % (n = 111)

Data from Shah et al. [21]

free from recent hospitalization of any cause, with no clinical cardiovascular disease or stage III or greater chronic kidney disease; the 99th percentile for men ranging 50–64 years-old was 28 ng/L, double than the standard manufacturer's package 99th percentile of 14 ng/L. In a separate study, Vasikaran and colleagues, assessed the distribution of hs-cTnT results in their laboratory including the first result only, on each of 19,998 patients and after removal of all results in the 2,159 patients that had a ≥50 % change from the first hs-cTnT; and demonstrated a steady increase in hs-cTnT concentration after 50 years of age [23]. Ninety nineth percentile URLs have also been shown to vary by specimen type (serum, plasma, or whole blood) [19]. Therefore, it is important to report details on how specimens are collected, handled and stored. As an example, in study by Apple and colleagues, the Abbott ARCHITECT cTnI assay showed marked differences in the reported 99th percentile when using plasma (0.012 µg/L) vs. serum (0.025 µg/L) [24, 25].

Contemporary, Point-of Care and High-Sensitivity Cardiac Troponin Assays

Contemporary cTn assays are defined as those assays that measure normal values below the 99th percentile in less than 50 % of a normal reference population [15]. Contemporary assays measure cTn above the limit of detection in less than 35 % of normal individuals [19]. Moreover, most contemporary cTn assays do not have a CV below 10 % at the 99th percentile [6]. A list of cTn assays, including contemporary assays is shown Table 2.2. High-sensitivity cTn assays are defined as assays that measure cTnI and cTnT above the LoD in ≥ 50 % of healthy subjects, with an analytical imprecision of ≤10 % at the 99th percentile URL. A list of hs-cTn assays is shown in Table 2.2. Using hs-assays, sex-specific cutoffs will be reported and results should be reported in nanograms per liter (whole numbers) to distinguish from contemporary or point of care (POC) assays.

POC cTn assays utilize rapid, simple, portable, instruments that are able to deliver rapid turn-around-time results in under 30 min, and require minimal sample handling and preparation, that waive the necessity for skilled laboratory personnel to operate the assays [26]. Ideally, POC devices should be sensitive to cTn at very low concentrations, maximize analytical specificity to cTn by minimizing

Table 2.2 Analytical characteristics of contemporary, point of care and high sensitivity cardiac troponin I and T assays

Company/platform/assay	LoD µg/L	99th µg/L	%CV at 99th	10% CV µg/L	Epitopes
Contemporary assays					
Abbott ARCHITECT	<0.01	0.028	15.0	0.032	C 87–91, 24–40: D: 41–49
Beckman Coulter Access 2	0.01	0.04	14.0	0.06	C: 41–49; D: 24–40
Roche E170	0.01	<0.01	18.0	0.03	C: 125–131; D: 136–147
Siemens Centaur Ultra	0.006	0.04	10.0	0.03	C; 41–49, 87–91; D: 27–40
Siemens VISTA	0.015	0.045	10.0	0.04	C: 27–32; D: 41–56
Tosoh AIA II	0.06	<0.06	8.5	0.09	C: 41–49; D: 87–91
Ortho Vitros ECi ES	0.012	0.034	10.0	0.034	C 24–40, 41–49; D 87–91
POC assays					
Abbott i-STAT	0.02	0.08	16.5	0.10	C: 41–49, 88–91; D: 28–39,62–78
Alere Triage	0.05	<0.05	NA	NA	C: NA; D: 27–40
bioMerieux Vidas Ultra	0.01	0.01	27.7	0.11	C: 41–49, 22–29; D: 87–91, 7B9
LSI Medience PATHFAST	0.008	0.029	5.1	0014	C: 41–49; D:71–116, 163–209
Radiometer AQT90 cTnI	0.0095	0.023	17.7	0.039	C: 41–49, 190–196; D: 137–149
Radiometer AQT90 cTnT	0.01	0.017	20.0	.03	C: 125–131; D:136–147
Response Biomedical RAMP	0.03	<0.1	18.5	0.21	C: 85–92; D: 26–38
Roche Cardiac Reader	<0.05	<0.05	NA	NA	C: 125–131; D:136–147
Siemens Stratus CS*	0.03	0.07	10.0	0.06	C: 27–32; D: 41–56
Trinity Meritas	0.019	0.036	17.0	NA	C: 24–40; 41–49, D: 88–90, 137–148, 190–196
High-sensitivity assays	**ng/L**	**M/F, ng/ LL**		**ng/L**	
Abbott ARCHITECT hs-cTnI	1.9	34/16	<6.0	3	C; 24–40; D: 41–49
Beckman Access hs-cTnI	2.1	11/9	<5.0	3.3	C; 41–49; D: 24–40
Ortho-Clin Diagnos hs-cTnI	1.0	19/16	<5.0	6.5	C 24–40, 41–49; D 87–91
Roche E170 hs-cTnT	5	20/13	<8.0	13	C: 136–147; D:125–131
Siemens Vista hs-cTnI	0.8	55/33	<5.0	3	C: 30–35; D: 41–56, 171–8
Singulex Erenna hs-cTnI	0.1	27/15	<5.0	0.9	C: 41–49; D: 27–41

LoD limit of detection. Sex specific 99th percentiles, *M* male, *F* female

interference and minimize the CV% at the 99th percentile; while being able to deliver a result in less than 30 min [26]. Conceptually, these are attractive assays, yet very few achieve the ideal imprecision of ≤10 % at the 99th percentile. A list of POC cTn assays is shown in Table 2.2.

IFCC Educational Efforts to Define High Sensitivity Assays

hs-cTn assays promise better diagnostic accuracy for AMI. This is why it is essential that laboratory medicine professionals and clinicians understand the performance of these tests and how to use them. An IFCC Task Force on Clinical Applications of Cardiac Bio-Markers collaborated with representatives from in vitro diagnostics companies who have expertise in hs-cTn troponin immunoassays on education materials addressing the question, how does an assay become designated high-sensitivity and how to implement them into clinical practice and research? [20] These educational guidelines focus on two main issues, the 99th percentile URL and calculating serial change values (delta cTn) in accord with the Third Universal Definition of Myocardial Infarction. This task force was a global collaboration reflecting a balanced perspective on hs-cTn assays from both clinical and laboratory viewpoints, providing guidance on the how and why of implementing hs-assays into practice, proving based definitions to the scientific and medical literature for consistency. The task force's primary priority was to address the potential for inconsistent use of the analytical characteristics of hs-cTn assays. The document is assay blind to whether cTnI or cTnT is measured for patient care, but proposes clear operational recommendations. Unfortunately, U.S.-based laboratories cannot put these recommendations into practice, as the Food and Drug Administration (FDA) has not yet cleared hs-cTn assays for clinical use. Table 2.3 shows the selected key recommendations from the IFCC educational materials.

Delta Troponin

Using a delta cTn value is critically important to improve the diagnostic specificity for AMI versus elevated levels due to a chronic myocardial injury that might be related to structural heart disease [20]. Numerous issues about delta cTn exist, including variation and timing of serial cTn measurements that impact delta change calculations [27]. It is important for both laboratorians and clinicians to understand that there is no universal delta cTn value for all hs-assays. Laboratory medicine professionals must prepare to educate clinicians on this point, emphasizing that one delta value does not fit all assays, that serial change delta values are assay dependent, and that the utility of hs-cTn is related to the onset of ischemic symptoms and the timing of presentation [20, 27]. For example, a patient presents with chest pain and a non-ischemic ECG and is admitted to the observation unit for serial cTn

Table 2.3 IFCC Task Force educational points regarding high sensitivity cardiac troponin assays

99th Percentile URL
Should be determined from a healthy population
Coefficient of variation (CV%) ≤10 % at 99th percentile
Measure cTn above the LoD in ≥50 %
Values will be reported as whole values, in ng/L units
Assays are not standardized and 99th percentiles are assay dependent
Sex-specific URLs established with minimum of 300 males and 300 females
Serial Change Delta Value
Best method to differentiate acute myocardial injury, including AMI, from those that have chronic cardiac troponin elevations; optimizes clinical specificity
Timing of presentation is an essential aspect for an accurate delta calculation
Delta change may be absent at or near peak values when the presentation is late after an acute event
Need to use fixed time intervals for sampling and measure
Absolute concentration delta change values must be developed for each assay

measurements every 3 h. His initial (baseline) contemporary cTnI is 0.012 μg/L (99th percentile: 0.034 μg/L). His 3- and 6-h results are as follows: 3-h sample: 0.029 μg/L and 6-h sample: 0.127 μg/L. In order to correlate the delta concepts mentioned above, the individual 6-h cTnI measurement with a value above the 99th percentile would likely provide an optimal clinical sensitivity for AMI. However, the individual value alone has a low specificity for AMI. Therefore in order to improve the diagnostic accuracy and improve clinical specificity for the diagnosis of AMI one includes the use of serial cTn changes to the interpretation of the results. In a simplistic fashion without taking into account timing of presentation, the presence of a significant delta would support the diagnosis of an AMI, whereas the absence of it would argue against an acute event. It is also important to emphasize that the use of serial cTn changes (delta) has been associated an increase in the specificity for AMI [28], however these dynamic changes are not specific exclusively for AMI, but rather indicative of acute myocardial injury with necrosis which could be due to numerous etiologies other than acute myocardial infarction [29].

When using delta cTn for hs-assays, absolute concentration changes have been shown to have significantly higher diagnostic accuracy for AMI than relative changes [30, 31]. Using serial changes investigators have categorized patients into three cohorts: 'rule-out MI' group, 'observational zone' group and 'rule-in MI' group [32]. The rule-out MI strategy integrates the use of baseline presentation hs-cTn levels in combination with minimal absolute changes, which if met, provide a very high NPV. In contrast, the rule-in MI strategy relies on the presence of significant absolute changes, which if present, provide a high diagnostic specificity for AMI. Finally, if none of the rule-in or rule-out MI criteria are met, then patients fall into a "observational zone", in which an individualized approach is utilized and clinical suspicious is important as there is an acute myocardial infarction prevalence of 8–19 % in this category [6].

Integration of Analytical Characteristics with Rule-out/ Rule-in Strategies

Based on the analytical characteristics described, four major diagnostic strategies have been studied and/or implemented in clinical practice with high-sensitivity assays: (1) use of undetectable values (cTn concentrations below the LoB or LoD); (2) use of accelerated serial cTn sampling (baseline 0-h cTn measurement and 1–3 h sampling); (3) use of hs-cTn measurements in combination with risk scores (accelerated diagnostic protocols); and (4) use of a cTn concentration threshold tailored to meet a specific clinical need [6]. The use of undetectable values refers to the rapid rule-out of acute myocardial infarction by using one-single measurement on presentation. If the initial measurement provides an undetectable concentration, defined as those below the LoB or LoD, then the patient falls into a very low risk category with a high negative predictive value for adverse events. This strategy relies on the ability of hs-assays to provide precise results at these low levels. Such approach is impossible with contemporary cTn assays. Importantly, studies have shown that this strategy has an inferior performance in early presenters. Therefore, in patients presenting early, serial sampling should be considered.

Accelerated serial sampling relies on hs-cTn measurements over time to rule-in and rule-out acute myocardial infarction. In contrast to the prolonged serial sampling required with contemporary assays, which requires several measurements every 3-h, often up to 9 or 12-h; with accelerated serial sampling using hs-assays, one can perform two measurements over time and expedite the rule-in/out of AMI. This can be achieved with hs-assays due the improved total imprecision and ability to measure low cTn concentrations. Most studies have used a baseline measurement at presentation (0-h) in combination with a second sample obtained at a range of 1–3 h (heterogeneity observed across studies in regards to the timing of the 2nd sample). These protocols categorize patients into either a rule-in, rule-out or observational group. Based on the numerous studies examining these protocols, the 2013 and 2015 European guidelines endorse as a Class I recommendation the use of both 0–1 h and 0–3 h protocols [33]. The decision to implement a protocol is directly linked to the ability of each healthcare setting to obtain the samples at the recommended timing intervals. For example, in hospitals that allow nurse to phlebotomize and obtain cTn samples, the 0–1 h protocol might be feasible due to the proximity of the nurse. Conversely, the 0 and 2–3 h protocols might appear more appropriate for hospitals that use laboratory personnel to obtain cTn samples. Accelerated diagnostic protocols, ADPs, refer to rule-out strategies that integrate cTn measurements with clinical risk scores (e.g.,: TIMI score) and 12-lead electrocardiography to determine whether patients are at low risk. Most studies examining ADPs have combined the use of serial hs-cTn measurements (e.g.,: 0 h and 2 h measurements) in combination with a selected risk-score and electrocardiography. ADPs increase the proportion of patients identified as low-risk, hence more attractive for clinicians seeking to expedite evaluation and potential discharge. For example, the TRUST-ADP, which uses hs-cTnT, identified 39.8 % as potentially suitable for immediate discharge, in contrast to 29.3 % using the LoD alone (<5 ng/L) and 7.9 % using the

Table 2.4 Short-term biological variation characteristics of high-sensitivity cardiac troponin assays

	Abbott	Beckman	Roche (E170)	Siemens	Singulex
CV_A, %	13.8	14.5	7.8	13.0	8.3
CV_I, %	15.2	6.1	15.0	12.9	9.7
CV_G, %	70.5	34.8	NA	12.3	57
Index of individuality	0.22	0.46	NA	0.11	0.21
RCV, %	NA	NA	47.0	NA	NA
RCV increase, %	69.3	63.8	NA	57.5	46.0
RCV decrease, %	−40.9	−38.9	NA	−36.5	−32
Within-subject mean, ng/L	3.5	4.9	NA	5.5	2.8

LoB alone (<3 ng/L) [34]. Lastly, based on the improved analytical precision at low concentrations, an alternative strategy explored in the HIGH-STEACS study, was to use a concentration threshold tailored to meet a clinical need. Investigators demonstrated that a hs-cTnI (Abbott ARCHITECT) concentrations below 5 ng/L provided a NPV of 99.6 % for the primary endpoint, hence potentially expediting the rule-out and discharge of two-thirds of patients with initial samples below the 99th percentile who present to the emergency department with possible ischemic symptoms [12].

Biological Variation

Biological variability is a type of pre-analytical variation due to changes over time in normal individuals, which may be secondary to circadian rhythm, monthly changes, or seasonal changes inherent to a species [35]. The determination of biological variation became possible until the development of hs-assays that allowed the measurement of cTn concentrations at low concentrations in healthy individuals [10]. Measurement of the biological variation of cTn allows determination of reference change values used for interpreting serial testing [10, 36] (Table 2.4). Reference change values represent that percent-change that the next test result must exceed before it exceeds the biomarker's biological variation.

Summary

The chapter has discussed the important role that analytical cTnI and cTnT assays play in clinical diagnostic decision making. Each cTnI and TnT assays is unique and no two assays should be assumed to be the same. With the global implementation of high sensitivity assays into clinical practice except in the us when one they not yet FDA cleared for clinical use as well as for research studies, improved diagnostics with better cost effective management of patients, with improved outcomes are already being realized.

References

1. Thygesen K, Alpert JS, Jaffe AS, et al. Third universal definition of myocardial infarction. J Am Coll Cardiol. 2012;60:1581–98.
2. Jaffe AS, Babuin L, Apple FS. Biomarkers in acute cardiac disease: the present and the future. J Am Coll Cardiol. 2006;48:1–11.
3. Cummins B, Auckland ML, Cummins P. Cardiac-specific troponin-I radioimmunoassay in the diagnosis of acute myocardial infarction. Am Heart J. 1987;113:1333–44.
4. Katus HA, Remppis A, Looser S, Hallermeier K, Scheffold T, Kübler W. Enzyme linked immune assay of cardiac troponin T for the detection of acute myocardial infarction in patients. J Mol Cell Cardiol. 1989;21:1349–53.
5. Armbruster DA, Pry T. Limit of blank, limit of detection and limit of quantitation. Clin Biochem Rev. 2008;29 Suppl 1:S49–52.
6. Sandoval Y, Smith SW, Apple FS. Present and future of cardiac troponin in clinical practice: a paradigm shift to high sensitivity assays. Am J Med. 2016;129(4):354–65.
7. Body R, Carley S, McDowell G, Jaffe AS, France M, Cruickshank K, Wibberley C, Nuttal M, Mackway-Jones K. Rapid exclusion of acute myocardial infarction in patients with undetectable troponin using a high-sensitivity assay. J Am Coll Cardiol. 2011;58:1332–9.
8. Bandstein N, Ljung R, Johansson M, Holzmann MJ. Undetectable high-sensitivity cardiac troponin T level in the emergency department and risk of myocardial infarction. J Am Coll Cardiol. 2014;63:2569–78.
9. Body R, Burrows G, Carley S, Cullen L, Than M, Jaffe AS, Lewis PS. High-sensitivity cardiac troponin T concentrations below the limit of detection to exclude acute myocardial infarction: a prospective evaluation. Clin Chem. 2015;61:983–9.
10. Apple FS, Collinson PO, IFCC Task Force on Clinical Applications of Cardiac Biomarkers. Analytical characteristics of high-sensitivity cardiac troponin assays. Clin Chem. 2012;58:54–61.
11. Apple FS, Hollander J, Wu AH, Jaffe AS. Improving the 510(k) FDA process for cardiac troponin assays: in search of common ground. Clin Chem. 2014;60:1273–5.
12. Shah AS, Anand A, Sandoval Y, et al. High-sensitivity cardiac troponin I at presentation in patients with suspected acute coronary syndrome: a cohort study. Lancet. 2015. doi:10.1016/S0140-6736(15)00391-8.
13. Dawson B, Trapp RG. Basic & clinical biostatistics. New York: Lange Medical – McGraw Hill, Medical Pub. Division; 2004.
14. Omar F. Essential laboratory knowledge for the clinician. Continuing medical education. 2012;30(7):244–48. ISSN 2078–5143. Available at: http://www.cmej.org.za/index.php/cmej/article/view/2524/2433.
15. Apple FS. A new season for cardiac troponin assays: it's time to keep a scorecard. Clin Chem. 2009;55:1303–6.
16. Sandoval Y, Smith SW, Schulz KM, Murakami MM, Love SA, Nicholson J, Apple FS. Diagnosis of type 1 and type 2 myocardial infarction using a high-sensitivity cardiac troponin I assay with sex-specific 99th percentiles based on the third universal definition of myocardial infarction classification system. Clin Chem. 2015;61:657–63.
17. Korley FK, Jaffe AS. Preparing the United States for high-sensitivity cardiac troponin assays. J Am Coll Cardiol. 2013;61:153–8.
18. Newby LK, Jesse RL, Babb JD, Christenson RH, De Fer TM, Diamond GA, Fesmire FM, Geraci SA, Gersh BJ, Larsen GC, Kaul S, McKay CR, Philippides GJ, Weintraub WS. ACCF 2012 expert consensus document on practical clinical considerations in the interpretation of troponin elevations: a report of the American College of Cardiology Foundation task force on Clinical Expert Consensus Documents. J Am Coll Cardiol. 2012;60:2427–63.
19. Sandoval Y, Apple FS. The global need to define normality: the 99th percentile value of cardiac troponin. Clin Chem. 2014;60:455–62.

20. Apple FS, Jaffe AS, Collinson P, et al. IFCC educational materials on selected analytical and clinical applications of high sensitivity cardiac troponin assays. Clin Biochem. 2015;48:201–3.
21. Shah AS, Griffiths M, Lee KK, et al. High sensitivity cardiac troponin and the under-diagnosis of myocardial infarction in women: prospective cohort study. BMJ. 2015;350:7873. doi:10.1036/bmj.g7873.
22. Gore MO, Seliger SL, Defilippi CR, et al. Age- and sex-dependent upper-reference limits for the high-sensitivity cardiac troponin T assay. J Am Coll Cardiol. 2014;63:1441–8.
23. Vasikaran SD, Bima A, Botros M, Sikaris KA. Cardiac troponin testing in the acute care setting: ordering, reporting, and high sensitivity assays—an update from the Canadian society of clinical chemists (CSCC); the case for age related acute myocardial infarction (AMI) cut-offs. Clin Biochem. 2012;45:513–4.
24. Apple FS, Murakami MM. Serum and plasma cardiac troponin I 99th percentile reference values for 3 2nd-generation assays. Clin Chem. 2007;53:1558–60.
25. Apple FS, Ler R, Murakami MM. Determination of 19 cardiac troponin I and T assay 99th percentile values from a common presumably healthy population. Clin Chem. 2012;58:1574–81.
26. Amundson BE, Apple FS. Cardiac troponin assays: a review of quantitative point-of-care devices and their efficacy in the diagnosis of myocardial infarction. Clin Chem Lab Med. 2015;53:665–76.
27. Jaffe AS, Moeckel M, Giannitsis E, et al. In search for the Holy Grail: suggestions for studies to define delta changes to diagnose or exclude acute myocardial infarction: a position paper from the study group on biomarkers of the Acute Cardiovascular Care Association. Eur Heart J Acute Cardiovasc Care. 2014;3:313–6.
28. Keller T, Zeller T, Ojeda F, et al. Serial changes in highly sensitive troponin I assay and early diagnosis of myocardial infarction. JAMA. 2011;306:2684–93.
29. Thygesen K, Mair J, Giannitsis E, et al. How to use high-sensitivity cardiac troponins in acute cardiac care. Eur Heart J. 2012;33:2252–7.
30. Reichlin T, Irfan A, Twerenbold R, et al. Utility of absolute and relative changes in cardiac troponin concentrations in the early diagnosis of acute myocardial infarction. Circulation. 2011;124:136–45.
31. Mueller M, Biener M, Vafaie M, et al. Absolute and relative kinetic changes of high-sensitivity cardiac troponin T in acute coronary syndrome and in patients with increased troponin in the absence of acute coronary syndrome. Clin Chem. 2012;58:209–18.
32. Reichlin T, Schindler C, Twerenbold R, et al. One-hour rule-out and rule-in of acute myocardial infarction using high-sensitivity cardiac troponin T. Arch Intern Med. 2012;172:1211–8.
33. Roffi M, Patrono C, Collet JP, et al. 2015 ESC Guidelines for the management of acute coronary syndromes in patients presenting without persistent ST-segment elevation: task force for the management of acute coronary syndromes in patients without persistent ST-segment elevation of the European Society of Cardiology (ESC). Eur Heart J. 2016;37(3):267–315.
34. Carlton EW, Cullen L, Than M, Gamble J, Khattab A, Greaves K. A novel diagnostic protocol to identify patients suitable for discharge after a single high-sensitivity troponin. Heart. 2015;101:1041–6.
35. Sherwood MW, Newby KL. High-sensitivity cardiac troponin assays: evidence, indications and reasonable use. J Am Heart Assoc. 2014;3:e000403.
36. Wu AH. Biological and analytical variation of clinical biomarkers testing: implications for biomarker-guided therapy. Curr Heart Fail Rep. 2013;10:434–40.

Chapter 3
Unique Aspects of High Sensitivity Assays: What Are They, Why Do We Need Them, and How Do We Use Them?

Paul Ormandy Collinson

Abstract The development of immunoassays for the cardiac troponins (cTn) either cardiac troponin T (cTnT) or cardiac troponin I (cTnI) resulted in a paradigm shift in biochemical testing for the diagnosis of patients presenting with chest pain. For the first time, the laboratory was able to offer a specific diagnostic test for acute myocardial infarction (AMI). Compared to the tests then in use, measurement of creatine kinase (CK) and its MB isoenzyme (CK-MB), the measurement of cTnT or cTnI offered not only superior diagnostic efficiency but also prognostic information and treatment guidance. The superiority of cTnT and cTnI measurement led initially to the redefinition of myocardial infarction. This stated that the preferred biomarker for diagnosis of AMI was serial troponin measurement [1]. This document first recommended that the 99th percentile should be used as decision limit and the analytical imprecision of the assay (the coefficient of variation, CV) should be $\leq 10\%$ at the 99th percentile. It is worth remembering that at this point the analytical sensitivity of the available assays, although clinically superior to that of CK and CK-MB measurement was significantly less than those currently in use.

Keywords Immunoassays for the cardiac troponins • Cardiac troponin immunoassays • Cardiac troponin T • Cardiac troponin I • High-Sensitivity Cardiac Troponin Assays • Delta Troponin

Why Were High Sensitivity Troponin Assays Developed?

The development of immunoassays for the cardiac troponins (cTn) either cardiac troponin T (cTnT) or cardiac troponin I (cTnI) resulted in a paradigm shift in biochemical testing for the diagnosis of patients presenting with chest pain. For the first

P.O. Collinson, MA, MB, BChir, FRCPath, MD
Clinical Blood Sciences and Cardiology, St George's Hospital and Medical School, London, UK
e-mail: paul.collinson@stgeorges.nhs.uk

© Springer International Publishing Switzerland 2016
A.S. Maisel, A.S. Jaffe (eds.), *Cardiac Biomarkers*,
DOI 10.1007/978-3-319-42982-3_3

time, the laboratory was able to offer a specific diagnostic test for acute myocardial infarction (AMI). Compared to the tests then in use, measurement of creatine kinase (CK) and its MB isoenzyme (CK-MB), the measurement of cTnT or cTnI offered not only superior diagnostic efficiency but also prognostic information and treatment guidance. The superiority of cTnT and cTnI measurement led initially to the redefinition of myocardial infarction. This stated that the preferred biomarker for diagnosis of AMI was serial troponin measurement [1]. This document first recommended that the 99th percentile should be used as decision limit and the analytical imprecision of the assay (the coefficient of variation, CV) should be $\leq 10\%$ at the 99th percentile. It is worth remembering that at this point the analytical sensitivity of the available assays, although clinically superior to that of CK and CK-MB measurement was significantly less than those currently in use. In addition, decision limits had been optimized to correspond with the previous WHO diagnosis of AMI. The net result was to produce assays which were not only very sensitive (when compared to CK and CK-MB) but also highly specific. A cTnT or cTnI measurement would provide a binary diagnosis of AMI or not. This had two consequences. First, the cardiospecificity of the assay led to rapid and enthusiastic adoption by Emergency Department physicians. The second, and unintended, consequence was an over reliance on a biochemical test for diagnosis and an erosion of the importance of clinical assessment of the patient. The publication of the universal definition of myocardial infarction first introduced the concept of the 20% change in troponin values [2]. For the clinical chemist a 20% change in troponin values can only be detected with an assay with an imprecision less than 10%. So the concept of a 99th percentile with a 10% imprecision goal is intrinsically self-contradictory. The ability to detect a 99th percentile in a healthy population and the need to perform measurements with an imprecision of significantly less than 10% at the 99th percentile value, together with a desire to progressively improve any product, encouraged the manufacturers of cTnT and cTnI assays to progressively enhance analytical performance.

Currently assays can be divided into four broad categories. There are those assays where the imprecision at the 99th percentile exceeds 20%. These are not considered suitable for use on their own for diagnosis. Second, there are those assays where the imprecision at the 99th percentile is in the range 10–20%. These are considered to be clinically usable. The third group is those where the imprecision at the 99th percentile is 10% or less and the assay is able to measure cardiac troponin in a proportion of the normal healthy population. These are considered to be contemporary sensitive troponin assays. The final category is the high sensitivity troponin assays.

What Is a High Sensitivity Troponin Assay?

Calling an assay a "high sensitivity" assay refers to the analytical performance characteristics of the assay itself (Table 3.1). The assay is not measuring a different form of troponin but is measuring troponin with a greater degree of analytical sensitivity.

Table 3.1 What makes an assay a high sensitivity assay?

A high sensitivity assay refers to the assays analytical characteristics, it does not mean a different form of troponin is being measured
Total imprecision at the 99th percentile should be ≤10%
The assay should detect at least 50% of healthy individuals above the LoD of the assay
Results should be reported in ng/L

A good analogy the distinction between an assay for C reactive protein (CRP) and a high sensitivity CRP assay. A conventional CRP assay will typically measure down to 10 mg/L whereas a high sensitivity CRP assay will measure down to 0.1 mg/L. A troponin assay which in a previous format would have had a limit of detection of around 20 ng/L but will now have a limit of detection of around 1 ng/L when redeveloped as a high sensitivity assay. The improvements in assay sensitivity also produces an improvement in assay imprecision. In this case moving from a 10% CV of 160 ng/L to a 10% CV of 5 ng/L.

There is no uniformly agreed definition of a high sensitivity troponin assay but the International Federation of Clinical Chemists (IFCC) working group on cardiac markers has proposed a definition which is broadly accepted [3]. A high sensitivity troponin assay should have a total imprecision at the 99th percentile of ≤10% or ideally better. In addition, the assay should detect at least 50% of healthy individuals above the limit of detection (LoD) of the assay.

The final criterion for a high sensitivity assay is that the results should be reported in nanograms/L. The main reason for this is that high sensitivity troponin assays report to three decimal places if the current units of micrograms/L are used. This creates a risk when results are viewed as human beings cope much better with numbers to the left of the decimal point. In addition there is a significant risk with electronic data transfer. There is an unfortunate tendency in some software packages (from electronic messaging to electronic patient record programs) to round decimal points. Potentially this might give a result of zero for an elevated troponin value.

Why Do We Need High Sensitivity Troponin Assays?

Although there are sound analytical reasons for developing sensitive troponin assays, as discussed above, there are significant clinical advantages as well. Initially, diagnosis utilizing troponin assays recommended a sample taken 10–12 h from admission. This was because the assays were relatively insensitive in the early time period following myocardial infarction. It was for this reason that the concept of a panel of cytoplasmic markers combined with cardiac troponin was developed. The idea was that the early diagnostic sensitivity of markers such as myoglobin and CK-MB would be combined with the cardiac specific troponin measurement. The need for rapid diagnosis was driven by the desire of ED physicians for rapid triage of chest pain patients. Presentations with chest pain account for the largest single category medical presentation to the ED. The need was for rapid biochemical diagnosis to supplement the electrocardiogram and clinical assessment. Progressive improvements in assay sensitivity have produced cardiac troponin assays that are diagnostically superior, even in the early time period after infarction, to measurement of cytoplasmic markers [4, 5]. High sensitivity assays take this further. Not only are high sensitivity assays diagnostically superior to cytoplasmic markers but they allow measurement of troponin within the reference interval. In the era of high sensitivity troponin assays there is no longer any place for measurement of the cytoplasmic markers myoglobin and CK-MB.

Measurement of troponin within the reference interval allows serial measurement across short time intervals and the calculation of a significant change in value, typically an increase (although a decrease can also be used), the use of a delta change value. The concept of a delta change of a cardiac biomarker was originally developed for serial measurement of CK and CK-MB. The objective was to increase diagnostic sensitivity and to decrease time to diagnosis by eliminating between subject variability (the major contributor to the size of the reference interval) and making the only contributors to the ability to distinguish between two consecutive measurements the analytical imprecision of the assay and the within individual biological variation. Within individual biological variation for cardiac troponin has been shown to be low, of the order of 50–60 % [3]. High sensitivity cardiac troponin assays allow calculation of a delta value for troponin and the use of very short sampling intervals.

The measurement of cTnT and cTnI in apparently healthy populations with high sensitivity assays has revealed a number of interesting clinical findings. First, it is apparent that the definition of a healthy reference population needs to be more exacting when using a high sensitivity troponin assay. A number of studies have shown that the 99th percentile is critically influenced by the population studied. Measurement of troponin levels in 545 individuals from a primary care population demonstrated that the 99th percentile, progressively fell for cTnT from 29.9 to 14.4 ng/L and for cTnI from 66.8 to 43.8 ng/L when individuals were progressively excluded from the population initially on the basis of a health questionnaire, then with the addition of simple biochemical tests and finally with normal cardiac imaging by echocardiography [6]. This finding has been confirmed by two other studies. One with a very similar design demonstrated a fall of cTnI from 20.4 to 11.1 ng/L and for cTnT from 20.4 to 15.9 ng/L [7]. The second study found that higher cTnI concentrations were predicted by hypertension, left ventricular mass, systolic and diastolic dysfunction and coronary artery disease [8]. How a healthy population should be defined is still a matter of debate. Recommended criteria are that healthy individuals would have no significant cardiac history, would not be taking any cardio active medication, would be normotensive, would have normal renal function, be non-diabetic and have a normal B type natriuretic peptide level. Ideally, cardiac imaging information would be available and there would be normal cardiac function by echocardiography or magnetic resonance imaging.

High sensitivity assays also show a male female difference. The 99th percentile limit in males is higher than that in females. It has been recognized that there is a gender imbalance in the diagnosis and management of cardiac disease. Women are relatively under diagnosed and undertreated. The use of gender specific cut-offs, which can only be achieved with high sensitivity, assays allows this problem to be addressed. In a prospective observational cohort study of consecutive patients admitted to a regional cardiac center in the UK a total of 1126 patients (46 % women) were studied [9]. The final diagnosis was based on the universal definition of myocardial infarction. Two cardiologists independently adjudicated the diagnosis of myocardial infarction using a high sensitivity cTnI assay sex specific diagnostic thresholds and compared this with the existing practice were a single diagnostic threshold (based on a contemporary assay) was used. The use of a high sensitivity cTnI assay increased the diagnosis of myocardial infarction in women from 11 to 22 % (p <0.001) but had a minimal effect in men (from 19 to 21 %, p=0.002). They noted that women were less likely than men to be referred to a cardiologist or undergo coronary revascularization. At 12 month follow up those women who were noted to have had an increased troponin detected only by the high sensitivity assay using a gender specific threshold or had a diagnosis of myocardial infarction based on the conventional assay had the highest rated death or reinfarction compared to women with a cTnI values below the gender specific 99th percentile.

Finally, high sensitivity troponin assays can be used outside of the conventional acute hospital setting. Large population based studies have shown that the level of cardiac troponin in a population will predict long-term cardiac risk. cTnT was measured in 4221 community dwelling adults aged ≥65 years with repeat measurement 2–3 years late. An increase in cTnT levels of greater than 50 % predicted an increased risk of death or heart failure [10]. The Dallas heart study measured cTnT in 3546 individuals from 30 to 65 years also had cardiac imaging. The quintile of cTnT value predicted risk of death from 1.9 to 28.4 % from the lowest to the highest quintile, despite adjustment for traditional risk factors, CRP, chronic kidney disease and levels of NT pro-BNP. Troponin elevation correlated with the presence of left ventricular hypertrophy and left ventricular systolic dysfunction. The Atherosclerosis Risk in Communities (ARIC) study of 9698 participants 54–74 years of age free of vascular disease at baseline measured cTnT [11]. From the lowest to the highest quintile of cTnT there was a progressive increase in risk of death from cardiovascular disease, all-cause mortality and risk of heart failure during the follow up period.

How Do We Use High Sensitivity Troponin Assays?

High Sensitivity Troponin Assays in the Acute Hospital Setting

High sensitivity assays for routine clinical use are no different from conventional assays. They are an additional diagnostic modality and must be used in conjunction with clinical assessment the patient. A brief case history from the early days of troponin measurement illustrates this.

A 25-year-old male was admitted to the ED following a fight. He complained of chest pain and gave a history of being stabbed in the chest. It was noted he had a penetrating wound in the 5th left intercostal space and a plain chest x-ray showed cardiac enlargement. Echocardiography confirmed the presence of a large pleural effusion around the heart and he was prepared for emergency surgery. As part of his routine work up in addition to a renal and clotting profile a cardiac profile was also requested requested. It was noted by the consultant ED physician that he had an elevated cTnT. As the test is only been recently introduced the consultant ED physician contacted the laboratory to request interpretive advice, specifically at the patient had a myocardial infarction. The head of the laboratory (the author) explained to the ED physician that as myocardial injury had occurred due to the penetrating chest wound (also the cause of the chest pain!) this would be the cause of the troponin release. The patient was extremely unlikely to have had a myocardial infarction.

The measurement of the cTnT and cTnI by high sensitivity methods offers the advantages of more rapid diagnosis, the use of delta change and the use of gender specific cut-offs.

Rapid Diagnosis Using Conventional or Gender Specific Cut-Offs and Rapid Sampling Regimes

The superior diagnostic sensitivity of high sensitivity assays can be utilized by using sampling strategies involving measurement on admission and 3 h from admission. The evidence to support this has recently been reviewed by the UK National Institute of Clinical and health Excellence who have endorsed the use of two high sensitivity troponin assays (https://www.nice.org.uk/guidance/dg15). Diagnosis is based on one or more values exceeding the 99th percentile together with a significant change in the troponin value. An example of such an algorithm is illustrated in Fig. 3.1. Addition of gender specific cut-offs will improve diagnostic accuracy in women. More accelerated diagnostic strategies based on measurement on admission and at 90 min or 2 h have also been proposed. The strategies are appropriate for low risk chest pain patients and are probably best when combined with a formal risk stratification tool.

Diagnostic Strategies Utilizing Limit of Blank or Limit of Detection of a High Sensitivity Assay

As high sensitivity troponin assays have a low value as limit of blank or limit of detection, a diagnostic strategy using a single troponin measurement on admission combined with clinical selection of a low risk group has been proposed as a means of rapid exclusion of MI. Patients who have a low risk score and a normal ECG and

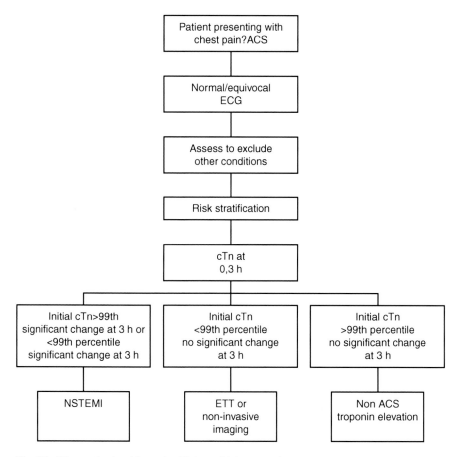

Fig. 3.1 Diagnostic algorithm using high sensitivity troponin measurement

a cardiac troponin below the limit of detection when measured using a high sensitivity assay are considered at low risk and discharged. Meta-analysis of existing studies has shown that the diagnostic accuracy of such an approach is probably clinically acceptable [12] but no prospective clinical trials have been undertaken of such a strategy.

Diagnostic Strategies Incorporating Delta Troponin

A very rapid rule out strategy based on a diagnostic discriminant plus the use of delta troponin has been proposed. This utilizes the low within individual imprecision combined with the low analytical imprecision of high sensitivity troponin assays. Current evidence suggests that an absolute value for delta troponin is diagnostically more efficient than a relative value (percentage change in troponin).

The value for this absolute delta needs to be established for each individual high sensitivity troponin assay. As it is known that within individual variation for cardiac troponin is of the order of 50–60 % the value corresponding to 50 % of the reference interval may be a useful pragmatic starting point. However, large-scale clinical validation of absolute troponin values remains a work in progress.

A preliminary study of such a strategy utilized measurement on admission and 1 h from admission [13]. Patients were then divided into three groups. The first group was those who had cTnT below 12 ng/L at presentation and an absolute delta less than 3 ng/L over 1 h. This corresponded to 56 % of the patients had a negative predictive value of 100 %. The second group was those who had an initial troponin greater than 52 ng/L and a Delta troponin of greater than 5 ng/L over 1 h. This accounted for 19 % of the patients and had a ruling positive predictive value 76 %. The remaining 24 % of patients were put in an intermediate category and went on for further diagnostic testing. The findings of this study have been confirmed in a subsequent multicenter evaluation.

Pitfalls of High Sensitivity Troponin Measurement

It has been recognized from the beginning of troponin measurements that elevation of cTnT and cTnI occur outside of the acute coronary syndrome population [14]. I improved sensitivity has proved to be a two-edged sword, as noted by Robert Jesse's insightful statement *"when troponin was lousy assay it was a great test, but now that it's a great assay it's a lousy test"* [15].

Although the range of other clinical conditions associated with a cardiac troponin above the 99th percentile is large and growing and may well be even larger with the advent of high sensitivity assays, these account for the minority of cases who present the chest pain where the differential diagnosis is of an acute coronary syndrome. It must be remembered that a troponin that remains below the 99th percentile and does not change is an excellent negative predictive test but must always be combined with clinical assessment. If this is remembered the majority of patients can be rapidly assessed and MI ruled out.

High Sensitivity Troponin in the Outpatient or Primary Care Setting

High sensitivity troponin has shown itself to be a prognostic marker in the community setting. The potential may well be there to use high sensitivity troponin measurements as a way of identifying apparently low-risk individuals who are at high risk the future for cardiovascular events for intervention with preventative strategies. Current risk scoring algorithms are known to be good at identifying high-risk individuals and low risk individuals but not very good for those at intermediate risk. It may be that measurement of cardiac troponin the high sensitivity assay will fulfil this role. Data (so far only published as an abstract and presented) has shown that in the context of a randomized controlled trial of a statin, those randomized to treatment that had a fall in troponin levels had the best outcome.

References

1. Myocardial infarction redefined–a consensus document of The Joint European Society of Cardiology/American College of Cardiology Committee for the redefinition of myocardial infarction. Eur Heart J. 2000;21:1502–13.
2. Thygesen K, Alpert JS, White HD, Jaffe AS, Apple FS, Galvani M, et al. Universal definition of myocardial infarction. Circulation. 2007;116:2634–53.
3. Apple FS, Collinson PO. Analytical characteristics of high-sensitivity cardiac troponin assays. Clin Chem. 2012;58:54–61.
4. Keller T, Zeller T, Peetz D, Tzikas S, Roth A, Czyz E, et al. Sensitive troponin I assay in early diagnosis of acute myocardial infarction. N Engl J Med. 2009;361:868–77.
5. Collinson P, Goodacre S, Gaze D, Gray A. Very early diagnosis of chest pain by point-of-care testing: comparison of the diagnostic efficiency of a panel of cardiac biomarkers compared with troponin measurement alone in the RATPAC trial. Heart. 2012;98:312–8.
6. Collinson PO, Heung YM, Gaze D, Boa F, Senior R, Christenson R, Apple FS. Influence of population selection on the 99th percentile reference value for cardiac troponin assays. Clin Chem. 2012;58:219–25.
7. Koerbin G, Abhayaratna WP, Potter JM, Apple FS, Jaffe AS, Ravalico TH, Hickman PE. Effect of population selection on 99th percentile values for a high sensitivity cardiac troponin I and T assays. Clin Biochem. 2013;46:1636–43.
8. McKie PM, Heublein DM, Scott CG, Gantzer ML, Mehta RA, Rodeheffer RJ, et al. Defining high-sensitivity cardiac troponin concentrations in the community. Clin Chem. 2013;59:1099–107.
9. Shah AS, Griffiths M, Lee KK, McAllister DA, Hunter AL, Ferry AV, et al. High sensitivity cardiac troponin and the under-diagnosis of myocardial infarction in women: prospective cohort study. BMJ. 2015;350:g7873.
10. deFilippi CR, de Lemos JA, Christenson RH, Gottdiener JS, Kop WJ, Zhan M, Seliger SL. Association of serial measures of cardiac troponin T using a sensitive assay with incident heart failure and cardiovascular mortality in older adults. JAMA. 2010;304:2494–502.
11. Saunders JT, Nambi V, de Lemos JA, Chambless LE, Virani SS, Boerwinkle E, et al. Cardiac troponin T measured by a highly sensitive assay predicts coronary heart disease, heart failure, and mortality in the Atherosclerosis Risk in Communities Study. Circulation. 2011;123:1367–76.
12. Zhelev Z, Hyde C, Youngman E, Rogers M, Fleming S, Slade T, et al. Diagnostic accuracy of single baseline measurement of Elecsys Troponin T high-sensitive assay for diagnosis of acute myocardial infarction in emergency department: systematic review and meta-analysis. BMJ. 2015;350:h15.
13. Reichlin T, Schindler C, Drexler B, Twerenbold R, Reiter M, Zellweger C, et al. One-hour rule-out and rule-in of acute myocardial infarction using high-sensitivity cardiac troponin T. Arch Intern Med. 2012;172:1211–8.
14. Collinson PO, Hadcocks L, Foo Y, Rosalki SB, Stubbs PJ, Morgan SH, O'Donnell J. Cardiac troponins in patients with renal dysfunction. Ann Clin Biochem. 1998;35(Pt 3):380–6.
15. Jesse RL. On the relative value of an assay versus that of a test: a history of troponin for the diagnosis of myocardial infarction. J Am Coll Cardiol. 2010;55:2125–8.

Chapter 4
Evaluation of Patients Presenting with Chest Pain in the Emergency Department: Where Do Troponins Fit In?

Martin Paul Than and Louise Cullen

Abstract Patients presenting to the Emergency Department with symptoms consistent with possible acute cardiac ischaemia, particularly chest pain, are one of the most common patient groups presenting to Emergency Departments in the developed world. These patients account for approximately 10% of Emergency Department presentations and up to 25% of hospital admissions (Goodacre et al., Heart 91:229–230, 2005). Up to 90% of these patients do not have a final diagnosis of an acute coronary syndrome (ACS). This large group of patients consumes considerable hospital resources with extensive investigations being common practice. Cardiac troponin is very important in this assessment process because traditionally, the large number of hospital admissions has been driven by a need to measure circulating cardiac troponin on arrival at hospital and then again at a delayed period afterwards. Historically, the second blood sample has been approximately 6 h or later after arrival or symptom onset. This timeframe has been used because early research on cardiac troponins suggested that troponin rises due to myocardial necrosis from acute myocardial infarction (AMI) were not reliably detectable until 6–12 h after symptom onset (Cooper et al., Chest pain of recent onset: assessment and diagnosis of recent onset chest pain or discomfort of suspected cardiac origin. London: National Clinical Guideline Centre for Acute and Chronic Conditions. http://publications.nice.org.uk/chest-pain-of-recent-onset-cg95. Accessed 15 Mar 2011, 2010).

Keywords Chest pain presenting in the ER • Troponins in chest pain in the ER • Emergency department use of troponins • Acute cardiac ischemia and troponins • Acute coronary syndrome and troponins

M.P. Than, MB, BS (✉)
Emergency Department, Chirstchurch Hospital, Christchurch, New Zealand
e-mail: martin@thanstedman.onmicrosoft.com

L. Cullen, MB, BS
Department of Emergency Medicine, Royal Brisbane and Women's Hospital, Herston, QLD, Australia
e-mail: louise-cullen@bigpond.com

© Springer International Publishing Switzerland 2016
A.S. Maisel, A.S. Jaffe (eds.), *Cardiac Biomarkers*,
DOI 10.1007/978-3-319-42982-3_4

Patients presenting to the Emergency Department with symptoms consistent with possible acute cardiac ischaemia, particularly chest pain, are one of the most common patient groups presenting to Emergency Departments in the developed world. These patients account for approximately 10 % of Emergency Department presentations and up to 25 % of hospital admissions [1]. Up to 90 % of these patients do not have a final diagnosis of an acute coronary syndrome (ACS). This large group of patients consumes considerable hospital resources with extensive investigations being common practice. Cardiac troponin is very important in this assessment process because traditionally, the large number of hospital admissions has been driven by a need to measure circulating cardiac troponin on arrival at hospital and then again at a delayed period afterwards. Historically, the second blood sample has been approximately 6 h or later after arrival or symptom onset. This timeframe has been used because early research on cardiac troponins suggested that troponin rises due to myocardial necrosis from acute myocardial infarction (AMI) were not reliably detectable until 6–12 h after symptom onset [2].

Most emergency departments are unable to keep such patients in acute resuscitation areas in which they are initially assessed for this prolonged period of testing, and will need to transfer them either to some form of observation ward, or to an inpatient ward for these delayed troponin tests to be performed. The consequence of this delay in the second blood sample is that such patients often remain in hospital overnight.

The sequence of events (highlighted by roman numerals) for assessment of patients is often as follows: (i) the patient is initially seen by a triage nurse, (ii) is then seen by a first emergency department nurse and (iii) assessed by an emergency department doctor. Following initial assessment and realisation that further, delayed, investigations are needed, the patient (iv) requires transfer to an observation area. If the patient is referred to an inpatient team they will be (v) moved to an inpatient ward where they will then be (vi) seen at some point by another acute in-patient doctor, sometimes two, such as the intern and the resident. The next morning the patient will then also be (vi) seen by an attending specialist on their ward round (with a resident and an intern) and a further plan will be made, often to initiate secondary testing such as Exercise Stress Test (EST) or Cardiac CT angiography CTCA). It may be felt these investigations are best dealt with immediately and therefore the (vii) patient remains in hospital even longer while these are performed. In addition to the steps described time multiple handovers occur between various doctors and many nursing shifts are involved with the patient care. Each of these handovers creates duplication and the potential for medical error through miscommunication. Thus, for the 85 % or more patients who will not finally have a diagnosis of AMI, there is considerable staff time, repetition and wastage occurring. Additionally, most hospitals in developed nations suffer from in-patient bed shortages, bed block and delayed patient flow, resulting in patients accumulating in the ED. Bed Block is the principle reason for ED overcrowding which has a proven association with a number of adverse patient outcomes, including increased mortality [3–7]. Recent data from 14 million patients showed an odds ratio of 1.79 for death in patients delayed in the ED for more than 6 h [8]. This problem also contributes to high costs. In the USA, ED overcrowding is associated with costs exceeding several billion dollars per year and is a significant health issue. A rapid, reliable and reproducible process to identify early-discharge candidates at low short-term risk of missed major adverse cardiac events amongst this patient group is a global need [9]. Later in this chapter we will discuss diagnostic strategies that that aim to achieve this by enabling testing for cardiac troponin at earlier time-points consequently avoiding prolonged observation of the patient.

As already mentioned, cardiac troponins are a cornerstone of this investigative process and the principal reason for prolonged observation in hospital. According to the first, second and third universal definitions of myocardial infarction [10], cardiac troponin are a vital component for the diagnosis of an AMI. Therefore the process of conducting serial troponin investigations principally relates to the detection of those patients presenting who do have myocardial necrosis and are diagnosed as having a non ST segment elevation myocardial infarction (NSTEMI). Acute Coronary Syndromes consist of ST-elevation myocardial infarction (STEMI), non-ST-elevation myocardial infarction (NSTEMI) and unstable angina (UA). The process of conducting serial troponin testing does not rule out the possibility of UA. This is why further tests are often ordered following the serial troponin sampling.

Cardiac Troponins and Other Diagnostic Tools in the Initial Assessment of Patients with Possible Cardiac Ischaemia (Excluding Stemi)

The principal diagnostic parameters available during the initial phase of assessment are (i) clinical assessment information, (ii) ECG and (iii) cardiac troponins.

(i) A history will be taken and a bedside examination performed to some extent in all patients. It is important to remember that based on Bayes theorem, the interpretation of any later test result is dependent upon the pre-test probability of the disease or outcome [11]. This is the rationale for always using pre-test probability or risk assessment in conjunction with an investigation.

Traditionally, the probability of AMI has been determined using clinical acumen primarily involving historical variables and risk factors learnt at medical school and reinforced during clinical practice. Unfortunately, evidence suggests that neither symptomatic history nor presence of chronic risk factors for coronary artery disease are as predictive as initially thought, when used in the emergency-department context [12–16]. In addition, the experience of the initial-assessing doctors in emergency departments may vary considerably depending on the hospital setting (i.e. an academic department or a rural hospital).

As a result of this, the other early investigations (ECG and cardiac troponin) are especially important to help with accurate assessment.

(ii) Patients with clear ST segment elevation on an initial ECG form a separate diagnostic group that will fast-tracked for emergent care. Acute ischemic changes on the ECG such as ST depression and T wave inversion can be useful indicators of an ACS but can occur in both NSTEMI and unstable angina.

More importantly ischemic ECG changes are often absent in AMI which limits the reliability of ECG in helping rule-out AMI.

(iii) Cardiac troponins form part of the definition of acute myocardial infarction and are both highly specific and highly sensitive for the assessment of AMI. The relative unreliability of both clinical and ECG findings makes the results of the cardiac troponin tests especially important.

This chapter will now focus on how cardiac troponins are utilised in the assessment of patients such as those with chest pain who are suspected of having an AMI.

Value of Combining Clinical Assessment with ECG and Cardiac Troponins

Given the relatively poor diagnostic performance of clinical findings and ECG compared to cardiac troponin in the assessment of patients with possible AMI one could be forgiven for wondering if these diagnostic parameters have any role at all apart from the detection of STEMI. ECG will always remain a key part of this assessment process as it is pivotal to the diagnosis of STEMI. What then of clinical assessment? Should one just rely upon ECG and cardiac troponin alone? Logic would suggest that no test should be used in isolation of the pre-test findings and clinical scenario. For example, considerable caution should exercised in using ECG and cardiac troponins alone to rule-out AMI in a patient whom the clinician believes subjectively to be at very high risk of AMI. In addition, UA will not be diagnosed by using ECG and troponin testing alone.

Purpose and Steps in Evaluation of Patients with Symptoms of Possible Cardiac Ischaemia in the Emergency Department

The four categories below summarise the process involved in assessing a patient with symptoms due to a possible AMI. Each step has a possible role for cardiac troponin testing.

Early Detection of ST Elevation Acute Myocardial Infarction (STEMI)

Patients with symptoms suggestive of acute cardiac ischaemia should have an electrocardiogram (ECG) performed almost immediately on arrival at hospital (and certainly within 10 min). This is to expedite the transfer of patients with STEMI to the catheter lab (or to initiate drug thrombolysis and/or patient transfer in centres without access to acute percutaneous intervention). Occasionally, the ECG (and the clinical findings) are inconclusive causing potential delays in transfer to the catheter lab.

> *Rapid testing for cardiac troponin (e.g. using point of care assays) may occasionally have a role in these patients if the diagnosis of STEMI is unclear from the patient presentation or ECG. However clinicians should be extremely cautious in interpreting these results due to delays to troponin elevation in very early presenters and imprecision of the POC assays.*

Assessment for the Possibility of Other Acute Potentially Life-Threatening Diagnoses

Other conditions can mimic the symptoms of acute cardiac ischaemia and early assessment of patients with symptoms of possible AMI such as chest pain should include screening for other serious diagnoses including (but not limited to) thoracic aortic dissection, pulmonary embolism and pancreatitis. Cardiac troponin may be raised in such conditions or indeed any cause of systemic stress but is not a principal diagnostic modality in such circumstances.

> *Cardiac troponin can provide useful prognostic information for such patients as a rising detectable troponin due to any other non-AMI condition is a poor prognostic sign.*

Assessment for Possible Non-ST Elevation Myocardial Infarction (NSTEMI)

Patients with a NSTEMI require monitoring for the possibility of cardiac arrhythmias, initiation of drug such as aspirin and beta blockers and usually angiography to detect critical coronary stenoses requiring intervention.

> Cardiac troponin (supported where necessary with imaging) is the key diagnostic modality for detecting NSTEMI. Consequently cardiac troponin is also the most important test in ruling-out NSTEMI. This is important because as already mentioned, most patients presenting to the ED with possible cardiac symptoms do not have an AMI or an ACS.

Assessment for Possible Unstable Angina and Underlying Coronary Artery Disease

After ruling out AMI further investigations are usually necessary to identify those patients likely to have unstable angina and/or needing further management interventions for underlying critical coronary artery stenosis. This group is almost defined by the fact that cardiac troponin levels are below the diagnostic cut-off for AMI (the 99th percentile of a healthy reference population).

> *It has become possible to detect very low levels of circulating cardiac troponin with increasing analytical accuracy and hence there has been increased identification of patients with NSTEMI. The cohort of patients with UA has become smaller but still certainly exists.*

Although troponin can provide useful information in all the scenarios described above, its principle role is in the detection of NSTEMI and this chapter will focus on this topic area.

Rule-out and Rule-in

In the introduction we discussed that most patients being assessed for possibly cardiac chest pain in the emergency department do not have an AMI or an ACS. This means that the initial assessment is predominately focused on rule-out. This chapter will focus on rule-out strategies, however accurate rule-in of AMI is also important.

Rule-in

Investigations such as angiography are expensive and carry a risk to the patient. Ideally, almost all patients with positive test results leading to angiography during chest pain work-up will be found to have critical coronary stenoses on angiography. Additionally, medications usually started after the diagnosis of AMI also have costs including side effects that make accurate rule-in of AMI important. The universal definition of myocardial infarction emphasises that a dynamic change in cardiac troponin levels should be present in order to diagnose AMI. This dynamic change is often described as the 'delta'. It is unclear exactly how much change is diagnostic and whether absolute or relative change in cardiac troponin levels should be used. Absolute

Fig. 4.1 (**a**) What currently happens in many hospitals in the developed world when patients with possible acute coronary syndrome are assessed in the emergency department. (**b**) The objective of an ADP is to facilitate the patient discharge as illustrated

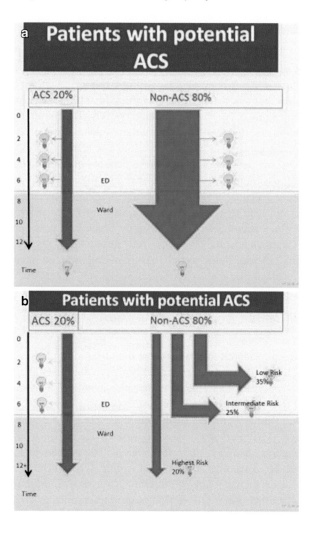

change may be preferable because and large and potentially misleading relative changes are possible at low detection levels. It should also be noted that such dynamic change criteria would be specific to the assay used and time between blood samples.

Rule-out

As mentioned, rule-out of AMI in patients with chest pain is often a protracted process. There has been considerable recent research on more rapid assessment strategies. We will discuss how cardiac troponin is integrated into such 'accelerated' diagnostic processes.

Rule-out: Traditional Management

Figure 4.1a demonstrates what currently happens in many hospitals in the developed world when patients with possible acute coronary syndrome are assessed in the emergency department. In this illustration it has been assumed that the prevalence rate of ACS is approximately 20 %. The lightbulbs represent decision-making points by the attending clinician in which a decision is made to proceed to another investigation (e.g. exercise stress test or angiography), and/or discharge the patient. One can see that amongst those patients that do have ACS (who really do require admission to hospital and further investigations), a small number of patients may have decisions made at earlier time points such as 2 or 4 h after arrival at the ED that could lead to essentially unsafe discharge decisions. The proportion of patients (80 %) without ACS is noticeably larger and traditionally most of these patients remain in hospital (in ED or elsewhere) undergoing prolonged observation and testing either on some sort of chest pain unit or on an inpatient ward.

Rule-out: Accelerated Decision Making for Rule-out of AMI

Initial research in this area use the terminology: 'accelerated diagnostic protocol'. This terminology is still used however there is some resistance to the concept of using protocols in medicine because it implies a certain rigidity. Subsequently, the expression accelerated diagnostic pathway has also been used and these processes are similar if not identical. Both these phrases are frequently abbreviated to the letters ADP. Perhaps the best phrase of all to use would be 'accelerated decision-making pathway', described below. The objective of an ADP is to facilitate the patient discharge as illustrated in Fig. 4.1b. In this scenario, strategies to identify those patients at low and intermediate risk of coming to short term harm have been identified. An ADP facilitates prompter diagnostic decisions through sampling blood at earlier time-points for cardiac troponin (cTn). This then allows clinicians to rapidly proceed to the same 'next step' in clinical management (such as cardiac stress test, imaging and/or discharge) as would have occurred using a more prolonged serial troponin testing time course to exclude AMI.

Case 1
A 64-year-old hospital porter who is fit and well had a single 50-min episode of chest pain following earthquake tremor 2 h previously. The chest pain self-resolved and he had no other episodes. He had a medical history of hypothyroidism only and no cardiac risk factors. He was not on any regular medications and had an allergy to penicillin. Initial ECGs were normal and he had a cTnI on arrival of <0.01 µg/L (assay 99th percentile at 0.028 µg/L and 10 % CV at 0.032 µg/L). His TIMI (Thrombolysis In Myocardial Infarction) score for unstable angina or non ST elevation myocardial infraction [17]) was zero (i.e. low-risk).

> *Usual management would have been for prolonged observation with blood taken for a second cTnI measurement 6–12 h after arrival but in this case he was managed using an accelerated diagnostic protocol as described in the ADAPT study [18].*
>
> *His repeat cTnI at 2 hours after arrival was also <0.01 µg/L. He was then discharged home approximately 4 h after arrival at hospital and returned to the outpatient department for an exercise stress test the next day; which was normal. There were no follow-up adverse events.*
>
> Comment
>
> Clearly this is a good outcome. Data from the ASPECT study [18] suggest that approximately 15 % of patients would be eligible for such an early discharge strategy using a central laboratory troponin assay as the only biomarker. This is a step forward but it would be of greater value if a higher proportion of patients were eligible for early discharge. Further research is in progress using later generation cTn assays. It is hoped that it will be possible to use a slightly higher pre-test probability level for new risk scores on the basis that the newer assays are more sensitive. This would allow the incorporation of a broader and larger risk group of patients in a rule-out strategy.

High Sensitivity Cardiac Troponin Assays

Do 'High Sensitive' Troponin Assays Provide an Advantage in the ED Over Analytically Less Sensitive Assays?

Patients *that do not have positive results using analytically less sensitive assays,* but that do have positive results (levels >99th percentile of a reference population) using highly sensitive (hs-cTn) assays are at an increased long-term risk of death and cardiac events [19]. Nonetheless, this is not necessarily of immediate and primary importance in the initial emergency department assessment for AMI.

Cardiac troponin assays with high sensitivity may more rapidly identify patients with an AMI, which may lead to the instigation of directed treatments at an earlier time point. However, it is still unproven that shortening the delay prior to targeted therapies will actually reduce morbidity and mortality in those with a non-diagnostic ECG (Non ST elevation AMI – NSTEMI).

What *is* of significant relevance for the initial assessment of patients with chest pain is the possibility of using cardiac troponin assays to assist with earlier discharge. Data suggests that using high sensitivity cardiac troponin assays may allow AMI to be detected earlier, i.e. 2–3 h after hospital attendance rather than more than 6 h after attendance [20]. In the United Kingdom the National Institute for Health Care and Excellence (NICE) has recently released a diagnostics guidance for high sensitivity cardiac troponin assays [21]. It recommends that "the assays are recommended for use with early rule-out protocols, which typically include a blood sample for cardiac troponin I or T taken at initial assessment in an emergency department and a second blood sample taken after 3 h". Also recommended is that high sensitivity cardiac troponin assays be used in conjunction with electrocardiogram (ECG) for diagnosis of NSTEMI. Using such strategies could lead to opportunities for earlier aggressive medical management and cardiac admission, as well as possible discharge. However a recent publication has suggested that testing for troponin at 0 and 4 h after arrival at hospital may not have sufficient sensitivity for safe rule-out in all patients even when used in conjunction with the ECG and without any pre-test probability scoring [22].

Challenges with Interpretation of High Sensitivity Cardiac Troponin

High sensitivity cardiac troponin provide assays more analytically reliable results below the 99th percentile of the assay. As often happens in medicine, extra information is usually a good thing but provide challenges too. This is illustrated by the cases below.

Case 2 (in 2 Parts)

(a) *A 63-year-old man presents to the ED with a history of 3 h of central chest pain radiating to left arm, starting at rest and sounding cardiac in nature. He has been pain-free after having some sublingual nitrate during a 15 min ambulance journey from his office. He had a similar episode of pain lasting 30 min the previous evening (10 h earlier) after running up some stairs. He is a current smoker with diabetes, and has a strong family history of early onset coronary artery disease. He has previously had a transient ischaemic attack and takes regular aspirin. His TIMI score is 3. His ECGs are normal. The local laboratory uses an hs-TnT assay and results at 0, 2 and 6 h after arrival at hospital are 4, 8 and 12 ng/L respectively (assay 99th percentile at 14 ng/L and 10% CV at 13 ng/L).*

What Should Happen Next?
He has three hs-TnT samples with values below the 99th percentile but hs-TnT shows a 8ng/L or 200% increase. Most emergency physicians would feel worried about the concerning presentation, risk profile and rising high sensitivity cardiac troponin levels, and would want further investigations before feeling comfortable with discharging the patient. Such testing could include further troponin measurement, a stress test or cardiac imaging.

(b) *Now let us suppose instead that the same patient has two hs-TnT tests done at arrival and 6 h later. The 0 and 6 h hs-TnT results are 15 and 16 ng/L respectively.*

Comment

Now there are levels above the 99th percentile but minimal dynamic change. Once again it is likely that further investigations would be requested, either further troponin measurement, stress test or cardiac imaging before discharging the patient. Such additional testing would also prove useful for deciding if AMI was present. Other investigation may be ordered to look for differential diagnoses. Sequential tests could be performed until more conclusive results were available.

Rises in High-Sensitivity Cardiac Troponin as a Result of Other Non-cardiac Diagnoses

It has been noted that a large number of causes of systemic and cardiac stress can lead to rises in cardiac troponin that are now detectable with the use of high-sensitivity cardiac troponin assays. As already mentioned, it is important the clinicians consider the possibility of other important diagnoses in the assessment of patients with chest pain. An example of this is illustrated by the case below:

Case 3

A 75 year-old man presents to the hospital with left-sided chest pain and shortness of breath. He is a vague historian and finds it hard to describe the nature of the chest pain although it seems to get worse on exertion. He is a smoker and suffers from bowel cancer, but following several operations he has been in remission for 3 months. He has mild lower leg pain but no swelling in his left calf. He is classified as intermediate probability (28%) of PE using the revised Geneva Score [18]. His initial investigations include both troponins and a d-dimer which is 1200 (cut-off <250). His hs-cTn results at 0 and 6 h are 15 and 25 ng/L (assay 99th percentile at 14 ng/L and 10% CV at 13 ng/L), respectively. He undergoes a CT pulmonary angiogram which shows multiple pulmonary emboli and mild cardiac septal bowing suggestive of right ventricular strain.

Comment

In this case a diagnosis of PE was made and further investigations for ACS will not be performed unless new symptoms or information arises. It is possibly useful to know that the presence of a raised cardiac troponin in conjunction with this patients pulmonary embolism put him at higher risk of complications from that pathology compared with a situation in which the cardiac troponin was not raised.

Unstable Angina and Underlying Coronary Artery Disease

It has already been mentioned that the proportion of patients diagnosed with unstable angina has gradually decreased as the 99th percentile of cardiac troponin assays has fallen but that also there will still be a small and important number of patients that still have unstable angina and underlying critical coronary artery stenosis. It is important to remember this because as illustrated by the Global Registry of Acute Coronary Events registry (GRACE) study, patients with unstable angina also have a significant medium-term risk of adverse event, and therapies including aggressive risk factor modification can improve patients longer term risk profile.

Two case examples of patients are described below:

Case 4
A 49 year old man attended the Emergency Department with a recent history of anterior central chest pain. The pain had started while he was at his desk at work and was not related to exertion. He had central anterior chest wall discomfort which are described as dull and heavy and also sharp in nature. He was an extremely fit man who participates in high level amateur cycling, exercising vigorously almost daily. His TIMI score was zero.

He had no significant past medical history, family history, or drug history.
Ongoing Management
He had blood drawn for contemporary cardiac troponin testing on arrival in the Emergency Department and 2 h later, with test results of 10 ng/L and 10 ng/L respectively. The doctor assessing the patient decided to admit the patient for a third delayed troponin, the result of which was 60 ng/L (99th percentile for assay 40 ng/L). As a result of this he was referred to cardiology services and underwent an angiogram which showed a 90 % stenosis of the circumflex artery. He underwent cardiac stenting and made a good recovery
Comment
This case was reviewed by faculty at the hospital to see if there are any clear lessons to learn from the case. The consensus was that apart from the physician's gestalt impression that the patient required a third troponin sample that there were no key features in the case that obviously indicated that such a third sample was needed. This case illustrates that there will always be some small number of patients for whom initial troponin levels will be negative but for whom there may be rises later due to a small NSTEMI, even in low risk patients. It is possible that one of the initial troponin tests may have been positive if a high-sensitivity troponin assay had been used.

Case 5

A 60-year-old man presented to the emergency department following a 30 min episode of heavy central chest pain. This occurred during a very stressful period of time at work but had not been related to exertion. He had had a similar episode approximately 3 days before, but none previously. The pain did not radiate and symptoms were not associated with diaphoresis. He was now feeling well. He had been previously well apart from mild hypothyroidism not requiring treatment. He had no family or significant drug history. The pain had occurred approximately 3.5 h prior to attendance at the emergency department. Other history and physical examination were unremarkable and is ECG was normal. He had blood drawn for troponin testing on arrival and after 3 h and the results of both these tests were the below the level of detection for the assay which was 10 ng/L. His Thrombolysis In Myocardial Infarction (TIMI) score was zero and he was discharged after approximately 4 h in hospital with an exercise treadmill test scheduled for the next day.

He remained asymptomatic until the treadmill which had to be stopped after 9 min because of heavy chest pain similar to the previous day. He had some early equivocal but non-diagnostic changes in his ST segments. A resident was called to review the test results and this doctor reported them as normal. The patient was discharged home.

Seven days later the patient be presented to hospital with more chest pain and an ECG showing an ST segment elevation myocardial infarction. Angiography showed a 90 % stenosis of his left anterior descending artery. During stenting there was a partial dissection of this artery which led to a ventricular fibrillation arrest which was terminated with a single DC shock. The patient spent 3 days in the cardiac intensive care unit subsequently made a good recovery and was completely well normal functionality and asymptomatic after 3 months.

Comment

This case again illustrates that even in low risk patients that the initial cardiac component tests can be negative in the presence of serious underlying coronary artery stenosis. It is not known if high-sensitivity cardiac troponins would have been raised this patient. It is also evident that the interpretation of the exercise treadmill test by the resident attending the patient was incorrect. Some ways, this case illustrates that secondary investigations: haemodynamic such as exercise stress tests or imaging based tests such as cardiac CT may still be necessary even in low risk patients. It is also worth noting that on case review hospital faculty felt that this patient should probably have been categorised as having crescendo angina because of the previous episode of chest pain 3 days before.

Summary

This chapter has described the process and difficulties associated with the initial assessment of patients with chest pain which is suspected to be due to acute cardiac ischaemia and possible AMI. Cardiac troponin is the most powerful diagnostic tool that a clinician has available and is used in conjunction with clinical pre-test probability assessment and ECG.

Traditionally, delayed troponin testing regimes have been used which have resulted in prolonged stays in hospital for patients. Recently, rapid diagnostic strategies have emerged along with high-sensitivity cardiac troponins which facilitate diagnostic pathways which allow earlier rule out of AMI.

High sensitivity cardiac troponins are more analytically reliable in low detection ranges blow the 99th percentile and research is ongoing as to how best use and integrate this information into optimal clinical practice. It is advised that the troponin results are always used in conjunction with a thorough clinical assessment including ECG testing and structured determination of pre-test probability preferably utilizing a validated risk score.

References

1. Goodacre S, Cross E, Arnold J, Angelini K, Capewell S, Nicholl J. The health care burden of acute chest pain. Heart. 2005;91:229–30.
2. Cooper A, Calvert N, Skinner J, et al. Chest pain of recent onset: assessment and diagnosis of recent onset chest pain or discomfort of suspected cardiac origin. London: National Clinical Guideline Centre for Acute and Chronic Conditions. 2010. http://publications.nice.org.uk/chest-pain-of-recent-onset-cg95. Accessed 15 Mar 2011.
3. Bernstein SL, Aronsky D, Duseja R, Epstein S, Handel D, Hwang U, et al. The effect of emergency department crowding on clinically oriented outcomes. Acad Emerg Med. 2009;16(1):1–10.
4. Richardson DB. Increase in patient mortality at 10 days associated with emergency department overcrowding. Med J Aust. 2006;184(5):213–6.
5. Sprivulis PC, Da Silva JA, Jacobs IG, Frazer AR, Jelinek GA. The association between hospital overcrowding and mortality among patients admitted via Western Australian emergency departments. Med J Aust. 2006;184(5):208–12.
6. Richardson DB. Increase in patient mortality at 10 days associated with emergency department overcrowding. Med J Aust [Comparative Study]. 2006;184(5):213–6.
7. Sprivulis PC, Da Silva JA, Jacobs IG, Frazer AR, Jelinek GA. The association between hospital overcrowding and mortality among patients admitted via Western Australian emergency departments. Med J Aust [Comparative Study Research Support, Non-U.S. Gov't]. 2006;184(5):208–12.
8. Guttmann A, Schull MJ, Vermeulen MJ, Stukel TA. Association between waiting times and short term mortality and hospital admission after departure from emergency department: population based cohort study from Ontario, Canada. BMJ [Research Support, Non-U.S. Gov't]. 2011;342:d2983.
9. Hollander JE, Robey JL, Chase MR, Brown AM, Zogby KE, Shofer FS. Relationship between a clear-cut alternative noncardiac diagnosis and 30-day outcome in emergency department patients with chest pain. Acad Emerg Med. 2007;14(3):210–5.

10. Thygesen K, Alpert JS, Jaffe AS, Simoons ML, Chaitman BR, Harvey D. White third universal definition of myocardial infarction. J Am Coll Cardiol. 2012;60(16):1581–98.
11. Diamond G, Kaul S. How would the Reverend Bayes interpret high-sensitivity troponin? Circulation. 2010;121:1172–5.
12. Goodacre SW, Angelini K, Arnold SR, Morris F. Clinical predictors of acute coronary syndromes in patients with undifferentiated chest pain. QJM. 2003;96(12):893–8.
13. Goodacre S, Locker T, Morris F, Campbell S. How useful are clinical features in the diagnosis of acute, undifferentiated chest pain? Acad Emerg Med. 2002;9(3):203–8.
14. Body R, McDowell G, Carley S, Mackway-Jones K. Do risk factors for chronic coronary heart disease help diagnose acute myocardial infarction in the emergency department? Resuscitation. 2008;79:41–5.
15. Body R, Carley S, Wibberley C, McDowell G, Ferguson J, Mackway-Jones K. The value of symptoms and signs in the emergent diagnosis of acute coronary syndromes. Resuscitation. 2010;81:281–6.
16. Han JH, Lindsell CJ, Luber S, Hoekstra KW, Hollander JE, Peacock WF, Pollack CV, Gibler WB. The role of cardiac risk factor burden in diagnosing acute coronary syndromes in the emergency department setting. Ann Emerg Med. 2007;49(2):145–52.
17. Antman EM, Cohen M, Bernink PJ, et al. The TIMI risk score for unstable angina/non-ST elevation MI: a method for prognostication and therapeutic decision making. JAMA. 2000;284:835–42.
18. Than M, Cullen L, Aldous S, Parsonage WA, Reid CM, Greenslade J, Flaws D, Hammett CJ, Beam DM, Ardagh MW, Troughton R, Brown AF, George P, Florkowski CM, Kline JA, Peacock WF, Maisel AS, Lim SH, Lamanna A, Richards AM. 2-Hour accelerated diagnostic protocol to assess patients with chest pain symptoms using contemporary troponins as the only biomarker: the ADAPT trial. J Am Coll Cardiol. 2012;5(59):2091–8.
19. Aldous SJ, Florkowski CM, Crozier IG, et al. High sensitivity troponin outperforms contemporary assays in predicting major adverse cardiac events up to two years in patients with chest pain. Ann Clin Biochem. 2011;48(Pt3):249–55. Epub 2011 Mar 25.
20. Reichlin T, Hochholzer W, Bassetti S, Steuer S, Stelzig C, Hartwiger S, et al. Early diagnosis of myocardial infarction with sensitive cardiac troponin assays. N Engl J Med. 2009;361:858–67.
21. National Institute of Health Care Excellence (NICE). Myocardial infarction (acute): early rule out using high-sensitivity troponin tests (Elecsys Troponin T high-sensitive, ARCHITECT STAT High Sensitive Troponin-I and AccuTnI + 3 assays)(DG15). 2015. http://nice.org.uk/guidance/dg15.
22. Pickering JW, Young JM, George P, Aldous S. The utility of presentation and 4-hour high sensitivity troponin I to rule-out acute myocardial infarction in the emergency department. Clin Biochem. 2015. pii: S0009-9120(15)00313-6. doi:10.1016/j.clinbiochem.2015.07.033.

Chapter 5
Using Cardiac Troponins in Patients with Acute Myocardial Infarction

Johannes Mair and Kristian Thygesen

Abstract Cardiac troponin I (cTnI) and cardiac troponin T (cTnT) have evolved as the new laboratory criterion standards for the diagnosis of myocardial injury with necrosis and thereby replaced creatine kinase isoenzyme MB (CKMB) as the bio-marker of choice in the Universal Definition of Myocardial Infarction. Over the last two decades the analytical sensitivities of troponin assays have been constantly improved which has resulted in an improved early diagnostic sensitivity of these cardiac biomarkers for the diagnosis of acute myocardial infarction (AMI). The most recent assays, the so called "high-sensitivity" cardiac troponin assays, have made it possible to introduce rapid rule-out and rule-in protocols for AMI in daily practice. Moreover, the time course of troponin release is greatly influenced by the situation depending on whether early reperfusion of the infarct-related coronary artery is achieved exposing an earlier cTn peak value around 12 h from symptom onset as an expression of emerged reperfusion of the myocardium supplied by this artery. Both cTnI and cTnT show a biphasic release pattern displaying a second peak 4–6 days after the onset of AMI. That is usually more pronounced for cTnT. Furthermore, the amount of troponin release correlates with infarct size and with the prognosis of AMI.

Keywords Cardiac troponins • High-sensitivity • Acute myocardial infarction • Diagnosis • Monitoring • Infarct size

J. Mair, MD
Department of Internal Medicine III – Cardiology and Angiology, Innsbruck Medical University, Innsbruck, Austria
e-mail: Johannes.mair@i-med.ac.at

K. Thygesen, MD, DSc (✉)
Department of Cardiology, Aarhus University Hospital, Aarhus, Denmark
e-mail: kristhyg@rm.dk; kthygesen@oncable.dk

© Springer International Publishing Switzerland 2016
A.S. Maisel, A.S. Jaffe (eds.), *Cardiac Biomarkers*,
DOI 10.1007/978-3-319-42982-3_5

Cardiac troponin I (cTnI) and cardiac troponin T (cTnT) are the biomarkers of choice for the diagnosis of myocardial injury with necrosis, because they are the most sensitive and cardiac-specific biomarkers currently available [1, 2]. Over the years the analytical sensitivity of cardiac troponin (cTn) assays has improved continuously and more recently, a new generation of cTn assays, i.e., the high-sensitivity (hs) cTn assays, have been introduced into routine clinical practice [2]. It is important to note, that these assays measure the same analyte as previous assay generations but with substantially improved analytical sensitivity and assay precision at a low measuring range [2]. From a clinical perspective it has been noted that the improved analytical performance of hs-cTn assays also increased their clinical ability to detect small amounts of myocardial injury with necrosis and to more precise identification of small differences in cTn concentrations in serial testing compared with previous cTn assay generations [2]. Thereby hs-cTn assays improve early diagnosis of acute myocardial infarction (AMI). However, hs-cTn is also more sensitive for the detection of myocardial injury unrelated to acute myocardial ischemia. Therefore, the increase in early diagnostic sensitivity of hs-cTn assays for AMI comes at the cost of a reduced AMI specificity, because more patients with other causes of acute or chronic myocardial injury without overt myocardial ischemia are detected than with previous cTn assays, which is a challenge in daily routine use.

Early Diagnosis of Acute Myocardial Infarction by Novel Rapid Algorithms

Patients presenting with suspected AMI are a major subset of patients presenting to the Emergency Department (ED). However, the majority will finally have other often benign disorders. Accordingly, rapid rule-out of AMI is an important task in chest pain patients. Assays of hs-cTn detect cTn release at an earlier time point than the previous generations of cTn assays and thus reduce the "troponin-blind" interval. This permits the implementation of more rapid algorithms for the evaluation of patients with clinically suspected AMI.

According to the recent European Society of Cardiology (ESC) guideline for the management of acute coronary syndrome (ACS), blood samples should be obtained at the time of the ED presentation and 3 h or alternatively even only 1 h after admission when using hs-cTn assays [3]. In low-risk patients presenting more than 6 h after chest pain onset, a single hs-cTn test result at presentation is considered to be sufficient for ruling out AMI. However, the exact onset of symptoms is often difficult to determine in clinical practice and ED physicians must be cautious about applying the 6 h threshold for single blood sampling. This strategy may be applied when the initial electrocardiogram (ECG) has ruled-out ST-segment elevation and all available clinical information (e.g., chest pain characteristics, ECG changes) including detailed clinical assessment and overall cardiovascular risk have been taken into consideration. Observation time in the ED may be reduced regarding rule-out of AMI in low-risk patients (without ongoing symptoms and a Global Registry of Acute Coronary Events [GRACE] score <140), because patients with an AMI can be reliably identified within 3 h after admission with close to 100 % sensitivity and negative predictive value when using a hs-cTn assay. As regards the decision limit for the AMI diagnosis it is recommended to apply the upper reference limit (URL) defined as the 99th percentile value of cTn concentrations measured in a healthy reference population [1, 2, 4].

It is worth noting that due to the higher sensitivity of hs-cTn assays for the detection of small myocardial injuries a significant number of patients with unstable angina migrates from that designation to the AMI category [5]. However, even by measurement with hs-cTn assays, cTn test results cannot rule out significant coronary artery disease (CAD), if it does not cause acute myocardial injury (Fig. 5.1). Consequently, if the clinical situation is ambiguous and the pre-test likelihood of CAD is high or in early presenters within 2 h from symptom onset, additional subsequent sampling (e.g., at 6 h and even beyond) and/or stress testing or CAD imaging (e.g., stress echocardiography, myocardial scintigraphy, computed tomography coronary angiography) is still necessary to rule out significant CAD. Provided that these conditions are met rapid AMI rule-out protocols with early discharge from the ED are safe and furthermore, other serious diseases causing chest pain, e.g., pulmonary embolism and aortic dissection may not be missed.

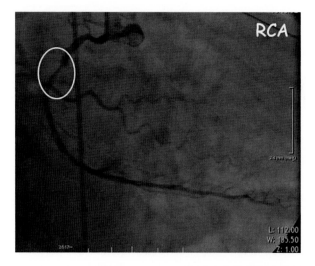

Fig. 5.1 A patient with 1-vessel coronary artery disease but normal admission high-sensitivity cardiac troponin T. This 59 year-old male had known arterial hypertension. He had a short episode of angina the day before admission. On admission he had no angina symptoms. The physical examination was normal except for a slightly elevated systolic blood pressure (150/80 mmHg). The resting ECG was normal. The high-sensitivity cardiac troponin T concentration was 8 ng/L (99th percentile URL = 14 ng/L). Elective coronary angiography revealed 1 vessel coronary artery disease with significant proximal stenosis of the RCA (marked with *white circle*). Abbreviations: *RCA* right coronary artery

Clinically Relevant Changes of hs-cTn Assay Concentration in Serial Testing

With respect to the clinical evaluation of chest pain patients serial testing of cTn is needed to evaluate the cTn kinetic [1, 2, 4]. According to the Universal Definition of Myocardial Infarction, at least two measurements of cTn are needed to verify a kinetic pattern [4]. Even in patients with pre-existing elevated hs-cTn values a significant change must be documented by serial measurements in order to demonstrate acute myocardial injury with necrosis. In general, most AMI patients have substantial changes of cTn values, i.e., the larger the cTn change, the higher the likelihood for the presence of AMI. However, it must be emphasized that dynamic cTn changes are not specific for AMI but are rather indicative of ongoing myocardial injury (Fig. 5.2).

Previously, the criteria for a significant change have only taken the analytical variation into account. Thus, based on a total analytical coefficient of variation (CV) <10 %, changes of serial cTn measurements >20 % have been considered to be significant for additional myocardial injury. This high analytical precision that is required to implement this approach is not present within the reference range for hs-cTn assays [2]. In addition, biological variation including diurnal rhythmicity needs to be considered for hs-cTn as well [2, 6]. Changes of hs-cTn measurements

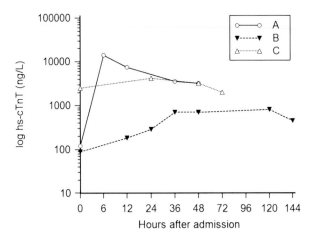

Fig. 5.2 The course of high sensitivity cardiac troponin T concentrations in a patient with and a patient without early reperfusion of the infarct-related coronary artery as compared to the troponin T kinetics in a patient with peri/myocarditis. (*A*) Successful primary PCI of a proximal LAD occlusion with a short delay from symptom onset of approximately 3 h. A rapid and very high early peak hs-cTnT value around 12 h is observed due to "wash-out" phenomenon. (*B*) Subacute successful primary PCI of an occlusion of a small LAD with a delay >24 h from symptom onset. Because of the late reperfusion of the infarct related coronary artery the peak of cTn values is delayed. The importance of an early tissue reperfusion of the infarcted myocardium for cTn release is obvious. (*C*) Pronounced myocardial injury with necrosis in a 31 year-old male with acute peri/myocarditis, which has been verified by magnetic resonance imaging of the heart. Coronary artery disease was ruled out by acute coronary angiography. Be aware of the log transformation of the presented cTnT values. Abbreviations: *hs-cTnT* high sensitivity troponin T, *PCI* percutaneous coronary intervention, *LAD* left anterior descending coronary artery

near the 99th percentile upper reference limit (URL) must exceed the conjoint analytical and biological variation to be of clinical significance. This is ensured by calculation of the so-called reference change values (RCV). These RCV values being assay and analyte specific must be obtained separately for each commercially available hs-cTn assay. For many of those the short-term RCVs are in the range of 40–60 % [2]. It is important to stress, that performance data for relative and absolute concentration changes are always hs-cTn assay specific.

However, there is a trade-off between sensitivity and specificity for the diagnosis of AMI when establishing the decision limit. Recently, it was demonstrated when evaluating serial changes using a pre-marketing version of the Abbott® hs-cTnI assay in pre-selected chest pain unit patients that an elevation of hs-cTnI values above the 99th percentile URL and with relative increases of >250 % over a 3 h period in patients with baseline values < URL as well as increases >50 % with modestly increased baseline values have optimized the specificity for the AMI diagnosis [7]. As expected, higher cTnI sensitivities were found at lower percentage changes of the cTnI concentrations. Hence, the selection of criteria for change limits for the AMI diagnosis will differ depending on whether there is a need for high specificity at the cost of lower sensitivity or increased sensitivity at the cost of lower specificity. Clinicians must be aware of this trade-off in evaluating individual patients.

As regards the evaluation of absolute versus relative changes in serial testing or whether the diagnostic performances of a percentage change would differ from an absolute change of hs-cTn concentrations, has been tested recently with the hs-cTnT assay. It was shown that in case of hs-cTnT values below or close to the 99th percentile URL, an absolute increase of hs-cTnT values (e.g., >7 ng/L over 2 h) is superior to a relative percentage changes from baseline [8]. In addition, the study design (e.g., AMI prevalence, blood sampling protocol) may influence the performance data of algorithms and optimal decision limits for absolute or relative changes in serial testing. Thus, there may be substantial differences if an algorithm, which has been developed in a high-risk population (e.g., a chest pain unit population or pre-selected ED chest pain patients), is applied in a low-risk everyday general ED population with an AMI prevalence in the range of 5–10 %.

Despite these limitations when gathering data from the literature into a solitary algorithm, the model in Fig. 5.3 is suggested to be applied for the evaluation of patients being suspect for AMI based on the use of hs-cTn serial testing. Although the algorithm pretends to bring all published clinical data for hs-cTnI and hs-cTnT together, it should be pointed out that an individually assay-specific algorithm may function better for special hs-cTn assays.

Timing of hs-cTn Measurements in Serial Testing

Although an interval of 3 h for cTn sampling is still recommended in patients who are admitted at the ED with chest pain, further algorithms with shorter periods of sampling (i.e. 2 h and even 1 h) have been examined:

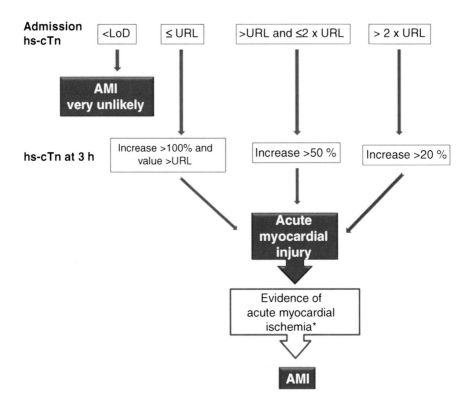

Fig. 5.3 Algorithm for rapid evaluation of clinically suspected acute myocardial infarction with high-sensitivity cardiac troponin testing. This approach assures that the changes will be at least above the analytical and biological variation of hs-cTnI and hs-cTnT values, respectively. *Evidence of acute myocardial ischemia by new ECG changes and/or new imaging corroborations. Abbreviations: *hs-cTn* high-sensitivity cardiac troponin, *URL* 99th percentile upper reference limit of healthy controls, *AMI* acute myocardial infarction, *LoD* lower limit of detection

Diagnostic Value of a Single hs-cTn Measurement

Undetectable hs-cTn concentration at admission has a very high negative predictive value (NPV) of (98–100%) for AMI [9, 10]. Besides, the aggregated sensitivities and specificities are 89.5% and 77.1%, respectively at the URL of 14 ng/L of hs-cTnT (Roche Diagnostics®) [10]. Likewise, the commercially available hs-cTnI assay (Abbott Diagnostics®) yields comparable values at the URL with an aggregated sensitivity of 80% and an aggregated specificity of 93%[11]. So, when evaluating a single admission sample of cTn a low rule-out limit and a higher rule-in threshold for the diagnosis of AMI could be used. Aside from this rule, a higher rule-in limit may be applied in the elderly (>70 years) and in case of hs-cTnT in patients with renal failure [12].

Diagnostic Value of hs-cTnT Measurements Based on a 2 h Algorithm

A study that included chest pain patients with hs-cTnT values <14 ng/L at 0 and 2 h with an increase <4 ng/L has revealed a very high NPV for AMI of 99.5–99.9 % (95 % confidence interval) [13]. Furthermore, it was shown that AMI could be ruled-out safely even in patients with mild, unspecific ECG abnormalities which often are pre-existing. These findings permit rapid rule-out of the diagnosis of AMI in up to 60 % of patients suspected as having AMI. Moreover, it also has a rule-in part (hs-cTnT values >52 ng/L at 0 or 2 h and an increase >10 ng/L from baseline to 2 h) that provides a high positive predictive value (PPV) of 85 % for the rule-in of AMI. However, a significant proportion (approximately 20 %) of "grey zone" patients remains standing in whom additional blood sampling is required. Even though this algorithm has been derived from a high-risk population (AMI prevalence of 16 %) it has been successfully validated in a low risk population (AMI prevalence of 9 %) as well [13].

Do We Need Additional Biomarkers Beyond hs-cTn for the Diagnosis of AMI?

The most marketed biomarkers beyond hs-cTn for the early diagnosis of AMI are heart-type fatty acid binding protein (H-FABP) and copeptin. However, the majority of studies regarding that have been comparisons with the prior less sensitive cTn assays only. More recent comparative data with hs-cTn assays do not support a clinical relevant benefit of these biomarkers when combined with hs-cTn measurements [14–16].

Monitoring and Risk Stratification by Serial hs-cTn Testing in AMI

In patients with AMI, cTn concentrations rise rapidly after symptom onset and remain elevated usually several days and even 1–2 weeks in more extended AMI due to ongoing proteolysis of the contractile apparatus [17]. The time course of cTn release is greatly influenced by the situation as to whether early reperfusion of the infarct-related coronary artery can be achieved with an earlier and higher peak value around 12 h from onset of symptom in case of emerged tissue reperfusion of the myocardium perfused by this artery (Fig. 5.2) [17]. It appears that cTnT as well as cTnI show a biphasic release pattern displaying a second peak several days (4–6d) after AMI, which usually are more pronounced for cTnT. This second peak should not be misinterpreted as a reinfarction in uncomplicated AMI patients. Furthermore, the amount of cTn release correlates with infarct size and with the prognosis of AMI patients [18].

Conditions with hs-cTn Elevations Other Than Caused by AMI

Given the high frequency of detectable elevated hs-cTn values in patients admitted to the ED [9], especially in patients with cardiovascular comorbidities, it is worth mentioning that an elevated hs-cTn concentration alone is insufficient to make the diagnosis of AMI [1, 2, 4]. Every hs-cTn elevations should be interpreted in the context of the clinical circumstances (Fig. 5.4). Regardless of the cut-off value used for ruling in AMI, the critical distinction that remains to be made is to determine whether there is a significant rising pattern of hs-cTn values in serial testing as an indicator of acute myocardial injury with necrosis (see above). Chronically elevated hs-cTn values without significant changes during the observation period are often detected in patients with cardiac diseases other than CAD [1, 2]. Slightly elevated stable hs-cTnT concentrations are commonly found in patients with renal failure [1, 12]. However, even if there is unequivocal evidence for acute myocardial injury, clinical judgement still remains essential to assess whether acute myocardial ischemia is the most likely underlying cause. Only if the latter condition is present an AMI may be diagnosed (Figs. 5.3 and 5.4) [1–4].

Type 2 MI Versus Non-ischemic Myocardial Injury with Necrosis

The categorization of patients into types of myocardial infarction was initiated in 2007 in an attempt to make sure that there was a distinction between individuals who might need urgent treatment from what is most often an event associated with acute plaque rupture (MI type 1) from those who could have ischemic myocardial necrosis in a clinical setting coexistent with an acute supply/demand oxygen imbalance without plaque rupture (MI type 2) [19]. However, to distinguish type 2 MI from non-ischemic myocardial injury with necrosis represents another challenging problem for the clinician. Non-ischemic myocardial injuries are common in patients with severe illness as for example sepsis [20].

It appears that the peak cTn concentrations are significantly lower in AMI type 2 compared with patients with type 1 AMI, independent of the type of biomarker used [21, 22]. On the other hand, patients with non-ischemic myocardial injury with necrosis often have modestly elevated cTn levels but usually without a rise and/or fall indicating protracted injurious effect to the myocardial tissue [20].

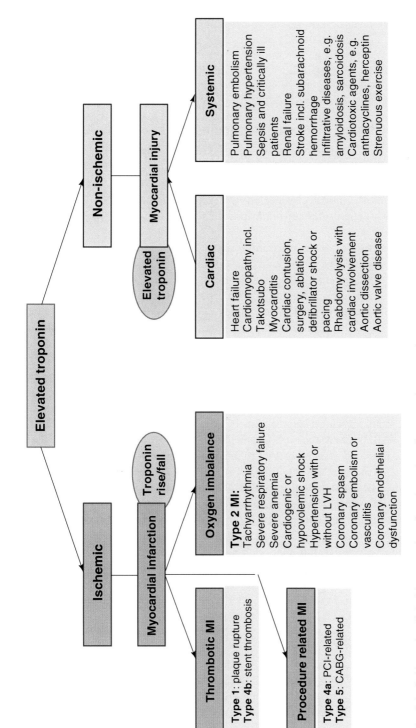

Fig. 5.4 Guidance for clinical interpretation of an elevated cardiac troponin test result

However, regardless of the cause, elevations of hs-cTn values are associated with an adverse clinical outcome in most clinical conditions, as in patients with AMI, stable CAD, heart failure, pulmonary embolism or chronic pulmonary arterial hypertension [2, 23, 24].

Critical Clinical Concepts Regarding the Use of cTn in AMI

1. The 99th percentile concentration of the reference population should be used as the cTn URL indicating the decision limit for the diagnosis of AMI. In patients with clinically suspected AMI, the lower detection limit (LoD) of hs-cTn assays is a useful cut-point for ruling-out AMI with a negative predictive value >99 %.
2. The detection of acute myocardial injury with necrosis requires a significant elevation of hs-cTn values with serial testing. At low cTn baseline concentrations (≤99th percentile URL) the change in serial testing in order to be clinically significant requires an elevation >100 % provided being above the URL. In case of borderline elevated baseline values (>URL and ≤2 times URL) a change >50 % should be considered clinical significant. In the event of markedly elevated baseline values (>2 times URL), a change >20 % in the serial testing is sufficient to be called clinical significant. However, it may turn out that for some hs-cTn assays an absolute assay-specific concentration change functions better than a relative change.
3. When hs-cTn assays are employed routinely, an additional testing using other biomarkers for acute detection of myocardial necrosis such as myoglobin, CKMB, or H-FABP is unnecessary. Copeptin testing adds very little as well, particularly if the LoD is used as an early AMI rule-out limit for the hs-cTn assays.
4. Blood sampling at a single time point only for cTn measurement is not recommended. Blood sampling for hs-cTn testing in patients with suspicion of AMI should be performed on admission and at an interval of 3 h later. However, recent studies show that algorithms based on shorter blood sampling intervals, e.g., on admission and after 1 or 2 h work as well. Nevertheless, measurements of hs-cTn must be repeated at 6 h after admission in patients of whom the 3 h (or 1-2 h) values are unchanged but in whom the clinical suspicion of AMI is still high. In patients with chest pain who are admitted after 6 h following onset of symptoms, subsequent blood sampling (e.g., after 12 h) is also needed to document a significant change of cTn [19]. In addition, serial cTn testing provides information as to whether tissue reperfusion has occurred and moreover, the amount of cTn release correlates with infarct size.
5. Cardiac troponin is a marker of myocardial injury with necrosis but not a specific marker for AMI, of which the criteria require a rise and/or fall of cTn values together with characteristic symptoms, and/or ECG changes indicative of ischemia or imaging evidence of acute myocardial ischemia. A number of non-

ischemic reasons for acute myocardial injury with necrosis are for example acute heart failure, myocarditis, pulmonary embolism or myocardial trauma [4].

6. Stable or inconsistently variable cTn elevations without significant dynamic changes are likely markers of chronic structural heart disease provided that analytical interferences (which are rare) have been ruled out.

Disclosure of Potential Conflicts of Interests In the past year Dr Mair has received minor consulting fees from Philips Health Care Incubator.

References

1. Thygesen K, Mair J, Katus H, Plebani M, Venge P, Collinson P, Lindahl B, Giannitsis E, Hasin Y, Galvani M, Tubaro M, Alpert JS, Biasucci LM, Koenig W, Mueller C, Huber K, Hamm C, Jaffe AS, Study Group on Biomarkers in Cardiology of the ESC Working Group on Acute Cardiac Care. Recommendations for the use of cardiac troponin measurement in acute cardiac care. Eur Heart J. 2010;31:2197–204.
2. Thygesen K, Mair J, Giannitsis E, Mueller C, Lindahl B, Blankenberg S, Huber K, Plebani M, Biasucci LM, Tubaro M, Collinson P, Venge P, Hasin Y, Galvani M, Koenig W, Hamm C, Alpert JS, Katus H, Jaffe AS, the Study Group on Biomarkers in Cardiology of the ESC Working Group on Acute Cardiac Care. How to use high-sensitivity cardiac troponins in acute cardiac care. Eur Heart J. 2012;33:2252–7.
3. Roffi M, Patrono C, Collet JP, Mueller C, Valgimigli M, Andreotti F, Bax JJ, Borger MA, Brotons C, Chew DP, Gencer B, Hasenfuss G, Kjeldsen K, Lancellotti P, Landmesser U, Mehilli J, Mukherjee D, et al.; Management of Acute Coronary Syndromes in Patients Presenting without Persistent ST-Segment Elevation of the European Society of Cardiology. Eur Heart J. 2016;37:267–315.
4. Thygesen K, Alpert JS, Jaffe AS, Simoons ML, Chaitman BR, White HD; Writing Group on the Joint ESC/ACCF/AHA/WHF Task Force for the Universal Definition of Myocardial Infarction, et al.; ESC Committee for Practice Guidelines (CPG), Alpert JS, Jaffe AS, Simoons ML, Chaitman BR, White HD on behalf of the Joint ESC/ACCF/AHA/WHF Task Force for the Universal Definition of Myocardial Infarction. Third universal definition of myocardial infarction. Eur Heart J. 2012;33:2551–67.
5. D'Souza M, Sarkisian L, Saaby L, Poulsen TS, Gerke O, Larsen TB, Diederichsen AC, Jangaard N, Diederichsen SZ, Hosbond S, Hove J, Thygesen K, Mickley H. The diagnosis of unstable angina pectoris has declined markedly with the advent of more sensitive troponin assays. Am J Med. 2015;128(8):852–60.
6. Klinkenberg LJJ, van Dijk J-W, Tan FES, van Loon LJC, van Dieijen-Visser MP, Meex SJR. Circulating cardiac troponin T exhibits a diurnal rhythm. J Am Coll Cardiol. 2014;63:1788–95.
7. Keller T, Zeller T, Ojeda F, Tzikus S, Lillpopp L, Sinning C, Wild P, Genth-Zotz S, Warnholtz A, Giannitsis E, Möckel M, Bickel C, Peetz D, Lackner K, Baldus S, Münzel T, Blankenberg S. Serial changes in highly sensitive troponin I assay and early diagnosis of myocardial infarction. JAMA. 2011;306:2684–93.
8. Reichlin T, Irfan A, Twerenbold R, Reiter M, Hochholzer W, Burkhalter H, Bassetti S, Steuer S, Winkler K, Peter F, Meissner J, Haaf P, Potocki M, Drexler B, Osswald S, Mueller C. Utility of absolute and relative changes in cardiac troponin concentrations in the early diagnosis of acute myocardial infarction. Circulation. 2011;124:136–45.
9. Hammerer-Lercher A, Ploner T, Neururer S, Schratzberger P, Griesmacher A, Pachinger O, Mair J. High-sensitivity cardiac troponin T compared with standard troponin T testing on

emergency department admission: how much does it add in everyday clinical practice? J Am Heart Assoc. 2013;2:e000204. doi:10.1161/JAHA.113.000204.

10. Zhelev Z, Hyde C, Youngman E, Rogers M, Fleming S, Slade T, Coelho H, Jones-Hughes T, Nikolaou V. Diagnostic accuracy of a single baseline measurement of Elecsys troponin T high sensitive assay for the diagnosis of acute myocardial infarction in emergency department: systematic review and metaanalysis. BMJ. 2015;350:h15. doi:10.1136/bmj.h15.

11. National Institute for Health and Care Excellence: Myocardial infarction (acute): early rule out using high sensitivity troponin tests (Elecsys troponin T high-sensitive; Architect STAT high sensitive troponin I and AccuTnI+3 assays), NICE. 2014. (Available at www.nice.org.uk/guidance/dg15).

12. Chenevier-Gobeaux C, Meube C, Freund Y, Wahbi K, Claessens YE, Doumenc B, Zuily S, Riou B, Ray P. Influence of age and renal function on high-sensitivity cardiac troponin T diagnostic accuracy for the diagnosis of acute myocardial infarction. Am J Cardiol. 2013;111:1701–7.

13. Reichlin T, Cullen L, Parsonage WA, Greenslade J, Twerenbold R, Moehring B, Wildi K, Mueller S, Zellweger C, Mosimann T, Gimenez MR, Rentsch K, Osswald S, Müller C. Two-hour algorithm for triage toward rule-out and rule-in of acute myocardial infarction using high-sensitivity cardiac troponin T. Am J Med. 2015;128:369–79.

14. Reiter M, Twerenbold R, Reichlin T, Mueller M, Hoeller R, Moehring B, Haaf P, Wildi K, Merk S, Bernhard D, Mueller CZ, Freese M, Freidank H, Campodarve Botet I, Mueller C. Heart-type fatty acid-binding protein in the early diagnosis of acute myocardial infarction. Heart. 2013;99:708–14.

15. Lipinski MJ, Escarcega RO, DÀscenzo F, Magalhaes MA, Baker NC, Torguson R, Chen F, Epstein SE, Miro O, Liorens P, Giannitsis E, Lotze U, Lefebre S, Sebbane M, Cristol JP, Chenevier-Gobeaux C, Meune C, Eggers KM, Charpentier S, Twerenbold R, Mueller C, Biondi-Zoccal G, Waksman R. A systematic review and collaborative meta-analysis to determine the incremental value of copeptin for rapid rule-out of acute myocardial infarction. Am J Cardiol. 2014;113:1581–91.

16. Collison P, Gaze D, Goodacre S. Comparison of contemporary troponin assays with novel biomarkers, heart fatty acid binding protein and copeptin, for the early confirmation or exclusion of myocardial infarction in patients presenting to the emergency department with chest pain. Heart. 2014;100:140–5.

17. Mair J. Progress in myocardial damage detection: new biochemical markers for clinicians. Crit Rev Clin Lab Sci. 1997;34:1–66.

18. Mayr A, Mair J, Klug G, Schocke M, Pedarnig K, Trieb T, Pachinger O, Jaschke W, Metzler B. Cardiac troponin T and creatine kinase predict mid-term infarct size and left ventricular function after acute myocardial infarction: a cardiac MR study. J Magn Reson Imaging. 2011;33:847–54.

19. Thygesen K, Alpert JS, White HD, Joint ESC/ACCF/AHA/WHF Task Force for the Redefinition of Myocardial Infarction. Universal definition of myocardial infarction. Eur Heart J. 2007;28:2525–38.

20. Alpert JS, Thygesen KA, White HD, Jaffe AS. Diagnostic and therapeutic implications of type 2 myocardial infarction: review and commentary. Am J Med. 2014;127:105–8.

21. Saaby L, Poulsen TS, Hosbond S, Larsen TB, Pyndt Diederichsen AC, Hallas J, Thygesen K, Mickley H. Classification of myocardial infarction: frequency and features of type 2 myocardial infarction. Am J Med. 2013;126:789–97.

22. Baron T, Hambraeus K, Sundström J, Erlinge D, Jernberg T, Lindahl B, TOTAL-AMI study group. Type 2 myocardial infarction in clinical practice. Heart. 2015;101:101–6.

23. Bjurman C, Larsson M, Johanson P, Petzold M, Lindahl B, Fu ML, Hammarsten O. Small changes in troponin T levels are common in patients with non-ST-segment elevation myocardial infarction and are linked to higher mortality. J Am Coll Cardiol. 2013;62:1231–8.

24. Saaby L, Poulsen TS, Diederichsen AC, Hosbond S, Larsen TB, Schmidt H, Gerke O, Hallas J, Thygesen K, Mickley H. Mortality rate in type 2 myocardial infarction: observations from an unselected hospital cohort. Am J Med. 2014;127:295–302.

Chapter 6
What Is a Type 2 Myocardial Infarction: How Is It Recognized and What Should One Do to Establish That Diagnosis?

Joseph S. Alpert and Allan S. Jaffe

Abstract In the 2007 Task Force for the Universal Definition of Myocardial Infarction document, published simultaneously in the Journal of the American College of Cardiology, the European Heart Journal, and Circulation, five subcategories of myocardial infarction (MI) were established (Thygesen et al., J Am Coll Cardiol 50:2173–2195, 2007). The 2007 document was an updated revision of the original document from this group that had first been published in 2000 (Alpert et al., J Am Coll Cardiol 36:959–969, 2000). As noted above, in this second communication the task force defined five subtypes of MI which were retained with modest changes in the 2012 revision (Thygesen et al., Eur Heart J 33:2551–2567, 2012).

Keywords Type 2 myocardial infarction • Myocardial infarction type 2 • Non-ischemic myocardial injury • Definition of myocardial infarction • Cardiac troponin assays

In the 2007 Task Force for the Universal Definition of Myocardial Infarction document, published simultaneously in the Journal of the American College of Cardiology, the European Heart Journal, and Circulation, five subcategories of myocardial infarction (MI) were established [1]. The 2007 document was an updated revision of the original document from this group that had first been published in 2000 [2]. As noted above, in this second communication the task force

J.S. Alpert, MD
Department of Medicine, Sarver Heart Center, University of Arizona College of Medicine, Tucson, AZ, USA

Mayo Clinic, Rochester, MN, USA
e-mail: jalpert@email.arizona.edu

A.S. Jaffe, MD (✉)
Cardiology Department and Department of Laboratory Medicine and Pathology, Mayo Clinic, Rochester, MN, USA
e-mail: Jaffe.Allan@mayo.edu

© Springer International Publishing Switzerland 2016
A.S. Maisel, A.S. Jaffe (eds.), *Cardiac Biomarkers*,
DOI 10.1007/978-3-319-42982-3_6

defined five subtypes of MI which were retained with modest changes in the 2012 revision [3].

Type 1 MI is most often the result of atherosclerotic coronary artery disease (CAD) with thrombotic coronary arterial obstruction secondary to an atherosclerotic plaque rupture or fissuring, with an occasional patient demonstrating normal luminal coronary anatomy at catheterization despite presenting with the clinical syndrome of a type 1 MI. Electrocardiographic abnormalities are usually present such as new ST segment elevation or depression. In contrast, patients with type 2 MI do not have atherosclerotic plaque rupture. In these individuals, myocardial cell necrosis develops because of an increase in myocardial oxygen demand and/or a decrease in myocardial blood flow such as vasoconstriction, embolus or coronary dissection. Rarely, patients with type 2 MI may demonstrate coronary arterial erosions with minimal or no overlying thrombus. This may be the result of embolization of the thrombus to the microvasculature. Type 3 MI is the result of coronary arterial thrombosis with early demise, and types 4 and 5 MI are related to complications of percutaneous coronary intervention and coronary bypass surgery.

Type 2 MI has been the subject of considerable clinical discussion and confusion throughout the world in part because the frequency of these events has risen as cardiac troponin assays have become more sensitive. Thus in some clinical series, 25–50 % of all MIs were found to be "type 2 AMIs." For that reason, all of the co-authors of the Task Force for the Universal Definition of Myocardial Infarction have received multiple questions from colleagues concerning the criteria for diagnosing this latter entity and distinguishing it first from type 1 MI and, second, from myocardial necrosis resulting from a variety of entities other than myocardial ischemia. This chapter will seek to clarify some of the confusion surrounding the distinction between type 1 and type 2 MI and non-ischemic myocardial necrosis.

Type 1 Versus Type 2 MI

Distinguishing patients with type 2 MI from those with type 1 MI is reasonably straightforward in most clinical situations. The clinical picture at presentation is usually definitive. Patients with type 1 MI commonly present with spontaneous symptoms such as chest discomfort usually associated ischemic ECG changes and without any evident cause for increased myocardial oxygen demand, e.g., tachycardia, or decreased myocardial blood flow, e.g., hypotension secondary to marked bradycardia. There is usually a rising and/or falling pattern of blood troponin values. Clinical presentation is important since a typical clinical picture combined with rising or falling troponin values has a very high likelihood of being an acute MI. Patients with type 1 MI, since they are in general larger events, usually have important ECG changes such as ST elevation or depression. During coronary angiography, type 1 MIs are often found to have a new or presumably new coronary arterial occlusion and/or the presence of an obstructing plaque rupture, fissure, or thrombus within a coronary artery (Tables 6.1 and 6.2). However, one may see

Table 6.1 Characteristics of a type 1 MI

Usually spontaneous in onset with discomfort developing often in morning;
The underlying pathological process is coronary arterial plaque erosion, fissuring, or rupture with subsequent thrombus formation.
Almost all ST elevation MIs are in this category.
Patients usually do not present with a serious medical illness or marked arrhythmia.
Troponin values tend to be higher than with type 2 MI.

Table 6.2 Characteristics of a type 2 MI

Onset of MI is usually in the setting of a serious medical illness, for example, respiratory failure with marked hypoxemia or a rapid tachycardia, for example, atrial fibrillation with a rapid ventricular response.
The underlying pathophysiological mechanism is not plaque rupture or fissuring with thrombosis, but markedly increased myocardial oxygen demand or markedly decreased myocardial oxygen supply, for example, severe anemia secondary to a gastrointestinal hemorrhage.
Troponin values are usually low although still abnormal.
In distinguishing a type 1 MI from a type 2 MI, it is helpful if one understands the underlying pathophysiologic mechanism that led to myocardial necrosis. If myocardial ischemia was felt to be secondary to an increase in myocardial oxygen demand or a decrease in perfusion secondary to systemic hypotension, then a type 2 MI is more likely than a type 1 MI.

apparently stable atherosclerotic lesions or even relatively normal coronary arterial luminal angiographic images despite a typical clinical picture of acute MI together with abnormal blood troponin values. Since plaque rupture can occur without the development of an acute coronary syndrome, the presence of such lesions on angiography does NOT necessarily mean that the patient is presenting with an acute coronary syndrome.

The peri-operative setting is a common clinical situation where it is important to attempt to distinguish whether the patient has had a type 1 or a type 2 MI. Observations from a number of clinical studies on the pathophysiology of MI following non-cardiac surgery have demonstrated that many post-operative patients (11.6 % in the recent Vision trial) [4] have elevated cTn values and it appears that many of these patients have had a non-ST-elevation MI, which in most cases represents a type 2 MI resulting from intra-operative hypotension or tachycardia. However, type 1 MIs can also occur during the perioperative period [5–7], and there are obviously multiple other causes for elevated cTn values. Autopsy studies in patients with perioperative MI suggest a higher prevalence of type 1 MI in this setting than would be suspected from the clinical findings, and recent data suggest that nearly 50 % of patients with perioperative MI have coronary arterial abnormalities including intra-coronary arterial thrombus that is consistent with an acute lesion [8]. Unfortunately, as noted earlier, similar acute lesions can be seen in individuals with stable coronary artery disease. Patients with perioperative MI as well as patients with clinically stable coronary arterial disease and elevated blood troponin values are known to be at higher risk for a subsequent myocardial ischemic event [9]. In conclusion, a type

1 MI can occur in the perioperative setting, although it appears that most perioperative MIs are type 2. In preliminary data from the ongoing Vision 2 trial, it appears that with high sensitivity troponin, up to 45 % of post-operative patients will have elevated cTn values and half will have a major rise from their baseline. Thus, these events are likely to increase in frequency over time [10].

Distinguishing a type 1 perioperative MI from a type 2 MI can be challenging. When the MI occurs during the postoperative period, particularly if there is ST elevation on the ECG, a type 1 MI is likely. On the other hand, if the patient has an ECG without ST segment elevation and has had a recognized alteration in hemodynamic status, for example, intraoperative hypotension, then a type 2 MI has probably occurred. A potentially confusing situation can arise when a type 1 perioperative MI results in hypotension and/or tachycardia thereby demonstrating some of the characteristics of a type 2 MI. Since these patients have had a larger MI with hemodynamic compromise, a type 2 MI is less likely since type 2 events tend to be smaller.

The Essence of a Type 2 MI

In the most recent publication from the task force for the universal definition of MI, type 2 MI was categorized as a myocardial infarction secondary to an imbalance between blood supply and myocardial oxygen demand thereby causing myocardial ischemia with resultant myocardial necrosis [2, 3]. Patients may or may not have atherosclerotic coronary artery disease.

Instances of myocardial injury with necrosis where an imbalance between myocardial oxygen supply and/or demand occur include coronary endothelial dysfunction, coronary artery spasm, coronary embolism, tachy- and bradyarrhythmias, anemia, respiratory failure, hypotension, and hypertension with or without left ventricular hypertrophy. Recently, Saaby and associates in Denmark studied more than 500 patients with a clinical diagnosis of acute myocardial infarction admitted to hospital during a one year period (2010–2011) [11]. They categorized these patients according to the five subsets described in the task force documents from 2007 and 2012 [1, 3] using criteria they developed.

Seventy-two per cent of the patients in this series had a type 1 MI and 26 % had a type 2 MI. Type 2 MI patients were older, more likely to be female, and had considerably more co-morbidities. Nearly 50 % of the patients with a type 2 MI had a normal coronary angiographic study [11]. However, when coronary artery disease was present, it was often diffuse and severe. Only 12 % of type 1 MI patients had normal coronary angiography. Not surprisingly, the patients with type 2 MI frequently had multiple co-morbidities and a considerably higher mortality rate compared with patients with a type 1 MI. The type 2 MI patients were also much less aggressively treated compared with those with type 1 events [11].

An example of a typical patient with a type 2 MI would be an individual with or without known coronary atherosclerosis who presents with or without ischemic symptoms during rapid atrial fibrillation, e.g., a heart rate > 150 beats per minute for a substantial period of time, e.g., at least 30–60 min and usually considerably longer. In such individuals with rapid atrial fibrillation (AF), one frequently observes ST segment depression and/or T wave abnormalities on the electrocardiogram accompanied by subsequent elevations in blood troponin levels. We usually classify these latter patients as having had a type 2 MI secondary to markedly increased myocardial oxygen demand as a result of the tachycardia. Unfortunately, it can be difficult to know whether the ischemia precipitated the episode of AF or the arrhythmia itself precipitated the ischemia. We usually assume that the later course has occurred in these patients. It can be challenging to make a diagnosis of acute myocardial infarction if the patient just described has less clear cut symptoms or less typical ischemic ECG findings accompanying elevated and rising blood troponin values. In that situation, excluding other etiologies for the cTn abnormalities such as pulmonary embolism and sepsis is often helpful [12–15].

Type 2 MI Versus Non-ischemic Myocardial Injury

Distinguishing type 2 MI from a non-ischemic myocardial injury represents yet another challenging problem for the clinician. Non-ischemic myocardial injuries are common in patients with severe illness, for example, sepsis accompanying pneumonia. Problems with the diagnosis of type 2 MI usually do not arise in relatively straightforward patients with a variety of severe illnesses such as respiratory failure with severe hypoxemia or even hypotension despite the fact that one might suspect coronary artery disease to be present in many of those individuals because of their history of smoking. Attempts to link elevations of cTn to the presence of coronary artery disease in patients with acute respiratory failure have not thus far been successful [15] . However, in complex medical and surgical patients with multiple co-morbidities, it is often difficult to decide if the patient has had a type 2 MI or rather a myocardial injury secondary to markedly elevated toxic levels of cytokines and/or catecholamines (Table 6.3). An example of such a complex patient with a probable non-ischemic myocardial injury would be a young or middle aged individual with no clinical history of coronary artery disease and without prominent atherosclerotic risk factors who is admitted to the hospital with a serious infection accompanied by systemic sepsis. An elevated troponin level is often noted in such individuals in the absence of ischemic symptoms or ECG changes and the clinical question often posed at this point is "Has this patient had an acute MI that requires

Table 6.3 Characteristics of a myocardial injury

A myocardial injury is diagnosed when an abnormal cTn value is noted but the underlying mechanism of cardiac injury is not ischemia, for example, cardiac trauma.
In many cases, for example, chronic renal failure and heart failure, the blood cTn values remain chronically elevated rather than rising and/or falling.

urgent therapeutic intervention?" It is our opinion that such patients have not had an MI but rather they have suffered a myocardial injury secondary to the humoral factors noted above that are almost invariably associated with serious illness (Table 6.3). Urgent therapy for an acute coronary syndrome is almost never indicated in such settings. Indeed, recent data suggest that an elevated cTn in patients with sepsis is strongly associated with diastolic abnormalities and right ventricular dilatation [16].

As already noted, factors that have been suggested as causative of myocardial necrosis in these situations include elevated circulating levels of catecholamines and inflammatory cytokines such as TNFα, combined with electrolyte abnormalities, acute renal insufficiency, and some degree of hypotension and tachycardia. Such patients should not be labelled as having had a type 2 MI, but rather the diagnostic label should be myocardial injury secondary to the direct toxic effects of factors elaborated with sepsis. An acute coronary arterial intervention in such a critically ill patient is undoubtedly high risk and almost certainly not prudent. Regardless of the diagnosis, patients with elevated blood troponin levels are at increased risk for cardiovascular and other complications both acutely and in the long term [13–15, 17].

The diagnosis of myocardial injury should be applied to patients with myocardial necrosis felt not to be secondary to ischemia in the setting of a critical illness. However, if the patient reports myocardial ischemic symptoms and/or ischemic ECG changes are present, or the patient is known to have clinically important coronary artery disease, it may be very difficult for the clinician to decide if this patient has had a myocardial injury alone and/or a type 2 myocardial infarction. If a biomarker were available that could accurately identify the presence of a ruptured plaque and the need, therefore, for angiography and possible intervention, or if standardized clinical criteria for diagnosing MI type 2 are developed in the future, it would be helpful in devising therapy for these patients. Unfortunately, such a biomarker is not available at present, but studies regarding clinical criteria are underway [16].

The distinction between a type 2 MI and a myocardial injury usually has less immediate therapeutic implications. Once the critical illness has resolved, it is up to the clinician to determine whether evaluation for possible underlying coronary artery disease is indicated. However, it is clear that some cardiovascular evaluation is often necessary since those patients who survive are at increased risk for mortality going forward. Thus, trying to define the presence of treatable cardiac disease, including possible coronary artery disease, is often indicated.

Additional diagnostic problems involved in making a correct diagnosis of a type 2 MI arise when the seriously ill patient has a history consistent with prior coronary artery disease or important atherosclerotic risk factors. Has such a patient had a myocardial injury or a type 2 MI? As already noted above, it is often very difficult to answer this question without lingering doubt as to the veracity of the eventual diagnosis applied. The 2012 definition of MI document suggests that careful clinical judgment should be applied in such settings [3]. Factors that should be taken into account include the likelihood of the patient having an acute coronary syndrome

[18], any associated symptoms consistent with the presence of myocardial ischemia and/or new electrocardiographic changes such as 0.5 mm or more of horizontal ST segment depression in two contiguous leads as well as serial troponin measurements demonstrating a rising and/or falling pattern as opposed to a plateaued elevation. In the latter circumstance (a plateaued elevation of troponin), the diagnosis is likely to be chronic myocardial injury, for example, in patients with chronic renal failure.

A definitive diagnostic answer for these challenging patients cannot be given as yet with a simple clinical algorithm. The clinician must weigh the totality of the clinical evidence and render a judgment: Has a type 2 MI occurred or is this an example of a myocardial injury secondary to the underlying pathophysiologic state? If a type 2 MI is suspected, another clinical conundrum develops. Should the patient undergo coronary angiography; should aspirin, a P2Y12 inhibitor and/or antithrombotic therapy be administered; should the patient be treated with, beta blockers, calcium channel blockers, angiotensin converting enzyme inhibitors, an angiotensin receptor blocker, a statin, ranolazine, and/or nitrates? At this time, there is a dearth of scientific information that can help physicians make clinical decisions in this challenging setting. Cardiac catheterization is almost certainly associated with significant risk in such critically ill patients as is anti-thrombotic therapy. Often, statins, beta blockers, nitrates, and low dose aspirin are given *but without a strong sense on the part of the clinician involved that this therapy is beneficial in this setting.* Clinical research involving patients with presumptive type 2 MI or myocardial injury is desperately needed to assist the clinician in differentiating these two entities and determining what if any specific therapy is indicated.

Diagnostic and Therapeutic Implications

Diagnostic and therapeutic interventions in patients with type 2 MI or a myocardial injury should be tailored to the critical nature of the patient's illness. Urgent coronary angiography in the absence of ST elevation, new left bundle branch block, marked ST depression or continuing ischemic symptoms, is almost certainly not indicated, however, control of symptoms and a test for inducible ischemia at a later date may be appropriate particularly since perioperative MI, for example, is associated with high risk and often a poor long term outcome. More than one troponin determination (at least two and occasionally more) should be obtained in these patients to assist in diagnosis and prognostication. Patients with the typical abnormal rising and/or falling pattern of blood troponin values have likely suffered a myocardial infarction [18, 19]. Although an acute myocardial injury can at times have a similar pattern of rising and falling blood troponin values. As noted earlier, patients with elevated blood troponin values that remain abnormal chronically at approximately the same level are more likely to have suffered a myocardial injury, for example, a patient with chronic renal or heart failure [18, 19]. The presence of an elevated troponin value should not be automatically equated with the presence of MI [18, 19].

The authors recently discussed therapeutic decision making in patients with type 2 MI or myocardial injury and felt that *no definitive therapeutic recommendations could be made at this time* given the lack of clinical trial information involving these patients. It would seem prudent to avoid attempting aggressive therapeutic interventions that might lead to harm, for example, coronary angiography or intensive anti-thrombotic therapy in a patient at high risk for bleeding early after an operation. Such measures may be indicated, however, if plaque rupture is thought to be the mechanism causing myocardial cell necrosis.

As noted above, therapeutic interventions for patients with type 2 MI have not been investigated as yet, and there is even less known about how to a treat myocardial injury that develops in the setting of serious illness. Administration of oral medications such as low dose aspirin, a statin drug, and a beta blocker would seem reasonable *but have not been proven to be beneficial in this setting.*

Following recovery, a clinical decision can be rendered concerning further diagnostic intervention such as some form of stress test for inducible ischemia or even coronary angiography which could lead to a change in the diagnosis. The authors feel that careful weighing of the clinical situation is important in guiding further diagnostic testing. Thus, a patient with a poor prognostic outlook might not undergo any further testing following recovery from an acute illness where blood troponin values were elevated. On the other hand, a patient with a reasonably good prognosis would be offered additional diagnostic evaluation to assess the likelihood of important underlying coronary artery disease.

Examples of a Type 2 Myocardial Infarction and a Myocardial Injury

Case 1

A 19 year old male student with WPW comes to the ED complaining of 6 h of a fast heart beat and a sense of chest heaviness under his sternum. His ECG reveals that he has an atrial tachycardia at 180 beats per minute. After he is cardioverted to normal sinus rhythm, his ECG demonstrates non-specific ST-T changes. He is admitted for observation. That night his blood troponin value is 0.88 ng/ml. Is this a type 1 MI, a type 2 MI, or a myocardial injury? This young man has undoubtedly suffered a small amount of myocardial necrosis secondary to markedly increased myocardial oxygen demand. As such, he might be labelled as having a type 2 MI. However, carrying such a diagnosis into the future might well harm this individual's chances of obtaining a number of jobs such as an airline pilot. Therefore, we usually label such events as a myocardial injury secondary to a cardiac arrhythmia.

Case 2

A 66 year old man with long-standing severe COPD is admitted to the hospital in severe respiratory distress without chest discomfort. His ECG reveals non-specific ST-T wave changes and his troponin is 1.2 ng/ml. His arterial oxygen saturation is 68 % and his heart rate is 124 beats per minute(bpm) in normal sinus rhythm. His blood pressure is 98/55 mmHg. Is this a type 1 MI, a type 2 MI, or a myocardial injury? This man has almost certainly suffered a type 2 MI secondary to the combination of hypoxemia, tachycardia, and hypotension. Whether or not he has underlying coronary artery disease is unknown at the time of his presentation to the hospital. Once he recovers from his present illness, a diagnostic evaluation for coronary artery disease would be appropriate.

Case 3

A 58 year old woman with chronic coronary artery disease and a previous MI treated with a drug eluting stent two years earlier comes to the Emergency Department in rapid atrial fibrillation (HR = 180 bpm). She is treated with intravenous diltiazem and beta blockade and 5 h later she converts to normal sinus rhythm. Her ECG reveals non-specific ST-T wave changes. Her troponin is 1.1 ng/ml. Is this a type 1 MI, a type 2 MI, or a myocardial injury? This patient has likely suffered a type 2 MI as a result of tachycardia. She has known coronary artery disease and will eventually need evaluation for progression of her atherosclerotic coronary artery disease.

References

1. Thygesen K, Alpert JS, White HD, et al.; Joint ESC/ACCF/AHA/WHF Task Force for the Redefinition of Myocardial Infarction. Universal definition of myocardial infarction. Eur Heart J. 2007;28:2525–38. J Am Coll Cardiol. 2007;50:2173–95. Circulation. 2007;116:2634–53.
2. Alpert JS, Thygesen K, et al. Myocardial infarction redefined – a consensus document. J Am Coll Cardiol. 2000;36:959–69.
3. Thygesen K, Alpert JS, White HD, Jaffe AS, Katus HA, Apple FS, et al. Third universal definition of myocardial infarction. Eur Heart J. 2012;33:2551–67.
4. Devereaux PJ, Chan MT, Alonso-Coello P, et al. Association between post operative troponin levels and 30 day mortality among patients undergoing noncardiac surgery. JAMA. 2012;307:2295–304.
5. Dawood MM, Gutpa DK, Southern J, Walia A, Atkinson JB, Eagle KA. Pathology of fatal perioperative myocardial infarction: implications regarding pathophysiology and prevention. Int J Cardiol. 1996;57:37–44.
6. van Waes JA, Nathoe HM, de Graaff JC, Kemperman H, de Borst GJ, Peelen LM, van Klei WA, on behalf of the CHASE investigators. Myocardial injury after noncardiac surgery and its association with short-term mortality. Circulation. 2013;127(23):2264–71.

7. Cohen MC, Aretz TH. Histological analysis of coronary artery lesions in fatal post-operative myocardial infarction. Cardiovasc Pathol. 1999;8:133–9.
8. Gualandro DM, et al. Coronary plaque rupture in patients with myocardial infarction after noncardiac surgery: frequent and dangerous. Atherosclerosis. 2012;222:191–5.
9. Korosoglou G, Lehrke S, Mueller D, Hosch W, Kauczor HU, Humpert PM, Giannitsis E, Katus HA. Determinants of troponin release in patients with stable coronary artery disease: insights from CT angiography characteristics of atherosclerotic plaque. Heart. 2011; 97:823–31.
10. Kavsak PA, Walsh M, Srinathan S, Thorlacius L, Buse GL, Botto F, et al. High sensitivity troponin T concentrations in patients undergoing non-cardiac surgery: a prospective cohort study. Clin Biochem. 2011;44:1021–4.
11. Saaby L, Poulsen TS, Hosbond S, Larsen TB, Pyndt Diederichsen AC, Hallas J, Thygesen K, Mickley H. Classification of myocardial infarction: frequency and features of Type 2 myocardial infarction. Am J Med. 2014;127:297–302.
12. Babuin L, Vasile VC, Rio Perez JA, Alegria JR, Chai HS, Afessa B, Jaffe AS. Elevated cardiac troponin is an independent risk factor for short- and long-term mortality in medical intensive care unit patients. Crit Care Med. 2008;36:759–65.
13. Vasile VC, Chai HS, Abdeldayem D, Afessa B, Jaffe AS. Elevated cardiac troponin T levels in critically ill patients with sepsis. Am J Med. 2013;126:1114–21.
14. Vasile VC, Babuin L, Rio Perez JA, Alegria JR, Song LM, Chai HS, Afessa B, Jaffe AS. Long-term prognostic significance of elevated cardiac troponin levels in critically ill patients with acute gastrointestinal bleeding. Crit Care Med. 2009;37:140–7.
15. Vasile VC, Chai HS, Khambatta S, Afessa B, Jaffe AS. Significance of elevated cardiac troponin T levels in critically ill patients with acute respiratory disease. Am J Med. 2010;123:1049–58.
16. Landesberg G, Jaffe AS, Gilon D, Levin PD, Goodman S, Abu-Baih A, Beeri R, Weissman C, Sprung CL, Landesberg A. Troponin elevation in severe sepsis and septic shock: the role of left ventricular diastolic dysfunction and right ventricular dilatation. Crit Care Med. 2014;42:790–800.
17. Jaffe AS, Moeckel M, Giannitsis E, Huber K, Mair J, Mueller C, Plebani M, Thygesen K, Lindahl B. In search of the Holy Grail: suggestions for studies to define delta changes to diagnose or exclude acute myocardial infarction: a position paper from the study group on biomarkers of the Acute Cardiovascular Care Association. Eur Heart J. 2014;3(4):313–6.
18. Jaskanwal SDS, Holmes DR, Jaffe AS. Fundamental concepts of effective troponin use: important principles for internists. Am J Med. 2015;128:111–9.
19. Apple FS, Jaffe AS, Collinson P, Moeckel M, Ordonez-Llanos J, Lindahl B, Hollander J, Plebani M, Than M, Chan MHM. IFCC educational materials on selected analytical and clinical applications of high sensitivity cardiac troponin assays. Clin Biochem. 2015;48(4–5): 201–3.

Chapter 7
Use of Cardiac Troponin in Patients with Heart Failure

Wayne L. Miller

Abstract The use of cardiac troponins, and particularly with the advent of new high-sensitivity troponins, has come without adequate discussion of the proper interpretation, limitation of values, and their best use in heart failure (HF) patients. The objective of this chapter is to provide a balanced assessment of how cardiac troponins are advocated for clinical use in HF patients and areas where there are gaps in knowledge that are important for clinicians to appreciate.

Although biomarkers such as troponin add to the magnitude of risk prediction, it is unclear how often their use leads to changes in treatment. The use of serial troponin testing over time would be helpful. To do this, it is necessary to take into account assay characteristics and the analytical and biological variability in addition to the ability to define normal values and effectively monitor therapy. These factors are often overlooked leading to conclusions that may not be clinically or analytically sound. An understanding of the value and limitations of troponin use is important to all clinicians who manage HF patients. If used optimally, troponin values will likely be helpful in defining when and how to effectively intervene clinically.

Keywords Chronic heart failure • Troponin T and I • Risk stratification and cardiac troponins • Heart failure and troponins • Troponins in chronic heart failure

The use of cardiac troponins has been well vetted in patients with acute coronary syndromes [1], but the role of troponins in the theater of acute and chronic heart failure (HF) is less well delineated and understood by clinicians. This is particularly confounded with the advent of high-sensitivity cardiac troponin assays where very low levels (ten-fold lower concentrations measured than standard assays) of circulating troponins can be detected. A role for cardiac troponins in the diagnosis of HF, in contrast to a prognostic role, has in general not been developed and generally over- shadowed in this role by the use of natriuretic peptides such as B-type

W.L. Miller, MD, PhD
Department of Cardiovascular Diseases, Mayo Clinic, Rochester, MN, USA
e-mail: miller.wayne@mayo.edu

© Springer International Publishing Switzerland 2016
A.S. Maisel, A.S. Jaffe (eds.), *Cardiac Biomarkers*,
DOI 10.1007/978-3-319-42982-3_7

natriuretic peptide (BNP) and NT-proBNP. The potent prognostic value of elevated troponins will be reviewed among other issues in the use of troponin values but ultimately the most important issue relates to the modification of treatment of HF based upon troponin values or changes in values in a manner that is timely for patient care and also cost-effective – can the monitoring of troponin values be used to guide therapy in HF patients is an unaddressed issue. The intent of this chapter is, thus, to provide a discussion into the effective use and caveats of use of cardiac troponin and high-sensitivity troponins in the context of patients with HF. The following are pertinent discussion points on the use and interpretation of troponin values that will provide background for the review of the clinical cases to follow.

The Importance of Knowing What Is a Normal Troponin Value

Fundamental to the use and interpretation of troponin values is the understanding of the importance of normal reference values and how such values are determined. What denotes an elevated or abnormal troponin value which in turn warrants an association with increased risk has been described using different cut-points which are highly dependent upon how robustly the normal reference population is evaluated and defined. There has been a desire to keep the definition process simple and, therefore, that the value used to define disease be arrived at simply. For some biomarkers the lowest detectable level that is different from zero is to identify the cut-point associated with increased risk. This is often the case when the assay for a given analyte is not particularly sensitive. A practical and more universally applicable approach is the use of the 99th percentile of the upper range limit of normal values to provide a cut-point that can be applied to different patient cohorts with a common basis for comparison [2, 3]. This is most applicable in the use of cardiac troponins, but not true for all biomarkers, and even for troponin values it depends upon what generation of assay is being used and factors such as age, gender, and ethnicity. So, attempts to keep it simple have confounders.

There has been ambiguity about how to define normal ranges and, therefore, appropriate cut off values to identify elevated values. Ideally, it should take a minimum of 300 subjects of each patient gender, ethnicity, and age grouping [4] to accurately define statistically each subset whether to determine normal ranges or elevated values indicative of disease. Doing this for a large number of subsets is generally cost prohibitive. However, if not done, it may mean ignoring differences that might be present due to age, sex, ethnicity, patient characteristics, medications, subtypes of disease, and comorbidities. Also, there are substantial issues related to how to define a normal population [5, 6]. Definitions of an elevated troponin value, as well as, other biomarkers should bear some relation to reference values of a normal population. However, it is uncommon that truly normal subjects are recruited for such analyses. Most "normal range" studies come from convenience cohorts and involve at most a medical questionnaire to identify disease. Very few studies include even a formal history and physical examination. As a result it is not surprising that adding other clinical measurements such a creatinine or eGFR lowers what is defined as normal values. Even more vigorous screening including imaging decreases values still further. This may not be important when analytes are used at high values but when the important metrics impinge on the upper limit of the normal range, as is the case with high-sensitivity (hs) troponins, they can become crucial. For analytes such as cardiac troponin where small differences may be important, clearly accounting for risk factors and obtaining imaging for each patient are essential elements to truly define normality [5, 7, 8]. These considerations may be lost in small studies defining normal ranges and in large clinical trials. These then in turn contribute to confusion in interpretation of what elevated troponin levels mean in the individual patient. These considerations generally are not important in those with overt HF but are critical to define at risk cohorts where values are generally very low and thus rely on truly "normal values". Also, whether the assay being used is for hs-troponin T or hs-troponin I makes a difference in that the sensitivities of the assays may differ significantly. In one community based study with a well characterized cohort, 93 % of the participants had detectable hs-troponin I levels [6], while in other population studies much lower levels of hs-troponin T were detected (25–66 %) [9, 10]. This may reflect differences in the cohort (i.e., how well were they characterized, age-gender mixes) or technical differences in the assays. However, important differences in assay sensitivities, age and gender differences in troponin concentrations in healthy reference vs. diseased individuals have important implications in defining clinically usable reference cut-point values.

In addition, a particular troponin cut-off value may not apply to every patient cohort with different clinical characteristics (different case mixes). ROC curve or median derived values of one patient cohort cannot necessarily be applied to other patient populations or other indications without losing the value of data comparison. Also, it is valuable to keep in mind that the concept of positive or negative cut-point of troponin or any other biomarker is an artifact of the need for clinical convenience. The reality is that most biomarkers are continuous variables of risk and cut-points should be viewed with that limitation in mind. Additionally, hs troponin cut-points may vary, for example in HF patients, according to age, gender, ethnicity, specific assay employed, acuity and duration of HF, severity of HF, penetration of appropriate treatment (presence and absence of established effective drug therapy), left ventricular ejection fraction (reduced or preserved), renal function, and co-morbidities (e.g., diabetes). Thus, troponin and other biomarker values must be interpreted in the proper clinical context and not per arbitrary fixed cut-off values. The concept of keeping it simple is reasonable for many situations but the concept that this means that one does not need to understand how biomarkers such as troponin work and when to recognize exceptions is nonetheless still critical if often ignored; this perhaps is more noted in the use of natriuretic peptides than troponins which have not yet been as universally adopted in the HF arena.

Analytical and Biological Variability of Troponin Values

The clinical significance of a biomarker level particularly during serial testing over time is in part dependent on the biomarker's analytical and biological variability. These factors in the performance of a biomarker are often over-looked and conclusions drawn based on changes in a biomarker concentration that may be statistically significant but not clinically or analytically significant. In general, values must be further apart than three standard deviations of the variation around the measures irrespective of the cause. This value which takes into account of both analytical and biological variability is the reference change value (RCV) [4, 11]. In theory biological variation can only be measured in normal subjects since pathologies that will influence the RCV are likely present in HF patients. The contemporary sensitive assays (i.e., non-hs-troponin assays) used in clinical practice cannot determine biological variation for either troponin T or troponin I because these assays cannot reliably detect and measure troponin values in healthy normal individuals. This caveat is often violated in the literature. Analytical variability relates to the performance of the biomarker assay in the laboratory and identifies the degree of imprecision of results obtained by the assay technique used to quantify the biomarker and by any issues related to the sample itself. If the quality of the sample, for example, is problematic then reliable values cannot be obtained. For example, hemolysis is common and can raise some troponin assay values and lower others [12]. These issues provide the reasons why most groups urge that precision be very high (<10 % imprecision), especially near critical values. However, imprecision does not often cause false positives [13, 14]. In comparison to analytical variability, biological variability can be substantial and commonly much greater than analytical variability alone. With the advent of hs-troponin assays measurable troponin concentrations can now be detected and measured in the general population without cardiovascular disease. This allows the determination of biological variability for hs-troponin T and I. The importance of taking these relationships into account is critical to the appropriate interpretation of serial biomarker measurements. Some identified changes, although statistically significant, may, therefore, be due to this combined variability alone. The RCV which reflects this combined variability and indicates the minimal percent change in serial troponin measurements required to reflect a clinically meaningful short-term change may vary, however, from a low of ±32–69 % for hs-troponin I assays and 47–85 % for hs-troponin T assays [4, 11]. Notable, however, is that for long-term serial monitoring of hs-troponin T to detect the onset of early cardiovascular disease, a >300 % change is necessary to achieve confidence that the RCV is clinically meaningful [11]. Thus, the magnitude of spontaneous change is important in interpreting changes in troponin values. In general, analytes with low RCV are likely to be much better at detecting changes in patients than those analytes with high RCVs.

Clinical Case 1

A 65 year-old male with a 5-year history of non-ischemic dilated cardiomyopathy with a reduced but stable ejection fraction of 37 % by echocardiography (most recently assessed 5 months previously) presents to the outpatient clinic with a complaint of worsening dyspnea, orthopnea, lower extremity edema, and a 10-lb weight gain over the past 2 weeks. He now experiences DOE with walking across the room. Furosemide dose has been stable at 40 mg in the AM and 20 mg in the PM. On physical exam there are no rales but JVD is approximately 14 cm H_2O at 60°, and there is soft 2+ pitting edema of the lower extremities focused mainly at the ankles. NT-proBNP was elevated at 2800 ng/mL; creatinine 1.6 mg/dL, K+ 3.9 mEq/L, sodium 138 mEq/L. ECG demonstrated SR at 64 BPM on beta-blocker therapy with LBBB but no acute changes. High-sensitivity troponin I was 123 pg/mL (gender specific 99th percentile URL value of 55 ng/mL). It was decided to admit the patient to hospital for intravenous diuretic therapy along with advancement of ACEi dose for afterload reduction. Repeat 6-h hs-troponin I was 130 pg/mL. Echocardiography demonstrated an estimated LVEF of 30 % with LVEDD 65 mm. Intravenous furosemide was initiated at 10 mg/h and after 12 h advanced to 20 mg/h due to low urine output. Urine output improved and over 4 days the patient lost 12 pounds with stable creatinine (1.8 mg/dL) and electrolyte values. NT-proBNP decreased to 1500 ng/mL, hs-troponin I was 118 pg/mL. Clinically, the patient felt improved with less DOE and no lower extremity edema after enforced bedrest with legs elevated. The patient was dismissed in the afternoon of hospital day 4 on an adjusted medical regimen of furosemide of 80 mg QD (in the AM) and re-education on fluid restriction to 2.0 l per day and sodium restriction to 2000 mg per day. One week follow up with PCP was unremarkable. Three-month post-hospital Heart Failure Clinic follow-up visit demonstrated sCr 1.6 mg/dL, K+ 3.6 mEq/L, and NT-proBNP of 750 ng/mL, and hs-troponin I 120 pg/mL (same lab and assays). How would you interpret the troponin I values?

Discussion

The patient presentation is a classic case of a patient presenting with an acute exacerbation of chronic heart failure. NT-proBNP was elevated at presentation secondary to increased myocardial stretch secondary to volume overload; however, hs-troponin I was also elevated. Both of these elevations are related to increased morbidity and mortality risk. Serial measurements of hs-troponin I demonstrated persistent elevations above the 99th percentile URL, but there was no pattern of rising values. While the persistent elevations in hs-troponin I reflect increased long-term risk, they do not support the presence of an acute ischemic event that warrants pursuing coronary angiography in this patient. The potent combination of both NT-proBNP and troponin elevation provides independent prognostic information

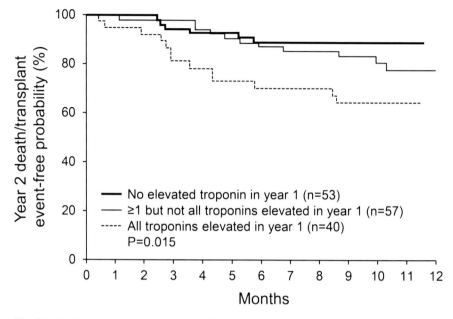

Fig. 7.1 Cardiac Troponin T Profiles and Risk of Events. Kaplan-Meier analysis of the risk of death or cardiac transplantation in year 2 of follow up based upon cardiac troponin T patterns from year 1 of clinical follow up (From Miller et al. [21] with permission)

and indicates a high risk of mortality or HF-related hospitalization (Fig. 7.1), [3]. The elevated hs-troponin I cannot be dismissed as due to renal dysfunction or CHF without associated consequence. This patient is in a high-risk category and merits close follow-up with titration to optimal medical therapy and the implantation of a biventricular pacemaker with defibrillator (CRT-D) capability would be appropriate if the patient meets criteria.

Significance of Elevated Troponin Levels in Heart Failure

Myocardial injury results from ischemia but can also occurs secondary to stresses and toxins on the myocardium such as inflammation, oxidative stress, catechol-amines, marked renin-angiotensin activation, and apoptosis [15, 16]. Plasma eleva-tions of troponins T and I have been shown to be highly sensitive and specific biomarkers of myocyte injury and death, regardless of the inciting event. Modest but persistent elevations of cardiac troponin have been demonstrated in patients with left ventricular systolic dysfunction of non-ischemic etiology (dilated cardiomyopathy, infiltrative cardiomyopathy) and in chronic HF patients with known coronary artery disease (ischemic cardiomyopathy) in the absence of acute ischemic events. With the availability of new generation hs-troponin assays, very low levels of circulating cardiac troponins can be detected with high precision. A high percentage of patients with HF have measureable cardiac troponin values at or just above the 99th percentile URL for a normal healthy population. Cardiac T elevations using contemporary standard assays have been shown to be detectable in 10–15 % of patients with chronic systolic HF, however, with the new high-sensitivity assays troponin T was detectable in over 90 % of the same patients [17]. These detected values were also predictive of increased risk of death in multivariate analyses adjusting for common HF related variables, as well as, BNP. These data and others support the conclusion that even small troponin "leaks" from the myocardium are indicative of heightened risk in the setting of chronic HF. Troponin elevations have also been shown to be predictive of outcome in hospitalized patients with acute decompensated HF [18]. In the large database from the ADHERE registry (N=67,924), elevations in either troponin T or I vs no elevations at hospital admission independently marked those patients at increased risk of in-hospital mortality (8.0 % vs 2.7 %, p<0.001).

Chronic persistent elevations in troponin levels detected in stable HF patients carry a short and long term risk of poor outcome [19, 20], but they do not reflect acute injury events but rather the ongoing chronic injury to the myocardium. The monitoring of serial measurements of troponins during hospitalization can also assist in determining the acuteness of myocardial injury and help differentiate chronic stable troponin release from that of acute ischemic events. A rising pattern of troponin elevations would help, along with clinical context, to distinguish between the chronic injury of established HF and acute ischemia or myocardial infarction. Serial monitoring in stable HF patients also can provide information on risk stratification and disease progression [3, 21]. Elevated troponin T levels have been shown to respond to medical therapy in patients with chronic HF (reductions of 25 % over 2 months, [22]) and in combination with parameters of clinical improvement associated with reduced risk; those patients who demonstrated persistent elevations in troponin T sustained higher risk of mortality.

Clinical Case 2

A 74 year-old female with a history of poorly controlled systemic hypertension presents to the ED with complaints of DOE associated with chest discomfort and lower extremity swelling. These have been intermittent for some time but worse over the last 3–4 weeks since she visited her daughter in New York City 5 weeks ago. The patient has 2+ lower extremity pitting edema and soft bilateral rales on pulmonary exam. The electrocardiogram shows a new finding of atrial fibrillation with ventricular rate of 98 bpm at rest, and LVH. Initial blood labs show sCr 1.3 mg/dL, K+ 4.0 mEq/L, BNP 2000 ng/mL and troponin T of 1.2 pg/mL (10 % CV with 99th percentile URL cut-point >0.01 pg/mL). Troponin T values at 6 and 12 h are 0.9 pg/mL and 1.1 pg/mL, respectively. Intravenous furosemide infusion at 5 mg/h is initiated with good diuresis and clinical improvement. Echocardiography reveals concentric left ventricular hypertrophy, an ejection fraction of 70 %, grade 3 out of

4 of left ventricular diastolic dysfunction, and no regional wall abnormalities. Do the elevated troponin T values support the need to obtain a pharmacologic myocardial perfusion nuclear imaging stress test?

Discussion

This patient presents with heart failure with preserved left systolic function (HFpEF) in the setting of concentric left ventricular hypertrophy secondary to long-standing systemic hypertension. This is a common presenting scenario in an elderly lady with this clinical history. HFpEF is a systemic disease and diastolic dysfunction is only one element accounting for the symptom complex. Ventricular-vascular mismatch is a prominent feature with patients being poorly tolerant of new onset atrial fibrillation with rapid ventricular response. This patient has a resting heart rate of 98 bpm but with little activity it quickly increases to 140 bpm with associated dyspnea on exertion. The atrial fibrillation with rapid ventricular response, left ventricular diastolic dysfunction, left ventricular hypertrophy, and probable intermittent subendocardial ischemia are all contributing factors to the elevation in troponin T values. Long-term this puts this patient at increased risk of more episodes of CHF and also increased mortality. HFpEF has a comparable poor outcome to HFrEF. Optimal therapy for HFpEF is still lacking but volume management and controlling hypertension are mainstays of care in this patient. A myocardial perfusion nuclear stress test was performed the following morning without evidence of inducible ischemia.

Single-Sample Values vs. Serial Measurements Over Time

Disease activity changes over time and this time frame can be quite variable between patients and within the same patient. Thus, serial measurements of a biomarker over time rather than single point-in-time measurements are needed to optimally manage patients. In contrast, however, most studies focus on the predictive value of an initial sample and the higher the value of a risk biomarker, the sicker the patient, and in general clinicians will be more aggressive with those patients in applying conventional therapies. Recent data relating to the application of recommended therapies such as mineralocorticoid antagonists (MRAs) suggest such a strategy is, however, not frequently pursued [23]. Additionally, in an apparently clinically stable patient does such an elevated biomarker such as troponin trump all other clinical information? This is why serial values over time should be more valuable [3, 21, 24, 25] An example is shown in Fig. 7.2 [21]. One might think that a biomarker level that decreases over time should reflect clinical improvement, while one that increases should reflect disease progression. Serial measurements thus provide information on which patients are at increasing risk but can also indicate which patients are responding to therapy or need a change in their treatment regimen to reduce the risk of adverse events. The specific subset of patients is also important in this arena. The

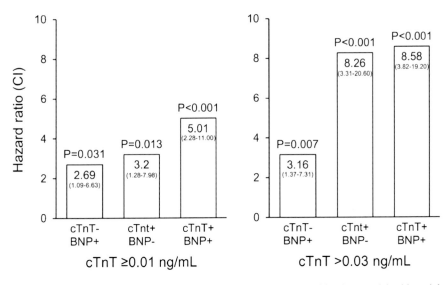

Fig. 7.2 Risk of death/cardiac transplantation. Time-dependent multivariate model with serial follow-up measurements of troponin T and BNP values. + indicates elevated troponin T or BNP; – indicates no elevation (From Miller et al. [3] with permission)

response of biomarkers in an acute HF patient may well be related to acute hemo-dynamics and may respond rapidly [26, 27] whereas those found in more chronic HF where biomarker pathways have been stimulated over time may not correlate nearly as well and may require more time to see change [28, 29]. Thus, the proper interpretation of change likely is clinical subset dependent.

Also, since deteriorations in chronic HF occur slowly, elevations or changes in troponin over time could potentially be used to provide an early indication of disease progression and myocardial remodeling and allow for earlier changes in therapy. Thus, biomarkers that have low levels of biological and analytical variability have an advantage. In addition, if changes in biomarkers can be used to demonstrate that risk is modified then such an approach might be used to test specific interventions rather than attempting to institute such interventions empirically through expensive RCTs. We have shown that the ability to monitor changes in serial troponin T measurements, adds significantly to the assessment of risk in ambulatory patients with chronic HF [3, 21, 24]. New elevations or changes in persistently elevated biomarkers measured serially any time during clinical follow-up independently predict increased risk of death or need for cardiac transplantation or HF-related hospitalization. These findings support the hypothesis that worsening HF is mediated by subclinical myocardial injury, and that increased frequency of myocardial injury results in further deterioration in myocardial function and worse clinical outcome. Therefore, the monitoring of serial changes in troponin values may well be the means, in the individual HF patient, to identify risk prospectively and to help determine which therapeutic modality would be most effective in that specific patient.

Clinical Case 3

A 70 year-old man with known ischemic cardiomyopathy (LVEF 40%), systemic hypertension, and diabetes presents to the emergency department. The patient has been stable NYHA Class II status for several years following an anterior STEMI for which he received a drug eluting stent without complications. Troponin T levels have been elevated but stable in the 0.08–1.4 ng/mL range over several 6 month interval visits in the past but the patient hasn't been seen for 3 years. He now describes the onset of increased SOB with exertion and intermittent chest pain beginning that morning but have resolved just prior to coming to the ED. Such episodes have been occurring over the past 2 months; no syncope. A grade III/IV harsh crescendo-decresendo systolic murmur is identified on auscultation (previous exams had indicated a soft systolic murmur and mild aortic valve stenosis). Electrocardiogram shows sinus rhythm with criteria for ventricular hypertrophy and non-specific ST-T wave changes. Initial labs show sCr 1.5 mg/dL, K+ 4.0 mEq/L, NT-proBNP 450 pg/mL, and troponin T 0.15 ng/mL. Over the next 6 h NT-proBNP increases to 900 pg/mL and troponin T increases to 0.36 ng/mL; 12-h troponin T is 0.28 ng/mL. Echocardiography reveals aortic stenosis with a mean gradient of 45 mmHg, calculated valve area of 0.70 cm/m^2, and an LVEF of 28%. Coronary angiography showed patent native vessels with no flow limiting stenosis and with a patent previously stented site in the LAD. How should the serial troponin T values be interpreted? Do they reflect worsening of the patient's heart failure, an acute ischemic event, or progression of aortic valve stenosis?

Discussion

The rising and falling pattern of troponin T in this clinical setting is consistent with a diagnosis of Type 2 myocardial infarction (ischemic coronary flow supply/demand mismatch) but can be easily missed if serial troponin measurements are not obtained and a pattern of change not assessed. Serial measurements are often ignored in patients with chronic heart failure who have a history of persistent troponin elevations. The clinical context should drive the decision to pursue serial troponin measurements. All of the factors identified with this patient have the potential to contribute to the mechanisms of myocardial injury and troponin release. Chronic heart failure with persistent elevations in troponin (myocyte apoptosis, catecholamine toxicity, subendocardial ischemia), increased transmural myocardial wall pressure producing subendocardial ischemia (decompensated aortic valve stenosis, ventricular hypertrophy from long-standing hypertension), small-vessel coronary obstruction (diabetes), and ischemia secondary to vascular endothelial dysfunction (chronic heart failure, diabetes) have been associated with troponin release in the absence of overt obstructive coronary artery disease. This patient underwent optimization of his medical regimen and underwent percutaneous replacement of the aortic valve (TAVR) with good result. LVEF returned to baseline level of 40%.

Value of Troponin as a Biomarker: Use for Diagnosis, Prognosis, and Guiding Treatment

While it is important to predict which patients are at increased risk due to their progression in HF, many times knowing that a patient who is clearly at risk does not require any biomarker data and in the absence of a specific path of therapy, is not cost effective. On the other hand, when we can identify individuals at risk where it was not anticipated clinically, troponin data might be even more important. Perhaps recent data concerning the importance of minor increases in hs cTnT and NT-proBNP in patients with left ventricular hypertrophy (LVH) might be an example of the latter [30]. It was only with the use of these biomarkers that the subset of individuals who were at risk was identified among those with LVH by MRI or ECG. Most important, however, is to provide information to guide therapeutic modifications based upon biomarker values or changes in biomarker values such as hs-troponins – this is the ultimate goal of biomarker-guided HF management. No trials pursuing such a goal with hs-troponin measurements are underway, but enthusiasm for identifying biomarkers of myocardial injury and fibrosis and the assessment of MRAs which retard the development of fibrosis [31], may advance the value of serial measurements of hs-troponin in identifying responders to therapy and guide the effective new use of this therapy. This is a reasonable extrapolation and there are data to suggest this may work [32], but RCT or well done registries and pathophysiological trials are needed to support the use of serial measurements of cardiac troponin in the guidance of HF therapy.

References

1. Newby LK, Jesse RL, Babb JD, Christenson RH, DeFer TM, ACCF, et al. Expert consensus document on the practical clinical considerations in the interpretation of troponin elevations. J Am Coll Cardiol. 2012;2012(60):2419–55.
2. Gore MO, Seliger SL, deFilippi CR, Namabi V, Christenson RH, Hashim IA, et al. Age and sex-dependent upper reference limits for the high-sensitivity cardiac troponin T assay. J Am Coll Cardiol. 2014;63:1441–8.
3. Miller WL, Hartman KA, Burritt MF, Grill DE, Rodeheffer RJ, Burnett Jr JC, Jaffe AS. Serial biomarker measurements in ambulatory patients with chronic heart failure – the importance of change over time. Circulation. 2007;116:249–57.
4. Apple FS, Collinson PO, IFCC task force on clinical applications of cardiac biomarkers. Analytical characteristics of high-sensitivity cardiac troponin assays. Clin Chem. 2012;58:54–61.
5. Collinson PO, Heung YM, Gaze D, Boa F, Senior F, Christenson R, Apple FS. Influence of population selection on the 99th percentile reference value of cardiac troponin assays. Clin Chem. 2012;58:219–25.
6. McKie PM, Heublein DM, Scott CG, Gantzer ML, Mehta RA, Rodeheffer RJ, Redfield MM, Burnett JC, Jaffe AS. Defining high-sensitivity cardiac troponin concentrations in the community. Clin Chem. 2013;59:1099–107.
7. Sandoval Y, Apple FS. The global need to define normality: the 99th percentile value of cardiac troponin. Clin Chem. 2014;60:455–62.

8. Hickman PE, Lindahl B, Potter JM, Venge P, Koerbin G, Eggers KM. Is it time to do away with the 99th percentile for cardiac troponin in the diagnosis of acute coronary syndrome and the assessment of cardiac risk? Clin Chem. 2014;60:734–6.

9. deLemos JA, Drazner MH, Omland T, Ayers CR, et al. Association of troponin T detected with a highly sensitive assay and cardiac structure and mortality risk in the general population. JAMA. 2010;304:2503–12.

10. deFillippi CR, deLemos JA, Christenson RH, Gottdiener JS, Kop WJ, Zhan M, Seliger SL. Association of serial measures of cardiac troponin T using a sensitive assay with incident heart failure and cardiovascular mortality in older adults. JAMA. 2010;304:2494–502.

11. Vasile VC, Saenger AK, Kroning JM, Jaffe AS. Biological and analytical variability of a novel high-sensitivity cardiac troponin T assay. Clin Chem. 2010;56:1086–90.

12. Bais R. The effect of sample hemolysis on cardiac troponin I and T assays. Clin Chem. 2010;56:1357–9.

13. Apple FS, Parvin CA, Buechler KF, Christenson RH, Wu AHB, Jaffe AS. Validation of the 99th percentile cutoff independent of assay imprecision (CV) for cardiac troponin monitoring for ruling out myocardial infarction. Clin Chem. 2005;51:2198–200.

14. Panteghini M, Pagani F, Yeo KT, Apple FS, Christenson RH, Dati F, et al. Evaluation of the imprecision at low-range concentrations of the assays for cardiac troponin determination. Clin Chem. 2004;50:327–32.

15. Kociol RD, Pang PS, Gheorghiade M, Fonarow GC, O'Connor CM, Felker GM. Troponin elevation in heart failure. J Am Coll Cardiol. 2010;56:1071–8.

16. Januzzi Jr JL, Filippatos G, Nieminen M, Gheorghiade M. Troponin elevation in patients with heart failure: on behalf of the third universal definition of myocardial infarction global task force: heart failure section. Eur Heart J. 2012;33:2265–71.

17. Latini R, Masson S, Anand IS, Missov E, Carlson M, Vago T, for the Val-HeFT Investigators, et al. Prognostic value of very low plasma concentrations of troponin T in patients with stable chronic heart failure. Circulation. 2007;116:1242–9.

18. Peacock WF, DeMarco T, Fonarow GC, Diercks D, et al. Cardiac troponin and outcome in acute heart failure. N Engl J Med. 2008;358:2117–26.

19. Sato Y, Yamada T, Taniguchi R, Nagai K, Makiyama T, et al. Persistently increased serum concentrations of cardiac troponin T in patients with idiopathic dilated cardiomyopathy are predictive of adverse outcomes. Circulation. 2001;103:369–74.

20. Perna ER, Macin SM, Canella JPC, Alvargenga PM, Rios NG, Pantich R, et al. Minor myocardial damage detected by troponin T is a powerful predictor of long-term prognosis in patients with decompensated heart failure. Int J Cardiol. 2005;99:253–61.

21. Miller WL, Hartman KA, Burritt MF, Grill DE, Jaffe AS. Profiles of serial changes in cardiac troponin T concentrations and outcomes in ambulatory patients with chronic heart failure. J Am Coll Cardiol-Heart Fail. 2009;54(18):1715–21.

22. Ishii J, Cui K, Kitagawa F, et al. Prognostic value of combination of cardiac troponin T and B-type natriuretic peptide after initiation of treatment in patients with chronic heart failure. Clin Chem. 2003;49:2020–6.

23. Maron BA, Leopold JA. Aldosterone receptor antagonists. Effective but often forgotten. Circulation. 2010;121:934–9.

24. Miller WL, Hartman KA, Grill DE, Struck J, Bergmann A, Jaffe AS. Serial measurements of mid-region-pro-ANP and C-terminal-pro-vasopressin (copeptin) in relation to B-type natriuretic peptide and troponin T in ambulatory chronic heart failure patients – incremental prognostic value. Heart (BHJ). 2012;98:389–94.

25. Miller WL, Hartman KA, Grill DE, Burnett JC, Jaffe AS. Only large reductions in natriuretic peptide concentrations (BNP and NT-proBNP) are associated with improved outcomes in ambulatory patients with chronic heart failure. Clin Chem. 2009;55(1):78–84.

26. Forfia PR, Watkins SP, Rame E, Stewart KJ, Shapiro EP. Relationship between B-type natriuretic peptides and pulmonary capillary wedge pressure in the intensive care unit. J Am Coll Cardiol. 2005;45:1667–71.

27. Cioffi G, Tarantini L, Stefenelli C, Azzetti G, Marco R, Carlucci S, Furlanello F. Changes in plasma N-terminal proBNP levels and ventricular filling pressures during intensive unloading therapy in elderly with decompensated congestive heart failure and preserved left ventricular systolic function. J Card Fail. 2006;12:608–15.
28. Latini R, Masson S, Wong M, Barlera S, Carretta E, et al. Incremental prognostic value of changes in B-type natriuretic peptide in heart failure. Am J Med. 2006;119:70e23–30.
29. Anand IS, Fisher LD, Chiang Y-T, Latini R, Masson S, Maggioni AP, Glazer RD, Tognoni G, Cohn JN. Changes in brain natriuretic peptide and norepinephrine over time and mortality and morbidity in the Valsartan Heart Failure Trial (Val-HeFT). Circulation. 2003;107:1278–83.
30. Neeland IJ, Dranzer MH, Berry JD, Ayers CR, de Filippi C, Seliger SL, Nambi V, McGuire DK, Omland T, de Lemos JA. Biomarkers of chronic cardiac injury and hemodynamic stress identify a malignant phenotype of left ventricular hypertrophy in the general population. J Am Coll Cardiol. 2013;61:187–95.
31. Li X, Qi Y, Li Y, Zhang S, Guo S, Chu S, Gao P, Zhu D, Wu Z, Lu L, Shen W, Jai N, Niu W. Impact of mineralocorticoid receptor antagonists on changes in cardiac structure and function of left ventricular dysfunction. Circ Heart Fail. 2013;6:156–65.
32. Weir RAP, Miller AM, Murphy GEJ, et al. Serum soluble ST2: a potential novel mediator in left ventricular and infarct remodeling after acute myocardial infarction. J Am Coll Cardiol. 2010;55:243–50.

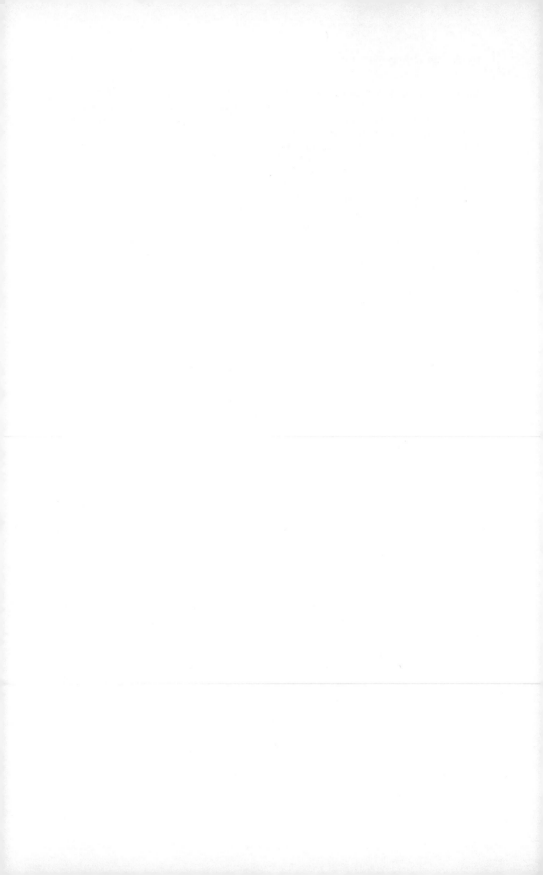

Chapter 8
Elevated cTn in Other Acute Situations Such as Atrial Fibrillation, Sepsis, Respiratory Failure, and Gastrointestinal Bleeding

Evangelos Giannitsis and Hugo A. Katus

Abstract Prevalence of elevated hs-cTnT (above the 99th percentile) with relevant concentration changes in patients without an ACS is high, and elevated hs-cTn is associated with adverse long-term outcomes, irrespective the exact underlying reason. Differentiation between ischemic and non-ischemic reasons is particularly challenging as ischemic and non-ischemic mechanisms frequently co-exist. Understanding the etiology of troponin elevation in critically ill patients is important to better target appropriate therapies for MI in this population.

Keywords Acute non-coronary • Cardiac troponin • Atrial fibrillation and cTn • Sepsis and cTn • Respiratory failure and cTn • Gastrointestinal bleeding and cTn • cTn and atrial fibrillation

Not all elevated troponin results represent an acute myocardial infarction (AMI) and even not all myocardial injury results are ischemic in etiology. The prevalence of elevated hs-cTnT, i.e. above the 99th percentile, in patients with non-MI diagnoses varies but single studies report rates above 50 % of patients in consecutive patients aged >40 years admitted to a district hospital [1, 2]. In the emergency department (ED) the prevalence of elevated hs-cTn in consecutively admitted patients may be 20 %, and most of them do not have an ACS [3, 4]. The challenge is to differentiate cardiac from systemic causes of myocardial injury as well as coronary from non-coronary and ischemic from non-ischemic causes [5] (Fig. 8.1).

As shown in Fig. 8.1 it is often difficult to identify the exact underlying pathomechanisms and to categorize patients accurately in clinical practice as

E. Giannitsis, MD (✉) • H.A. Katus, MD
Department of Internal Medicine III, Cardiology, University Hospital Heidelberg,
Medizinische Klinik III, Heidelberg, Germany
e-mail: Evangelos.Giannitsis@med.uni-heidelberg.de

© Springer International Publishing Switzerland 2016
A.S. Maisel, A.S. Jaffe (eds.), *Cardiac Biomarkers*,
DOI 10.1007/978-3-319-42982-3_8

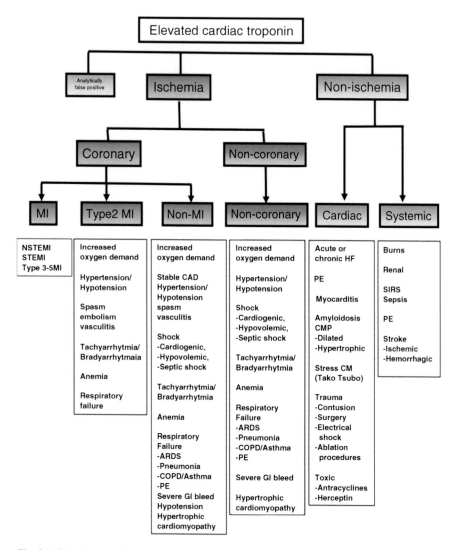

Fig. 8.1 Distribution of reasons of elevated cardiac troponin. Often causes for troponin elevation are multifactorial with myocardial ischemia (coronary, non-coronary, cardiac) contributing to variable extent (Data from references 5 and 19)

reasons may be multi-factorial and some acute diseases may be found in different categories.

In the following, an overview is given on prevalence, potential mechanisms and clinical relevance of elevated cTn in patients with atrial fibrillation, sepsis, respiratory failure, or gastrointestinal bleeding. Clinical cases are exemplified to illustrate presentation, clinical work-up and interpretation in clinical practice.

Case 1

A 76-year old male presents to an ED with dizziness and palpitations. He reported recent onset of exercise intolerance and shortness of breath when climbing more than 1 stair. Symptoms progressively worsened culminating the day of admission. There is a history of arterial hypertension, but otherwise no coronary risk factors and no cardiovascular disease. Physical examination revealed tachycardia with a heart rate of 123 bpm with an irregular pulse, no additional heart sounds, no murmurs on heart auscultation, normal lung auscultation, no signs of heart failure. Blood pressure was elevated at 160/100 mmHg. The standard ECG showed atrial fibrillation at a rate of 123 bpm, signs of LV hypertrophy but was otherwise unsuspicious.

On laboratory testing, all parameters were normal except for an elevated NT-pro BNP at 650 ng/L and an elevated hs-cTnT at 37 ng/L at presentation. Laboratory values were normal for thyroid function, renal function and haemoglobin, differential blood count, and C-reactive protein. After 3 h, hs-cTnT increased from 37 ng/L to 49 mg/L (>35 % rise).

Diagnostic work-up included a transthoracic echocardiography and blood gas analysis. On echocardiography there was a moderate LV hypertrophy with evidence for impaired LV relaxation on tissue Doppler. Otherwise echocardiography showed normal LV function, valvular function, no pericardial effusion and no regional wall motion abnormality. On blood gas analysis there was normal oxygenation and oxygen saturation.

Based on all clinical informations, the patient received a diagnosis of lone atrial fibrillation and acute myocardial injury as suggested by elevated hs-cTnT with a relevant rise at serial testing. Given the absence of signs or symptoms suggestive of MI acute myocardial injury was causally related to atrial fibrillation with inadequate rate control. The patient was given metoprolol to reduce heart rate below 70 bpm and was continued with 100 mg metoprolol OD. Based on a CHA$_2$DS$_2$-Vasc score of 3 points and a low bleeding risk, the patient was started on an oral Factor Xa inhibitor (20 mg Rivaroxaban OD). An electrical cardioversion was scheduled after 3 weeks of continuous intake of the oral anticoagulant, and a coronary MS-CT was planned to rule-out significant CAD 2 weeks after successful electrical cardioversion.

Cardiac Troponin and Atrial Fibrillation

Atrial fibrillatin (AF) has become a relevant public health burden due to increasing prevalence and its sequelae of TIA/stroke and peripheral thrombembolism [6, 7]. The exact pathomechanism for AF has not been fully elucidated. The most likely process of the most prevalent form of lone atrial fibrillation involves an age-related structural remodelling with connective tissue deposition and fibrosis as well as electrophysiological alterations that facilitate initiation and perpetuation of AF [8, 9]. Several additional mechanisms are being discussed to contribute, e.g. inflammation, oxidative stress and neurohumoral activity [10–12].

With introduction of more sensitive cTn assays it becomes increasingly evident that elevated hs-cTn level are also associated with the prevalence and incidence of AF [13–18]. Various mechanisms in patients with atrial fibrillation are believed to lead to release of cardiac troponin. The 3rd version of the Joint ESC/ACCF/AHA/WHF definition of MI designate acute or chronic cTn elevations outside the clinical context of myocardial ischemia as myocardial injury [19]. The exact pathomechanism for release of cTn has not been fully understood but is believed to include myocardial ischemia that is exaggerated by oxidative stress, impaired microvascular flow including the effect of elevated cardiac and systemic angiotensin II and endothelin-1 levels leading to vasoconstriction, impaired intracellular calcium handling, and activation of redox-sensitive signalling pathways [20]. Troponin elevation has been reported to occur in the absence of MI or manifest coronary artery disease [21–23]. Potential reasons include uncontrolled ventricular rate causing oxygen demand/supply mismatch, pressure overload, impaired microvascular flow, atrial calcium overload, oxidative stress, or alterations in tissue structure [24–26].

A small retrospective multicentre study on 662 patients demonstrated that patients presenting with AF and elevated cTn receive more cardiac testing and have more positive tests than those with normal cTn or those in whom cTn is not being measured [27].

In large epidemiological studies [16–18, 28] higher baseline levels of hs-cTn were associated with incident AF in covariate-adjusted analyses. In the CHS study [16] 4262 older adults free of AF with hs-cTnT measured at enrolment. During a follow-up of 11.2 years, 32 % developed AF. There was a concentration dependent risk to develop AF with a HR of 1.75 in the highest tertile vs undetectable. This risk of incident AF was independent of traditional risk factors, incident heart failure and biomarkers of inflammation and hemodynamic strain [16]. In the ARIC study [17], a prospective community cohort that included 10,584 middle aged adults free of AF. Over a follow-up duration of up to 12 years, incidence of AF was associated with increasing baseline hs-cTnT concentrations. Participants with hs-cTnT > 14 ng/L had a n adjusted HR of 1.78 compared to those with undetectable hs-cTnT concentrations (<5 ng/L). In the population-based Gutenberg Health Study on the first 5000 participants [18], several novel biomarkers measured and related to a history or a documented presence of AF. In adjusted multivariate analyses strongest associations were detected between per standard deviation increase of NT-pro BNP (HR2.89). In the Framingham Heart Study [28], levels of ST2, GDF-15 and hs-cTnI were measured at enrolment in 3217 participants without prevalent AF and subjects were followed for 10 years for incidence of AF and other outcomes [28]. After adjustment for AF risk factors, C-reactive protein and BNP, only hs-cTnI remained significantly associated with incident AF. The importance of troponin in an AF population was first reported from the Randomized Evaluation of Long-term Anticoagulant Therapy (RE-LY) biomarker substudy [13]. It was demonstrated that detectable level of cTnI were observed in 55 % of 6189 patients randomized to warfarin or Dabigatran, and that cTnI improved prediction of stroke or systemic embolism, cardiovascular death, and improved risk prediction for stroke and CV death when added to the CHADS$_2$ or CHA$_2$DS$_2$-Vasc Score [13]. The results of the RE-LY substudy were confirmed in the ARISTOTLE trial [14, 15]. In the ARISTOTLE Study [14] hs-cTnI was measured in 14,821 atrial fibrillation patients. Detectable rates were found in 98.5 % and levels exceeding the 99th percentile in 9.2 %. After adjustment, hs-cTnI was associated with a raised risk of stroke, cardiac death, and major bleeding and improved the C-statistics of the CHA$_2$DS$_2$-Vasc Score for stroke or systemic embolism, and for cardiac death [14]. Similar results were found for hs-cTnT albeit the proportion of patients with level close to and slightly above the 99th percentile were higher than with hs-cTnI (50 % had values >11 ng/L and 25 % had level >16.7 ng/L). Elevated level of hs-cTnT were independently predictive of stroke or systemic embolisation, cardiac death, and major bleeding, and improved the predictive value of the CHA$_2$DS$_2$vasc Score for stroke and death [15].

Another RE-LY substudy [29] evaluated the prognostic importance of persistent elevation of cTn in 2514 patients with AF with cTnI levels measured at randomisation and after 3 months. Patients with detectable cTnI level at both time points had higher rates of stroke, death and thrombembolic events than those with transient elevations or those without elevations. Interestingly, persistent elevation achieved a C-statistic of 0.644 for stroke as compared to 0.611 for the CHADS$_2$ score [29].

Cardiac troponin elevations in patients with AF has been reported to be associated with higher all-cause and CV mortality [13, 14, 30]. In addition, cTn has been found to predict subsequent AF in patients with or without stroke and undiagnosed AF, following CABG [31] and has been related to early incidence of early recurrence of AF in patients with AF [32].

The CHADS$_2$ and CHA$_2$DS$_2$-Vasc Score are the most commonly used scores. Both scores have a modest predictive value for identifying high risk subjects for stroke with C-statistics ranging from 0.6 to 0.8 (median 0.683) for CHADS$_2$ and 0.64 to 0.79 (median 0.673) for CHA$_2$DS$_2$ Vasc suggesting a need for improvement [33, 34].

Troponin is being detected very often in patients with AF and are being related to adverse outcomes. However, little is known about the effect of therapeutic interventions such as electrical or pharmacological cardioversion, rhythm control using antiarrhythmic agents or rate control on cTn levels. A recent small study on 60 patients reported that improved rate control reduced cTnT levels in patients with permanent AF [35].

Reduction of baseline heart rate from 95 ± 15 bpm to mean heart rates between 77 and 82 bpm by diltiazem, verapamil, metoprolol, or carvedilol decreased cTnT significantly from 11.8 (±6.8) to concentrations between 10.8 and 11.7 ng/L.

Given the association between detectable cTn and manifest or incident AF, it is anticipated that an elevated cTn is being measured in patients presenting with TIA or stroke, and may be useful to predict CV risk after cerebrovascular ischemia [36, 37]. In a registry on 193 consecutive patients admitted for acute stroke, an elevated hs-cTnT was measured in 33.7 % of patients previously tested negative with a conventional sensitive cTnT assay [37].

Table 8.1 Troponin and AF: key points to remember

In patients admitted with AF to an ED elevated hs-cTn/cTn is highly prevalent
Elevated hs-cTn indicates higher risk for incident and recurrent AF, and occurrence of AF post surgery
Higher risk for incident TIA/stroke and CV death
Reasons for cTn release multi-factorial indicating complex co-morbidities
Elevated cTn associated with tachycardia
Risk stratification for TIA/stroke and CV death, treatment according to underlying reason (MI, non-MI)

Case Annotation

This patient presented with lone atrial fibrillation with uncontrolled high heart rate. Along with elevated hs-cTnT at presentation there was a relevant rise on subsequent blood sampling but without additional clinical criteria to diagnose a type I or type II MI. Accordingly, the findings of elevated hs-cTnT at baseline with a relevant concentration change at serial sampling were classified as acute myocardial injury. Due to low level of suspicion for MI, invasive coronary angiography was not considered for the acute evaluation but a CT angiography was scheduled for a later time point. However, evaluation of patients with AF require further diagnostic workup since these patients were found to have a higher risk of stroke, recurrent AF, and higher risk of CV death. In the present case, echocardiography did not reveal evidence for regional wall motion abnormality or structural heart disease. Acute treatment of tachyarrhythmia has to be individualized according to findings from subsequent diagnostic work-up taking into consideration several acute and chronic conditions that may explain acute or chronic troponin elevations (Table 8.1).

Case 2

A 63-year old male is admitted to ED with new onset of fever (39 °C), coughing, and tachycardia. Blood pressure on admission is 110/75 mmHg. Chest X ray shows pneumonia of the right lower lobe with pleural effusion. Blood gas analysis shows hypo-oxygenation with 90 % oxygen saturation and a PO$_2$ of 89 mmHg under 2 liter oxygen supply. ECG is unsuspicious except for a heart rate of 95 bpm on admission. Laboratory testing reveals leukocytosis of 14,000/nl, a moderately elevated C-reactive protein (13 mg/dl) but highly elevated procalcitonin level (4 µg/L, decision cutoff 0.2 µg/L), normal serum creatinine (0.9 mg/dl), normal liver function. Patient received immediately antibiotic treatment for pneumonia with criteria of severe inflammatory response syndrome. During the next hours, the patient developed hypotension requiring fluid replacement and inotropic support and also developed acute renal failure. Hs-cTnT level on admission were slightly above the 99th percentile value on admission (23 ng/L) and increased to 157 ng/L during the next

24 h. There is no history of cardiovascular disease and no risk factors including diabetes or smoking. After adjustment of initial antibiotic therapy to the antibiogram that identified Pseudomonas aeruginosa as the pathogen, patients recovered to normal within several days. At discharge, hs-cTnT has declined to normal values (9 ng/L).

Cardiac Troponin and Sepsis

Severe sepsis and septic shock can be complicated by myocardial dysfunction even in patients without pre-existing CAD, and cardiac failure may contribute to poor outcome in these patients [38]. Obstructive CAD is frequently absent [39–41] and the mechanism for release of cTn is not fully elucidated. Several factors have been found to contribute to cTn release including cytokine-mediated cardiac cell injury with transient loss of membrane integrity, diastolic dysfunction and microvascular thrombotic injury [42, 43]. A recent meta-analysis on 17 studies with a total sample size of 1857 patients found that to be significantly associated with an almost two-fold increased risk of death [44]. In another meta-analysis of conventional troponin T or I and sepsis, including 1227 patients, elevated cTn that was present in 61 % and was found to be an independent predictor of mortality [45].

Troponin as a risk factor for mortality in critically ill patients without acute coronary syndromes [41].

Few studies have assessed the clinical utility of hs-cTn in patients with sepsis and septic shock. Wilhelm et al. [46] studied 313 patients with sepsis and septic shock in the ED, of whom 63 % had elevated hs-cTnT at admission. Among the 125 patients with severe sepsis or septic shock, nearly 80 % of patients had hs-cTnT above the 99th percentile of 14 ng/L. Although non-survivors showed significantly higher values of hs-cTnT than survivors, in the multivariate logistic regression model, the only variables independently related to 30-day mortality were Acute Physiology And Chronic Health Evaluation II (APACHE II) score, creatinine levels and history of CAD Røsjø et al. [38] measured hs-cTnT levels in 207 patients with severe sepsis/septic shock, of whom 80 % had hs-cTnT values above the normal 99th percentile cut-off value. High hs-cTnT levels on inclusion were associated with severity of disease, multiple organ dysfunction, creatinine levels and peak 24-h dose of dobutamine and noradrenaline. However, hs-cTnT did not provide independent prognostic information for in-hospital mortality after adjustment for potential confounders. Landesberg et al. [47] studied 106 patients with sepsis and septic shock, of whom 88 % had hs-cTnT above the 99th percentile cutoff of 14 ng/L. In patients with low APACHE II score, hs-cTnT independently predicted mortality. De Groot et al. [48] evaluated 292 patients with suspected sepsis in the ED and found that hs-cTnT was an independent predictor of in-hospital mortality. Bergenzaun et al. [49] studied 49 critically ill patients (two-thirds with septic shock), of whom 92 % had elevated hs-cTnT above the 99th percentile cut-off value of 14 ng/l, and found that hs-cTnT was an independent predictor of 1-year mortality. After performing a

Table 8.2 Sepsis, acute respiratory failure, GI bleed: points to remember

Elevated troponin highly prevalent in critically ill patients (>50%)
cTn release multi-factorial including ischemic, cardiac and systemic reasons
Exclude acute MI, if large spontaneous MI is likely weigh-out risk and benefits of conservative vs invasive therapy taking into account general condition and co-morbidities
Elevated troponin level indicate higher short-term and long-term mortality
Treat the acute underlying disease (GI bleed, respiratory failure, SIRS/sepsis) immediately and start to search for underlying reasons of troponin elevation

receiver operating characteristic curve for hs-cTnT and 1-year mortality [area under the receiver operating characteristics curve (AUC) 0.76], the cut-off value with best accuracy was 118 ng/l, which yielded a sensitivity of 72% and specificity of 82%.

Values of hs-cTn at ED presentation and changes over time are significantly higher in patients with AMI than in patients with acute cardiac non-coronary disorders, and absolute changes of hs-cTn over time are superior to relative changes in this setting [50]. Unfortunately, it is often very difficult, if not impossible, to differentiate among these different causes with our current non-invasive clinical tools. At present, however, routine troponin testing in septic patients is not recommended [5].

Case Annotation

Troponin elevation in SIRS or sepsis is common and often not associated with significant CAD or structural heart disease. The mechanism for release of cTn in SIRS, sepsis or septic shock is not fully understood but may be multifactorial. In the case presented several factors may have contributed such as a combination of inflammatory mediators in conjunction with a myocardial oxygen demand-supply mismatch (Table 8.2). Troponin elevation in SIRS and sepsis is associated with a worse prognosis. However, it is unclear whether any cardiovascular intervention could improve outcomes.

Case 3

A 26-year old female presents to ED with increasing coughing and greyish expectoration for several days, no fever, history of shortness of breath for several months with a recent increase in intensity. She also complains chest pain during exercise. She reported a history of bronchial asthma and a previous infection with pertussis on two consecutive years. She also reported a family history of MI, and is ex-smoker with 7 pack-years total cigarette exposure. No diabetes mellitus, no hypercholesterolemia, no arterial hypertension. Physical examination including neurological, cardiac and lung examination did not reveal any relevant findings including a normal blood pressure.

Standard-ECG showed a normal axis, sinus rhythm with a rate of 96 bpm, no signs of LV hypertrophy, no previous MI, and no right ventricular strain. Chest X-ray revealed no infiltrates or effusion, no pneumothorax and no other suspicious findings. On blood gas analysis, there was a marked hypo-oxygenation with an oxygen saturation of 87 %, a pO2 of 49 mmHg, a pCO2 of 51 mmHg, and a pH 7.29. Angio-CT of the lung was performed to exclude the presence of pulmonary embolism given a moderate pretest probability of pulmonary embolism. However, 256 MS-CT angiography excluded pulmonary embolism and detected only mild signs of acute bronchitis without lung infiltrates or other lung abnormalities.

On echocardiography there was a mildly depressed LV function with a hypokinesia of the apical segment of the anterior, septal and lateral wall. Laboratory testing showed a marked leukocytosis without detectable C-reactive protein (<5 mg/dl) and a procalcitonin level < 0.1 μg/L. In addition, D-dimer was elevated more than 3-times above the decision cutoff for VTE. The value of hs-cTnT at baseline was below the limit of detection but increased after 3 h to 37 ng/L and to 143 ng/L after 6 h. In the presence of an elevated hs-cTnT with a relevant rise from a normal baseline value to a hs-cTnT > 10-fold the 99th percentile value, chest pain and regional wall motion abnormality on echocardiography, the patient was diagnosed as NSTEMI and underwent a coronary angiography immediately after reporting of the last blood test result. However, coronary angiography did not find a significant obstruction of an epicardial coronary artery, except for a 30 % circumscipt atherosclerotic plaque on the right coronary artery. Therefore differential diagnoses were suspected and the patient received a contrast-enhanced cardiac MRI for exclusion of Tako Tsubo cardiomyopathy or myocarditis. In the absence of an unequivocal diagnosis of Tako Tsubo cardiomyopathy or myocarditis, acute myocardial injury was related to acute respiratory failure.

Cardiac Troponin and Respiratory Failure

Critically ill patients with cardiac involvement are at higher risk than others. Large numbers of investigations have documented elevations in 30–50 % of patients [51]. The mechanism depends on the clinical circumstances. Patients who have acute respiratory failure have a 30-fold increase in mortality when cTn is elevated. There are a number of potential pathophysiological mechanisms that could explain the interaction between COPD and cardiovascular disease. These include spill-over of pulmonary inflammation directly leading to development of atheromatous plaque formation and arterial re-modelling, development of pulmonary hypertension in COPD leading to right ventricular systolic failure, smoking as a shared risk factor, and lung hyperinflation reducing intra-thoracic blood volume and left ventricular performance [52]. The relationship between CV morbidity and COPD is supported by the beneficial effects of medications such as statins and β-blockers in patients with COPD [53, 54].

Vasile et al. [51] reported on a consecutive series of patients with respiratory failure admitted to an intensive care unit (ICU). Among 4433 patients, 2078 patients (46.9 %) had a cTnT value on admission constituting the study cohort. Of these, 878 (42.3 %) had elevated cTnT and 1200 patients (57.7 %) had undetectable cTnT. An elevated cTnT elevations was found to be independently associated with in-hospital, short-term and long-term mortality. The majority of patients had bacterial pneumonia, aspiration pneumonia, respiratory arrest, pulmonary edema and pulmonary embolism. There were several specific subsets of patients with severe acute respiratory disease including 1018 patients who met the clearly defined criteria for a diagnosis of acute respiratory failure, 1586 patients with acute lung injury, and 34 patients with an acute respiratory distress syndrome. In all subsets, the presence of an elevated cTnT in-hospital and long-term mortalities were more than 30-times higher than in patients with undetectable cTnt [51]. Consistently, Bajwa et al. [55] studied 248 patients with adult respiratory distress syndrome (ARDS) and blood results of whom 89 patients (35 %) had at least one elevated cardiac marker level. The presence of an elevated cardiac marker was associated with significantly higher mortality (p=0.01) and was an independent predictor of mortality (p=0.02) among patients with lower severity of illness (APACE III <79 points). A significant association between increasing quintiles of troponin I level and mortality rate was observed.

Patients with at least one elevated cardiac marker also had significantly more organ system derangement, including non-cardiovascular organ system failures (p=0.02).

Saaby et al. [56] included a series of 4499 patients of whom 553 patients received a diagnosis of AMI. Sub-classified by infarct subtype according to the Universal MI definition, 386 (72 %) had a type 1 myocardial infarction and 144 (26 %) had a type 2 myocardial infarction. In an analysis of mechanisms underlying a type 2 MI anemia, tachy-arrhythmias, and respiratory failure (30 of 144) were the most prevalent conditions [56].

Lee et al. [57] studied 152 patients with community-acquired pneumonia (39.5 %), health care-associated pneumonia (40.8 %), and hospital-acquired pneumonia (19.7 %). Eighty-eight (58 %) patients had detectable cTnI levels (median, 0.049 ng/ mL. There was a strong association between elevated cTnI levels and mortality with an adjusted HR of 1.398. Sparse data are available for acute exacerbation of COPD. In a meta-analysis on 37 studies including 189,772 study subjects [58] requiring hospitalization for acute exacerbation of chronic obstructive pulmonary disease, cardiac troponin was found to predict short-term mortality with a HR of 3.16.

Case Annotation

The present case demonstrates nicely the challenge to correctly interpret hs-cTnT. In presence of an equivocal clinical presentation driven by signs and symptoms of acute respiratory failure that are not explained by LV function clinical judgement and experience is paramount to initiate a diagnostic work-up that enables an early and accurate diagnosis. Given the clinical presentation, the diagnosis of acute respiratory failure of unknown reason was made after exclusion of other life-threatening acute diseases including pulmonary embolism, acute MI, or traumatic lung injury. Critical reduction of oxygen saturation may cause myocardial ischemia resulting in myocardial injury, even in the absence of underlying significant CAD or structural heart disease.

Case 4

A 54-year old male presents to ED with weakness and hypotension. ECG shows sinus rhythm with tachycardia at 105 bpm. Physical examination is normal except for a mild resistance of the upper abdomen. There is a history of rheumatoid arthritis and the patient takes continuously non-steroidal anti-inflammatory drugs for several months. The patient developed diabetes mellitus 5 years ago that is treated with metformin. In addition there is a history of arterial hypertension and hyperlipidemia, and the patient takes ramipril 10 mg OD and simvastatin 20 mg OD. No known cardiovascular disease or previous coronary intervention. Laboratory testing revelead a haemoglobin of 7.5 mg/dl and a haematocrit of 27. There is a mild leucocytosis and a small elevation of C-reactive protein. Serum creatinine is slightly increased to 1.4 mg/dl corresponding to a eGFR of 64 ml/min. Hs-cTnT was 22 ng/L on admission and remained stable at 24 ng/l after 3 and after 6 h. The patient received urgently endoscopy that showed active gastric bleeding presumably due to non-sterioidal drug. Patient received an endoscopic intervention with clipping of the arterial ulcer and recovered after blood transfusion. The patients remained hemodynamically stable and was discharged home.

Cardiac Troponin and GI Bleeding

Vasile et al. [59] evaluated cardiac cTnT levels of 1076 critically-ill patients consecutively hospitalized with a diagnosis of acute GI bleeding. Admission troponin measurements were available in 70.1 % of cases. Of these, 43.6 % had cTnT above the 99th percentile cutoff. The investigators found that albeit elevated cTn was predictive for long-term outcomes but not independently predictive for short-term outcomes when the severity of the acute illness was adjusted. The association between troponin elevations and long-term survival persisted even after adjustment for severity of illness as evaluated by APACHE III prognostic system, cardiovascular co-morbidities, and risk factors [59]. An important finding of this study was that endoscopy was safe for patients with acute GI hemorrhage seen in the ICU even when troponin levels upon admission are elevated. The study suggests that initial management should be focused on the GI bleeding. After successful treatment there is an opportunity to intervene in these patients at a later time point, particularly when the underlying mechanism has been identified [59]. In another series of patients with signs of gastrointestinal bleeds, a total of 19% demonstrated cTnI release. Age greater than 65 years, signs of hemodynamic instability at presentation, a recent history of cardiac disease, cardiovascular compromise following endoscopy, and re-bleeding were associated with troponin release [60].

Possible reasons for elevated troponin in the presence or absence of a relevant coronary stenosis include a type 2 MI due to the imbalance between oxygen demand and supply in the light of anemia, hypovolemia, tachycardia, cardiac toxicity of catecholamine use [61, 62]. A common mechanism between bacterial infection leading to gastric ulcer and a systemic inflammatory state that leads to the vulnerability of atherosclerotic plaque within coronary arteries has been described [63]. The coincidence of severe bleeding and a spontaneous type 1 MI, or a type IVb MI due to stent thrombosis after interruption of antiplatelet or anticoagulant therapy in the prodromal phase of bleeding event has to be considered, as well.

Case Annotation

Troponin elevation in critically ill patients with severe GI bleeds is not uncommon occurring in about 40% of cases. Elevated troponin is associated with an adverse long-term outcome. The acute risk is rather predicted by severity of illness (APACHE score) and baseline characteristics and not by troponin elevation. The primary clinical efforts should be directed toward care of the GI bleeding. After successful treatment and discharge, there is an opportunity to intervene in these patients if a significant CAD or another treatable reason for elevated cTn can be detected.

Summary

Prevalence of elevated hs-cTnT (above the 99th percentile) with relevant concentration changes in patients without an ACS is high, and elevated hs-cTn is associated with adverse long-term outcomes, irrespective the exact underlying reason.

Differentiation between ischemic and non-ischemic reasons is particularly challenging as ischemic and non-ischemic mechanisms frequently co-exist. Understanding the etiology of troponin elevation in critically ill patients is important to better target appropriate therapies for MI in this population.

References

1. Iversen K, Køber L, Gøtze JP, Dalsgaard M, Nielsen H, Boesgaard S, Bay M, Kirk V, Nielsen OW. Troponin T is a strong marker of mortality in hospitalized patients. Int J Cardiol. 2013;168(2):818–24.

2. Lindner G, Pfortmueller CA, Braun CT, Exadaktylos AK. Non-acute myocardial infarction-related causes of elevated high-sensitive troponin T in the emergency room: a cross-sectional analysis. Intern Emerg Med. 2014;9(3):335–9.

3. Javed U, Aftab W, Ambrose JA, Wessel RJ, Mouanoutoua M, Huang G, Barua RS, Weilert M, Sy F, Thatai D. Frequency of elevated troponin I and diagnosis of acute myocardial infarction. Am J Cardiol. 2009;104(1):9–13.

4. Mueller M, Biener M, Vafaie M, Blankenberg S, White HD, Katus HA, Giannitsis E. Prognostic performance of kinetic changes of high-sensitivity troponin T in acute coronary syndrome and in patients with increased troponin without acute coronary syndrome. Int J Cardiol. 2014;174(3):524–9.

5. Newby LK, Jesse RL, Babb JD, Christenson RH, De Fer TM, Diamond GA, Fesmire FM, Geraci SA, Gersh BJ, Larsen GC, Kaul S, McKay CR, Philippides GJ, Weintraub WS. ACCF 2012 expert consensus document on practical clinical considerations in the interpretation of troponin elevations: a report of the American College of Cardiology Foundation task force on Clinical Expert Consensus Documents. J Am Coll Cardiol. 2012;60(23):2427–63.

6. Stefansdottir H, Aspelund T, Gudnason V, Arnar DO. Trends in the incidence and prevalence of atrial fibrillation in Iceland and future projections. Europace. 2011;13(8):1110–7.

7. Holstenson E, Ringborg A, Lindgren P, Coste F, Diamand F, Nieuwlaat R, Crijns H. Predictors of costs related to cardiovascular disease among patients with atrial fibrillation in five European countries. Europace. 2011;13(1):23–30.

8. Frustaci A, Chimenti C, Bellocci F, Morgante E, Russo MA, Maseri A. Histological substrate of atrial biopsies in patients with lone atrial fibrillation. Circulation. 1997;96(4):1180–4.

9. Daoud EG, Bogun F, Goyal R, Harvey M, Man KC, Strickberger SA, Morady F. Effect of atrial fibrillation on atrial refractoriness in humans. Circulation. 1996;94(7):1600–6.

10. Wijffels MC, Kirchhof CJ, Dorland R, Power J, Allessie MA. Electrical remodeling due to atrial fibrillation in chronically instrumented conscious goats: roles of neurohumoral changes, ischemia, atrial stretch, and high rate of electrical activation. Circulation. 1997;96(10):3710–20.

11. Matsukida K, Kisanuki A, Toyonaga K, Murayama T, Nakashima H, Kumanohoso T, Yoshifuku S, Saigo M, Abe S, Hamasaki S, Otsuji Y, Minagoe S, Tei C. Comparison of transthoracic Doppler echocardiography and natriuretic peptides in predicting mean pulmonary capillary wedge pressure in patients with chronic atrial fibrillation. J Am Soc Echocardiogr. 2001;14(11):1080–7.

12. Carnes CA, Chung MK, Nakayama T, Nakayama H, Baliga RS, Piao S, Kanderian A, Pavia S, Hamlin RL, McCarthy PM, Bauer JA, Van Wagoner DR. Ascorbate attenuates atrial pacing-induced peroxynitrite formation and electricalremodeling and decreases the incidence of post-operative atrial fibrillation. Circ Res. 2001;89(6):E32–8.

13. Hijazi Z, Oldgren J, Andersson U, Connolly SJ, Ezekowitz MD, Hohnloser SH, Reilly PA, Vinereanu D, Siegbahn A, Yusuf S, Wallentin L. Cardiac biomarkers are associated with an increased risk of stroke and death in patients with atrial fibrillation: a Randomized Evaluation of Long-term Anticoagulation Therapy (RE-LY) substudy. Circulation. 2012;125(13):1605–16.

14. Hijazi Z, Siegbahn A, Andersson U, Granger CB, Alexander JH, Atar D, Gersh BJ, Mohan P, Harjola VP, Horowitz J, Husted S, Hylek EM, Lopes RD, McMurray JJ, Wallentin L, ARISTOTLE Investigators. High-sensitivity troponin I for risk assessment in patients with atrial fibrillation: insights from the Apixaban for Reduction in Stroke and other Thromboembolic Events in Atrial Fibrillation (ARISTOTLE) trial. Circulation. 2014;129(6):625–34.

15. Hijazi Z, Wallentin L, Siegbahn A, Andersson U, Alexander JH, Atar D, Gersh BJ, Hanna M, Harjola VP, Horowitz JD, Husted S, Hylek EM, Lopes RD, McMurray JJ, Granger CB, ARISTOTLE Investigators. High-sensitivity troponin T and risk stratification in patients with atrial fibrillation during treatment with apixaban or warfarin. J Am Coll Cardiol. 2014;63(1):52–61.

16. Hussein AA, Bartz TM, Gottdiener JS, Sotoodehnia N, Heckbert SR, Lloyd-Jones D, Kizer JR, Christenson R, Wazni O, deFilippi C. Serial measures of cardiac troponin T levels by a highly sensitive assay and incident atrial fibrillation in a prospective cohort of ambulatory

older adults. Heart Rhythm. 2015. pii: S1547-5271(15)00070-3. doi:10.1016/j. hrthm.2015.01.020. [Epub ahead of print].

17. Filion KB, Agarwal SK, Ballantyne CM, Eberg M, Hoogeveen RC, Huxley RR, Loehr LR, Nambi V, Soliman EZ, Alonso A. High-sensitivity cardiac troponin T and the risk of incident atrial fibrillation: the Atherosclerosis Risk in Communities (ARIC) study. Am Heart J. 2015;169(1):31–8.

18. Schnabel RB, Wild PS, Wilde S, Ojeda FM, Schulz A, Zeller T, Sinning CR, Kunde J, Lackner KJ, Munzel T, Blankenberg S. Multiple biomarkers and atrial fibrillation in the general population. PLoS One. 2014;9(11):e112486.

19. Thygesen K, Alpert JS, Jaffe AS, Simoons ML, Chaitman BR, White HD, Writing Group on the Joint ESC/ACCF/AHA/WHF Task Force for the Universal Definition of Myocardial Infarction, Thygesen K, Alpert JS, White HD, Jaffe AS, Katus HA, Apple FS, Lindahl B, Morrow DA, Chaitman BA, Clemmensen PM, Johanson P, Hod H, Underwood R, Bax JJ, Bonow RO, Pinto F, Gibbons RJ, Fox KA, Atar D, Newby LK, Galvani M, Hamm CW, Uretsky BF, Steg PG, Wijns W, Bassand JP, Menasché P, Ravkilde J, Ohman EM, Antman EM, Wallentin LC, Armstrong PW, Simoons ML, Januzzi JL, Nieminen MS, Gheorghiade M, Filippatos G, Luepker RV, Fortmann SP, Rosamond WD, Levy D, Wood D, Smith SC, Hu D, Lopez-Sendon JL, Robertson RM, Weaver D, Tendera M, Bove AA, Parkhomenko AN, Vasilieva EJ, Mendis S, ESC Committee for Practice Guidelines (CPG). Third universal definition of myocardial infarction. Eur Heart J. 2012;33(20):2551–67.

20. Goette A, Bukowska A, Lillig CH, Lendeckel U. Oxidative stress and microcirculatory flow abnormalities in the ventricles during atrial fibrillation. Front Physiol. 2012;3:236.

21. Zellweger MJ, Schaer BA, Cron TA, Pfisterer ME, Osswald S. Elevated troponin levels in absence of coronary artery disease after supraventricular tachycardia. Swiss Med Wkly. 2003;133(31–32):439–41.

22. Bakshi TK, Choo MK, Edwards CC, Scott AG, Hart HH, Armstrong GP. Causes of elevated troponin I with a normal coronary angiogram. Intern Med J. 2002;32(11):520–5.

23. Nunes JP, Silva JC, Maciel MJ. Troponin I in atrial fibrillation with no coronary atherosclerosis. Acta Cardiol. 2004;59(3):345–6.

24. Eggers KM, Lind L, Ahlström H, Bjerner T, Ebeling Barbier C, Larsson A, Venge P, Lindahl B. Prevalence and pathophysiological mechanisms of elevated cardiac troponin I levels in a population-based sample of elderly subjects. Eur Heart J. 2008;29(18):2252–8.

25. Dobrev D, Nattel S. Calcium handling abnormalities in atrial fibrillation as a target for innovative therapeutics. J Cardiovasc Pharmacol. 2008;52(4):293–9.

26. Hijazi Z, Oldgren J, Siegbahn A, Granger CB, Wallentin L. Biomarkers in atrial fibrillation: a clinical review. Eur Heart J. 2013;34(20):1475–80.

27. Gupta K, Pillarisetti J, Biria M, Pescetto M, Abu-Salah TM, Annapureddy C, Ryschon K, Dawn B, Lakkireddy D. Clinical utility and prognostic significance of measuring troponin I levels in patients presenting to the emergency room with atrial fibrillation. Clin Cardiol. 2014;37(6):343–9.

28. Rienstra M, Yin X, Larson MG, Fontes JD, Magnani JW, McManus DD, McCabe EL, Coglianese EE, Amponsah M, Ho JE, Januzzi Jr JL, Wollert KC, Fradley MG, Vasan RS, Ellinor PT, Wang TJ, Benjamin EJ. Relation between soluble ST2, growth differentiation factor-15, and high-sensitivity troponin I and incident atrial fibrillation. Am Heart J. 2014;167(1):109–15.

29. Hijazi Z, Oldgren J, Andersson U, Connolly SJ, Ezekowitz MD, Hohnloser SH, Reilly PA, Siegbahn A, Yusuf S, Wallentin L. Importance of persistent elevation of cardiac biomarkers in atrial fibrillation: a RE-LY substudy. Heart. 2014;100(15):1193–200.

30. van den Bos EJ, Constantinescu AA, van Domburg RT, Akin S, Jordaens LJ, Kofflard MJ. Minor elevations in troponin I are associated with mortality and adverse cardiac events in patients with atrial fibrillation. Eur Heart J. 2011;32(5):611–7.

31. Leal JC, Petrucci O, Godoy MF, Braile DM. Perioperative serum troponin I levels are associated with higher risk for atrial fibrillation in patients undergoing coronary artery bypass graft surgery. Interact Cardiovasc Thorac Surg. 2012;14(1):22–5.

32. Latini R, Masson S, Pirelli S, Barlera S, Pulitano G, Carbonieri E, Gulizia M, Vago T, Favero C, Zdunek D, Struck J, Staszewsky L, Maggioni AP, Franzosi MG, Disertori M, GISSI-AF Investigators. Circulating cardiovascular biomarkers in recurrent atrial fibrillation: data from the GISSI-atrial fibrillation trial. J Intern Med. 2011;269(2):160–71.

33. Lip GY, Nieuwlaat R, Pisters R, Lane DA, Crijns HJ. Refining clinical risk stratification for predicting stroke and thromboembolism in atrial fibrillation using a novel risk factor-based approach: the euro heart survey on atrial fibrillation. Chest. 2010;137(2):263–72.

34. Mahajan R, Lau DH, Sanders P. Biomarkers and atrial fibrillation: is it prime time yet? Heart. 2014;100(15):1151–2.

35. Ulimoen SR, Enger S, Norseth J, Pripp AH, Abdelnoor M, Arnesen H, Gjesdal K, Tveit A. Improved rate control reduces cardiac troponin T levels in permanent atrial fibrillation. Clin Cardiol. 2014;37(7):422–7.

36. Stahrenberg R, Niehaus CF, Edelmann F, Mende M, Wohlfahrt J, Wasser K, Seegers J, Hasenfuß G, Gröschel K, Wachter R. High-sensitivity troponin assay improves prediction of cardiovascular risk in patients with cerebral ischaemia. J Neurol Neurosurg Psychiatry. 2013;84(5):479–87.

37. Jensen JK, Ueland T, Aukrust P, Antonsen L, Kristensen SR, Januzzi JL, Ravkilde J. Highly sensitive troponin T in patients with acute ischemic stroke. Eur Neurol. 2012;68(5):287–93.

38. Røsjø H, Varpula M, Hagve TA, FINNSEPSIS Study Group, et al. Circulating high sensitivity troponin T in severe sepsis and septic shock: distribution, associated factors, and relation to outcome. Intensive Care Med. 2011;37:77–85.

39. Ver Elst KM, Spapen HD, Nguyen DN, et al. Cardiac troponins I and T are biological markers of left ventricular dysfunction in septic shock. Clin Chem. 2000;46:650–7.

40. Ammann P, Fehr T, Minder EI, et al. Elevation of troponin I in sepsis and septic shock. Intensive Care Med. 2001;27:965–9.

41. Ammann P, Maggiorini M, Bertel O, et al. Troponin as a risk factor for mortality in critically ill patients without acute coronary syndromes. J Am Coll Cardiol. 2003;41:2004–9.

42. Vasile VC, Chai HS, Abdeldayem D, et al. Elevated cardiac troponin T levels in critically ill patients with sepsis. Am J Med. 2013;126:1114–21.

43. Landesberg G, Gilon D, Meroz Y, Georgieva M, Levin PD, Goodman S, Avidan A, Beeri R, Weissman C, Jaffe AS, Sprung CL. Diastolic dysfunction and mortality in severe sepsis and septic shock. Eur Heart J. 2012;33:895–903.

44. Sheyin O, Davies O, Duan W, Perez X. The prognostic significance of troponin elevation in patients with sepsis: a meta-analysis. Heart Lung. 2015;44(1):75–81.

45. Bessière F, Khenifer S, Dubourg J, Durieu I, Lega JC. Prognostic value of troponins in sepsis: a meta-analysis. Intensive Care Med. 2013;39:1181–9.

46. Wilhelm J, Hettwer S, Schuermann M, et al. Elevated troponin in septic patients in the emergency department: frequency, causes, and prognostic implications. Clin Res Cardiol. 2014;103:561–7.

47. Landesberg G, Jaffe AS, Gilon D, et al. Troponin elevation in severe sepsis and septic shock: the role of left ventricular diastolic dysfunction and right ventricular dilatation. Crit Care Med. 2014;42:790–800.

48. De Groot B, Verdoorn RC, Lameijer J, van der Velden J. High-sensitivity cardiac troponin T is an independent predictor of inhospital mortality in emergency department patients with suspected infection: a prospective observational derivation study. Emerg Med J. 2014;31(11):882–8.

49. Bergenzaun L, Ohlin H, Gudmundsson P, et al. High-sensitive cardiac Troponin T is superior to echocardiography in predicting 1-year mortality in patients with SIRS and shock in intensive care. BMC Anesthesiol. 2012;12:25.

50. Mueller M, Biener M, Vafaie M, Doerr S, Keller T, Blankenberg S, Katus HA, Giannitsis E. Absolute and relative kinetic changes of high-sensitivity cardiac troponin T in acute coronary syndrome and in patients with increased troponin in the absence of acute coronary syndrome. Clin Chem. 2012;58(1):209–18.

51. Vasile VC, Chai HS, Khambatta S, et al. Significance of elevated cardiac troponin T levels in critically ill patients with acute respiratory disease. Am J Cardiol. 2010;123:1049–58.
52. Stone IS, Barnes NC, Petersen SE. Chronic obstructive pulmonary disease: a modifiable risk factor for cardiovascular disease. Heart. 2012;98:1055–62.
53. Short PM, Lipworth SI, Elder DH, Schembri S, Lipworth BJ. Effect of beta blockers in treatment of chronic obstructive pulmonary disease: a retrospective cohort study. BMJ. 2011;342:d2549.
54. Mancini GB, Etminan M, Zhang B. Reduction of morbidity and mortality by statins, angiotensin-converting enzyme inhibitors and angiotensin receptor blockers in patients with chronic obstructive pulmonary disease. J Am Coll Cardiol. 2006;47:2554–60.
55. Bajwa EK, Boyce PD, Januzzi JL, Gong MN, Thompson BT, Christiani DC. Biomarker evidence of myocardial cell injury is associated with mortality in acute respiratory distress syndrome. Crit Care Med. 2007;35:2484–90.
56. Saaby L, Poulsen TS, Hosbond S, Larsen TB, Pyndt Diederichsen AC, Hallas J, Thygesen K, Mickley H. Classification of myocardial infarction: frequency and features of type 2 myocardial infarction. Am J Med. 2013;126:789–97.
57. Lee YJ, Lee H, Park JS, Kim SJ, Cho YJ, Yoon HI, Lee JH, Lee CT, Park JS. Cardiac troponin I as a prognostic factor in critically ill pneumonia patients in the absence of acute coronary syndrome. J Crit Care. 2015;30(2):390–4.
58. Singanayagam A, Schembri S, Chalmers JD. Predictors of mortality in hospitalized adults with acute exacerbation of chronic obstructive pulmonary disease. Ann Am Thorac Soc. 2013;10:81–9.
59. Vasile V, Babuin L, Perez J, Alegria J, Song L, Chai H, et al. Long-term prognostic significance of elevated cardiac troponin levels in critically ill patients with acute gastrointestinal bleeding. Crit Care Med. 2009;37:140–7.
60. Iser DM, Thompson AJV, Sia KK, Yeomans ND, Chen RYM. Prospective study of cardiac troponin I release in patients with upper gastrointestinal bleeding. J Gastroenterol Hepatol. 2008;23:938–42.
61. Wu AH. Etiologies of troponin elevation in critically ill patients with gastrointestinal bleeding. Crit Care Med. 2009;37:347–8.
62. Yunge L, Bruneval P, Cokay MS, et al. Pertubation of the sarcolemmal membrane inisoproterenol-induced myocardial injury of the rat. Permeability and freeze-fracture studies in vivo and in vitro. Am J Pathol. 1989;134:171–85.
63. Miyazaki M, Baabazono A, Kadowaki K, et al. Is Helicobacter pylori infection a risk factor for acute coronary syndromes? J Infect. 2006;52:86–91.

Selected References

Hijazi Z, Oldgren J, Andersson U, Connolly SJ, Ezekowitz MD, Hohnloser SH, Reilly PA, Vinereanu D, Siegbahn A, Yusuf S, Wallentin L. Cardiac biomarkers are associated with an increased risk of stroke and death in patients with atrial fibrillation: a Randomized Evaluation of Long-term Anticoagulation Therapy (RE-LY) substudy. Circulation. 2012;125(13):1605–16.
Iversen K, Køber L, Gøtze JP, Dalsgaard M, Nielsen H, Boesgaard S, Bay M, Kirk V, Nielsen OW. Troponin T is a strong marker of mortality in hospitalized patients. Int J Cardiol. 2013;168(2):818–24.
Mueller M, Biener M, Vafaie M, Doerr S, Keller T, Blankenberg S, Katus HA, Giannitsis E. Absolute and relative kinetic changes of high-sensitivity cardiac troponin T in acute coronary syndrome and in patients with increased troponin in the absence of acute coronary syndrome. Clin Chem. 2012;58(1):209–18.

Newby LK, Jesse RL, Babb JD, Christenson RH, De Fer TM, Diamond GA, Fesmire FM, Geraci SA, Gersh BJ, Larsen GC, Kaul S, McKay CR, Philippides GJ, Weintraub WS. ACCF 2012 expert consensus document on practical clinical considerations in the interpretation of troponin elevations: a report of the American College of Cardiology Foundation task force on Clinical Expert Consensus Documents. J Am Coll Cardiol. 2012;60(23):2427–63.

Saaby L, Poulsen TS, Hosbond S, Larsen TB, Pyndt Diederichsen AC, Hallas J, Thygesen K, Mickley H. Classification of myocardial infarction: frequency and features of type 2 myocardial infarction. Am J Med. 2013;126:789–97.

Sheyin O, Davies O, Duan W, Perez X. The prognostic significance of troponin elevation in patients with sepsis: a meta-analysis. Heart Lung. 2015;44(1):75–81.

Thygesen K, Alpert JS, Jaffe AS, Simoons ML, Chaitman BR, White HD, Writing Group on the Joint ESC/ACCF/AHA/WHF Task Force for the Universal Definition of Myocardial Infarction, Thygesen K, Alpert JS, White HD, Jaffe AS, Katus HA, Apple FS, Lindahl B, Morrow DA, Chaitman BA, Clemmensen PM, Johanson P, Hod H, Underwood R, Bax JJ, Bonow RO, Pinto F, Gibbons RJ, Fox KA, Atar D, Newby LK, Galvani M, Hamm CW, Uretsky BF, Steg PG, Wijns W, Bassand JP, Menasché P, Ravkilde J, Ohman EM, Antman EM, Wallentin LC, Armstrong PW, Simoons ML, Januzzi JL, Nieminen MS, Gheorghiade M, Filippatos G, Luepker RV, Fortmann SP, Rosamond WD, Levy D, Wood D, Smith SC, Hu D, Lopez-Sendon JL, Robertson RM, Weaver D, Tendera M, Bove AA, Parkhomenko AN, Vasilieva EJ, Mendis S, ESC Committee for Practice Guidelines (CPG). Third universal definition of myocardial infarction. Eur Heart J. 2012;33(20):2551–67.

Vasile V, Babuin L, Perez J, Alegria J, Song L, Chai H, et al. Long-term prognostic significance of elevated cardiac troponin levels in critically ill patients with acute gastrointestinal bleeding. Crit Care Med. 2009;37:140–7.

Vasile VC, Chai HS, Khambatta S, et al. Significance of elevated cardiac troponin T levels in critically ill patients with acute respiratory disease. Am J Cardiol. 2010;123:1049–58.

Vasile VC, Chai HS, Abdeldayem D, et al. Elevated cardiac troponin T levels in critically ill patients with sepsis. Am J Med. 2013;126:1114–21.

Chapter 9
Use of cTn for Detection of More Chronic Disease States

Ravi H. Parikh and Christopher R. deFilippi

Abstract Progressively higher levels of cTn measured by new high sensitive assays, typically well below the range of detection by contemporary cTn assays, are associated with a pattern of both abnormal cross-sectional findings with cardiac imaging and risk factors as well as adverse prognostic consequences in a wide range of chronic settings ranging from the asymptomatic general populations to subjects with known coronary or structural heart disease. However, as of this writing the role for high sensitive cTn assays outside the evaluation and management of acute coronary syndromes is still a work in progress. Both data and hence guidelines are not ready to provide direction for the evaluation of the asymptomatic patient. This remains an area of intense research and ultimately after the completion of appropriately powered and designed intervention trials based on patient selection by high sensitive cTn level, the role for cTn testing may extend well beyond the patient with AMI.

Keywords cTn for detection of chronic disease states • Troponins in chronic CAD • cTn and chronic kidney disease • Chronic kidney disease and cTn • Cardiac troponin T • cTn IN ACC/AHA STAGE B HEART FAILURE

With the recent introduction of high sensitive assays, it has become apparent that even small elevations of cardiac troponin (cTn) levels are strong prognostic risk markers across a spectrum of acute and chronic cardiovascular diseases. This chapter will explore the use and interpretation of cTn in those without acute myocardial infarction (AMI), particularly with respect to chronic kidney disease (CKD), stable coronary artery disease (CAD), and American College of Cardiology (ACC)/American Heart Association (AHA) stage B heart failure (HF) consisting of asymptomatic structural heart disease, specifically those with

R.H. Parikh, MD (✉)
Department of Medicine, University of Maryland School of Medicine, Baltimore, MD, USA
e-mail: rparikh@medicine.umaryland.edu

C.R. deFilippi, MD
Department of Medicine, University of Maryland School of Medicine, Maryland Heart Center University of Maryland Medical Center, Baltimore, MD, USA

© Springer International Publishing Switzerland 2016
A.S. Maisel, A.S. Jaffe (eds.), *Cardiac Biomarkers*,
DOI 10.1007/978-3-319-42982-3_9

left ventricular systolic dysfunction (typically a low left ventricular ejection fraction [LVEF]), left ventricular hypertrophy (LVH), and valvular disease [1]. Improving low-end accuracy of cardiac troponin measurement in order to increase the sensitivity for detection of AMI has come at the cost of lower specificity for AMI with many other conditions (cardiac and systemic) being associated with elevated levels. In longitudinal studies, these non-AMI associated cTn elevations are usually associated with poor prognosis irrespective of the underlying etiology for their elevation [2]. Examples of these conditions are as diverse as sepsis [3], pulmonary hypertension [4], and sleep apnea [5] among many others. Furthermore, progressively higher cTn levels in asymptomatic community based populations using the newest generation of high sensitive assays have shown significant associations with cardiac risk factors, structural cardiac abnormalities, and longitudinal associations with adverse events including cardiovascular/all-cause mortality and HF [6–15].

cTn in CKD/ESRD

Clinical Case 1

A 58 year old African American man with history of CKD stage III secondary to long-standing HTN and diabetes is admitted to the hospital for right lower extremity cellulitis and was found to have two elevated cardiac troponin T (cTnT) levels in the emergency department (presentation 60 ng/L and 7 h later, 65 ng/L). Based on the absence of change (loosely defined as ≥20%) in cTn levels and no diagnostic ECG changes or symptoms of cardiac ischemia, he was "ruled-out" for AMI. Although he does not meet criteria for an AMI, what is the significance of these elevated troponin concentrations?

Many studies have evaluated the prognostic significance of elevated cTnT and cardiac troponin I (cTnI) with both the contemporary and high sensitive assays in patients with CKD (defined as an estimated glomerular filtration rate [eGFR] <60 mL/min/1.73 m^2) and end-stage renal disease (ESRD, defined as the requirement for renal replacement therapy [RRT]). It is well-known that patients with kidney disease have both detectable and elevated (above the 99th percentile of the general population) baseline levels of circulating cTn. With high sensitive assays, the percentage of those with a detectable and elevated level increases, with virtually all subjects having detectable levels [16–18]. Elevated levels in CKD patients not on RRT, irrespective of symptoms or known cardiovascular disease, have a poor prognosis. In this population, a recent meta-analysis by the Agency for Healthcare Research and Quality focusing on the contemporary, non-high sensitive cTn assays, found cTnT associated with all-cause mortality (pooled adjusted hazard ratio [HR] 3.4, 95 % CI 1.1–11.0 and pooled odds ratio [OR] 3.0, 95 % CI 1.4–6.7) and major adverse cardiac events (MACE; pooled adjusted HR 2.7, 95 % CI 1.1–7.6). cTnI also was associated with all-cause mortality (pooled adjusted HR 1.7, 95 % CI 1.2–2.7) but not MACE [19]. Studies with high sensitive cTnT and cTnI in patients not on RRT have shown similar prognostic results. The large National Institute of Health (NIH)-sponsored multicenter chronic renal insufficiency cohort (CRIC) study with 3243 well-characterized participants showed strong associations between baseline high sensitive cTnT levels and cardiovascular risk factors, structural cardiac pathology, and longitudinal outcomes [16, 17, 20]. Eighty-four percent of participants in the cohort had detectable levels of high sensitive cTnT with higher levels strongly associated with LVH, older age, African American and Hispanic race, male gender, diabetes, higher blood pressure, among other factors [16]. Longitudinal outcomes in this cohort showed increased new-onset (incident) HF (adjusted HR 4.8, 95 % CI 2.5–9.1, median follow-up 6 years) when comparing the groups with undetectable cTnT (<3 ng/L) and those in the highest quartile of cTnT [17]. These findings were congruent with the large PREVEND observational study involving 1505 patients with mostly mild CKD where cTnT, also measured with the high sensitive assay, was a significant prognostic marker of cardiovascular events [21].

For patients on RRT, elevated cTn levels are also associated with a poorer prognosis. A meta-analysis of studies conducted from 1999 to 2004 found that non high sensitive cTnT was associated with all-cause mortality (relative risk [RR] 2.64, 95 % CI 2.17–3.20) and cardiac death (RR 2.55; 95 % CI 1.93–3.37) and cTnI was associated with all-cause mortality (RR 1.74, 95 % CI 1.27–2.38) [22]. A more recent meta-analysis focusing mostly on studies using more contemporary, but still not high sensitive, cTn assays found similar results in dialysis patients [19].

The etiology of persistently elevated levels of troponin in patients with CKD regardless of whether or not they are on RRT remains incompletely explained, whether it is from increased cardiac production or decreased renal clearance. However, the preponderance of evidence suggests that simultaneous ongoing cardiac injury and not decreased clearance of cTn as the main etiology for detectable levels in this population. Potential mechanisms of cardiac injury including ongoing myocyte damage from uremic toxicity [23], oxidative injury [24, 25], supply/demand mismatch with resulting ischemia [26], inflammation [27, 28], and dialysis related physiologic changes [29]. A small post-mortem anatomic study specifically focusing on patients with ESRD and elevated pre-mortem cTnT levels showed that all 6 patients had underlying cardiac pathology regardless of the cause of death [30].

Both cTnI and cTnT are detectable in most patients with CKD and ESRD and are associated with an increased presence of cardiovascular risk factors and underlying structural heart disease with increased risk of progressing to symptomatic heart disease and cardiovascular death.

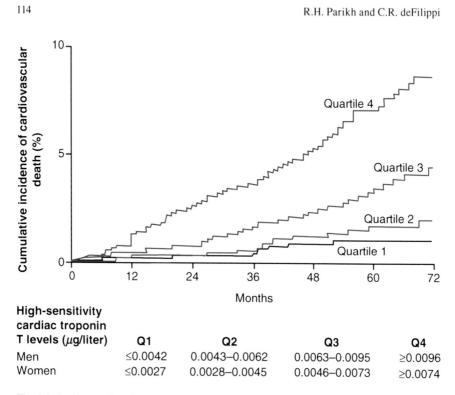

Fig. 9.1 Incidence of cardiovascular death by quartile of hs-cTnT in population with stable CAD (From Ref. [34], with permission)

cTn IN Chronic CAD

Clinical Case 2

A 68 year old Caucasian asymptomatic man with history of hypertension, hyperlipidemia, and known CAD on prior angiogram has an elevated cTn. What is the significance of this finding?

Several studies have reported cross-sectional and prognostic implications of elevated cTn in patients with stable CAD. Omland et al. showed in 3679 patients with stable CAD enrolled in the PEACE trial (a study of trandolapril versus placebo in subjects with chronic CAD), there was cross-sectional and prognostic information in elevated levels of cTnT using the high sensitive assay. Patients in the study at baseline all had stable CAD with a mean age of 63.6 years, majority Caucasian, male, and frequently had co-morbidities including diabetes, hypertension, and stroke. Figure 9.1 shows the cumulative incidence of cardiovascular death divided by quartile of cTnT. There was increased risk of cardiovascular death (HR 2.1, 95 % CI 1.6–2.7), HF (HR 2.2, 95 % CI 1.7–2.9) but not AMI (HR 1.16, 95 % CI 0.97–1.40) in the lowest compared to highest cTnT quartiles [31]. Furthermore, the addition of cTnT to NT-proBNP (a biomarker already established to provide prognostic information in this cohort and others with stable CAD in addition to those with HF) modestly but significantly improved prediction for cardiovascular mortality. In the HOPE study, another study of patients with known vascular disease or diabetes with at least one other cardiovascular risk factor, investigators found higher cTnT levels (also measured with the high sensitive assay) associated with subsequent AMI, HF, and cardiovascular mortality [32]. A third study, the HEART and SOUL study of veterans with known CAD, has also confirmed these findings [33].

The prognostic role of cTnI, again measured with a high sensitive assay, was also evaluated in patients enrolled in the PEACE trial. Almost all of the patients (98.5 %) had cTnI levels above the limit of detection of the assay and increasing quartiles of cTnI were associated with traditional clinical and laboratory risk factors. Prognostically, there was an increased risk of cardiovascular death or nonfatal HF (HR 1.3, 95 % CI 1.2–1.5) and nonfatal MI (HR 1.2, 95 % CI 1.0–1.4) per 1-standard deviation increase in the log of cTnI. Interestingly the association between levels of cTnI and cTnT was only moderate ($R = 0.44$) with each being independently predictive of HF and cardiovascular death. The fact that only cTnI was predictive for AMI suggests the presence of differing underlying biological properties among cTn assays which may account for their different prognostic information [34]. This finding will need to be further explored in other studies of at-risk chronic heart disease populations.

cTn IN ACC/AHA Stage B Heart Failure

Clinical Case 3

A 74 year old African American patient with a long-standing history of HTN is being evaluated for the first time in clinic. Despite being asymptomatic, a routine ECG is diagnostic for LVH and echocardiography confirms this finding. Does the measurement of cardiac troponin in the blood assist in further risk stratifying this patient?

The 2013 ACC/AHA guidelines define stage B HF as the presence of asymptomatic structural heart disease which includes LVH, asymptomatic left ventricular systolic dysfunction, asymptomatic valvular disease, and prior MI [1]. This patient qualifies as having ACC/AHA Stage B HF as defined in the introduction based on the presence of LVH. Stage B HF is also associated with a high prevalence of traditional cardiovascular risk factors and longitudinal studies have shown increased progression to symptomatic HF (stages C and D) [35–37]. The role of cTn, especially when measured with a high sensitive assay, in the prognostication of patients with stage B HF is gaining recognition as a powerful independent risk-factor with population-based, epidemiological studies [6–9].

LVH is typically a byproduct of multiple factors including pressure load, volume load, demographics which includes genetic factors, and co-morbidities. In the

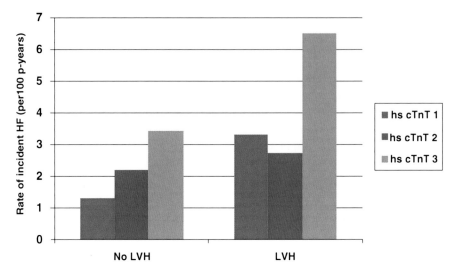

Fig. 9.2 Incidence rate of HF by LVH and tertile of high sensitive cTnT (From Ref. [41], with permission)

Framingham Offspring Study, increase in LV mass (LVM) was associated with age, gender, body mass index (BMI), systolic blood pressure, antihypertensive medications, smoking, and diabetes over a period of 16 years [38]. As a corollary, increased LVM is a risk factor for developing asymptomatic decreased LVEF and HF including subtypes with preserved and reduced LVEF [35]. Similar findings were observed in a prospective older community dwelling cohort in whom LVH was associated with increased risk of progression to a decreased LVEF with or without symptoms [39].

Three studies have evaluated the association of high sensitive cTn with LVH and risk of progression to HF and death in the general population. In the Dallas Heart Study, 9.2 % of the 2413 participants in the total cohort had LVH and among those, 45.7 % had detectable (>3 ng/L) cTnT. During a median follow-up of 8 years, those with LVH and a detectable cTnT level had over a 2-fold increase in the risk of HF or cardiovascular death compared to the group with LVH and undetectable cTnT [40]. Similar findings were observed in older adults from the Cardiovascular Health Study using cTnT also measured with the high sensitive assay. In this study subjects could frequently be differentiated between HF with reduced versus preserved LVEF (HFrEF and HFpEF, respectively). Similar to the Dallas cohort, but now with a median follow-up of over 13 years, the presence of LVH and higher levels of cTnT was associated with the highest incidence and risk of HF (Fig. 9.2). Elevated levels of cTnT at baseline appeared particularly good at differentiating which patients with LVH would develop HFrEF (HR 7.8, 95 % CI 4.4–13.8) versus HFpEF (HR 2.6, 95 % CI 1.4–4.8) when comparing the highest tertile of cTnT with LVH versus the lowest tertile without LVH. [41] The association of LVH and cardiac troponin is not unique to cTnT. A study of 2460 Framingham Offspring participants without HF and complete echocardiographic assessment found cTnI, measured with a high sensitive assay, associated with LVH or a low LVEF (adjusted OR 1.2, 95 % CI 1.1–1.3). In this same cohort cTnI was also a significant predictor of HF and cardiovascular death [14]. In conclusion, detectable levels of circulating cTnT and cTnI portend a poor prognosis in those with underlying LVH.

Given the high incidence and significant economic burden of HF, there has been recent interest in developing screening tests to identify those with asymptomatic low LVEF ($\leq$50 %) in an attempt to diagnose and initiate treatments earlier to prevent progression to clinical HF. The prevalence of an asymptomatic low LVEF in the Framingham Heart Study was reported at 6.0 % in men and 0.8 % in women and was associated with incident HF and mortality [35]. However, cTn alone, even when using a highly sensitive assay, is not an accurate screening test for a low LVEF. Further insight into the detection of asymptomatic structural heart disease may be provided with the combination of cTn testing, natriuretic peptide testing, and longitudinal outcomes. Levels of NT-proBNP and high sensitive cTnT in a cohort from the Cardiovascular Health Study found a significant association between the upward trajectories of both biomarkers over 2–3 years and development of an abnormal LVEF (<50 %) [42]. While two studies have shown that natriuretic peptide levels can be useful to guide therapy in general populations with risk factors to prevent HF hospitalizations and death, no such study has yet been conducted with cTn assays [43, 44].

Valvular heart disease is a field where the application of cTn may begin to assist in short-term management and long-term prognostication. Current ACC/AHA guidelines recommending surgery in those patients who have symptoms or who are asymptomatic with structural heart disease [45] are problematic in determining surgical necessity in those who have asymptomatic disease with risk factors for progression. A cross-sectional study evaluating 131 patients with mostly symptomatic, hemodynamically severe aortic stenosis (AS) found cTnI detectable (using a non-high sensitive assay) in 56 % and associated with symptoms of HF [46]. Two studies evaluated the prognostic role of cTnT and cTnI measured with high sensitive assays in patients with AS. The first study offers a comparison between the contemporary and high sensitive cTnT assay in 57 patients with moderate or severe AS. All patients had detectable cTnT when measured by the high sensitive assay (median 180 ng/L) compared to only 9 patients having detectable cTnT with the 4th generation test. High sensitive cTnT was associated with larger left ventricular dimensions, higher peak velocities across aortic valve (AV), and greater LVM. After a median follow-up of 769 days, there were 8 deaths and 30 patients underwent AV replacement surgery. Prognostically, cTnT levels >27 ng/L was independently associated with all-cause mortality [47]. The second study evaluated cTnI, measured with a high sensitive assay, in two different cohorts with AS. One cohort (n = 122) with mild to severe AS was used to determine cross-sectional associations between cTnI and structural and functional heart disease while the other cohort (n = 131) consisting of asymptomatic participants with moderate to severe AS was used to determine longitudinal associations with cTnI levels. cTnI levels above 1.2 ng/L (lower limit of detection) were present in 98 % of patients with AS. Cross-sectionally, cTnI was independently associated with greater left ventricular mass and myocardial fibrosis

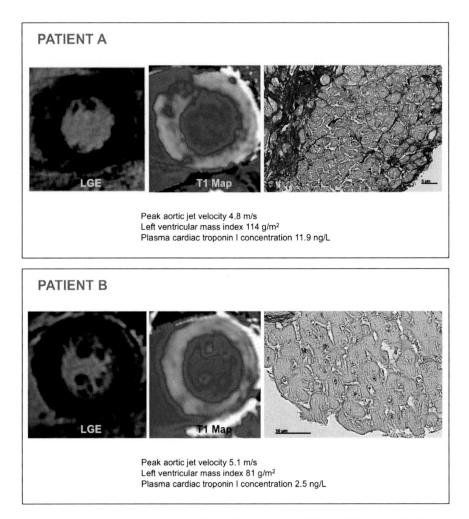

Fig. 9.3 Comparison of two patients with similar severity of AS but differing hs-cTnI levels. Patient A with the higher troponin level was found to have higher LVMI, extent of fibrosis on cardiac MRI, and more collagen deposition on myocardial biopsy (From Ref. [48], with permission)

on cardiac MRI (Fig. 9.3). Over a median follow-up of 10.6 years, there were 24 cardiovascular deaths and 60 patients who underwent AV replacement surgery in the longitudinal cohort. Figure 9.4 shows the survival curves of the outcomes divided by tertile of cTnI. On multivariate analysis, cTnI level was associated with both AV replacement and cardiovascular mortality [48]. In summary, cTn measured by a high sensitive assay provides insight into the severity of myocardial pathology and morbidity/mortality with AS. Measurement of cTn may ultimately become incorporated into algorithms to determine necessity of AV replacement prior to the onset of severe symptoms.

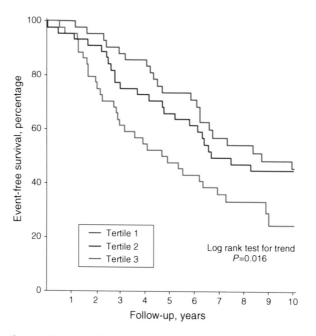

Fig. 9.4 Event-free survival or cardiovascular death or aortic valve replacement by tertile of cTnI in population with asymptomatic AS (From Ref. [48], with permission)

Conclusion

Progressively higher levels of cTn measured by new high sensitive assays, typically well below the range of detection by contemporary cTn assays, are associated with a pattern of both abnormal cross-sectional findings with cardiac imaging and risk factors as well as adverse prognostic consequences in a wide range of chronic settings ranging from the asymptomatic general populations to subjects with known coronary or structural heart disease. However, as of this writing the role for high sensitive cTn assays outside the evaluation and management of acute coronary syndromes is still a work in progress. Both data and hence guidelines are not ready to provide direction for the evaluation of the asymptomatic patient. This remains an area of intense research and ultimately after the completion of appropriately powered and designed intervention trials based on patient selection by high sensitive cTn level, the role for cTn testing may extend well beyond the patient with AMI.

References

1. Yancy CW, Jessup M, Bozkurt B, Butler J, Casey Jr DE, Drazner MH, et al. 2013 ACCF/AHA guideline for the management of heart failure: a report of the American College of Cardiology Foundation/American Heart Association Task Force on practice guidelines. Circulation. 2013;128(16):e240–319.

2. Newby LK, Jesse RL, Babb JD, Christenson RH, De Fer TM, Diamond GA, et al. ACCF 2012 expert consensus document on practical clinical considerations in the interpretation of troponin elevations: a report of the American College of Cardiology Foundation task force on Clinical Expert Consensus Documents. J Am Coll Cardiol. 2012;60(23):2427–63.
3. Bessiere F, Khenifer S, Dubourg J, Durieu I, Lega JC. Prognostic value of troponins in sepsis: a meta-analysis. Intensive Care Med. 2013;39(7):1181–9.
4. Velez-Martinez M, Ayers C, Mishkin JD, Bartolome SB, Garcia CK, Torres F, et al. Association of cardiac troponin I with disease severity and outcomes in patients with pulmonary hypertension. Am J Cardiol. 2013;111(12):1812–7.
5. Einvik G, Rosjo H, Randby A, Namtvedt SK, Hrubos-Strom H, Brynildsen J, et al. Severity of obstructive sleep apnea is associated with cardiac troponin I concentrations in a community-based sample: data from the Akershus Sleep Apnea Project. Sleep. 2014;37(6):1111–6, 6A-6B.
6. deFilippi CR, de Lemos JA, Christenson RH, Gottdiener JS, Kop WJ, Zhan M, et al. Association of serial measures of cardiac troponin T using a sensitive assay with incident heart failure and cardiovascular mortality in older adults. JAMA. 2010;304(22):2494–502.
7. de Lemos JA, Drazner MH, Omland T, Ayers CR, Khera A, Rohatgi A, et al. Association of troponin T detected with a highly sensitive assay and cardiac structure and mortality risk in the general population. JAMA. 2010;304(22):2503–12.
8. Saunders JT, Nambi V, de Lemos JA, Chambless LE, Virani SS, Boerwinkle E, et al. Cardiac troponin T measured by a highly sensitive assay predicts coronary heart disease, heart failure, and mortality in the Atherosclerosis Risk in Communities Study. Circulation. 2011;123(13):1367–76.
9. Wallace TW, Abdullah SM, Drazner MH, Das SR, Khera A, McGuire DK, et al. Prevalence and determinants of troponin T elevation in the general population. Circulation. 2006;113(16):1958–65.
10. Zethelius B, Berglund L, Sundström J, Ingelsson E, Basu S, Larsson A, et al. Use of multiple biomarkers to improve the prediction of death from cardiovascular causes. N Engl J Med. 2008;358(20):2107–16.
11. Sundstrom J, Ingelsson E, Berglund L, Zethelius B, Lind L, Venge P, et al. Cardiac troponin-I and risk of heart failure: a community-based cohort study. Eur Heart J. 2009;30(7):773–81.
12. Zeller T, Tunstall-Pedoe H, Saarela O, Ojeda F, Schnabel RB, Tuovinen T, et al. High population prevalence of cardiac troponin I measured by a high-sensitivity assay and cardiovascular risk estimation: the MORGAM Biomarker Project Scottish Cohort. Eur Heart J. 2014;35(5):271–81.
13. Otsuka T, Kawada T, Ibuki C, Seino Y. Association between high-sensitivity cardiac troponin T levels and the predicted cardiovascular risk in middle-aged men without overt cardiovascular disease. Am Heart J. 2010;159(6):972–8.
14. Wang TJ, Wollert KC, Larson MG, Coglianese E, McCabe EL, Cheng S, et al. Prognostic utility of novel biomarkers of cardiovascular stress: the Framingham Heart Study. Circulation. 2012;126(13):1596–604.
15. Neumann JT, Havulinna AS, Zeller T, Appelbaum S, Kunnas T, Nikkari S, et al. Comparison of three troponins as predictors of future cardiovascular events--prospective results from the FINRISK and BiomaCaRE studies. PLoS One. 2014;9(3):e90063.
16. Dubin RF, Li Y, He J, Jaar BG, Kallem R, Lash JP, et al. Predictors of high sensitivity cardiac troponin T in chronic kidney disease patients: a cross-sectional study in the chronic renal insufficiency cohort (CRIC). BMC Nephrol. 2013;14:229.
17. Bansal N, Hyre Anderson A, Yang W, Christenson RH, deFilippi CR, Deo R, et al. High-sensitivity troponin T and N-terminal Pro-B-type natriuretic peptide (NT-proBNP) and risk of incident heart failure in patients with CKD: the Chronic Renal Insufficiency Cohort (CRIC) study. J Am Soc Nephrol. 2015;26(4):946–56.
18. deFilippi CR, Thorn EM, Aggarwal M, Joy A, Christenson RH, Duh SH, et al. Frequency and cause of cardiac troponin T elevation in chronic hemodialysis patients from study of cardiovascular magnetic resonance. Am J Cardiol. 2007;100(5):885–9.

19. Michos ED, Wilson LM, Yeh HC, Berger Z, Suarez-Cuervo C, Stacy SR, et al. Prognostic value of cardiac troponin in patients with chronic kidney disease without suspected acute coronary syndrome: a systematic review. Ann Intern Med. 2014;161(7):491–501.
20. Mishra RK, Li Y, DeFilippi C, Fischer MJ, Yang W, Keane M, et al. Association of cardiac troponin T with left ventricular structure and function in CKD. Am J Kidney Dis. 2013;61(5):701–9.
21. Scheven L, de Jong PE, Hillege HL, Lambers Heerspink HJ, van Pelt LJ, Kootstra JE, et al. High-sensitive troponin T and N-terminal pro-B type natriuretic peptide are associated with cardiovascular events despite the cross-sectional association with albuminuria and glomerular filtration rate. Eur Heart J. 2012;33(18):2272–81.
22. Khan NA, Hemmelgarn BR, Tonelli M, Thompson CR, Levin A. Prognostic value of troponin T and I among asymptomatic patients with end-stage renal disease: a meta-analysis. Circulation. 2005;112(20):3088–96.
23. Dikow R, Hardt SE. The uremic myocardium and ischemic tolerance: a world of difference. Circulation. 2012;125(10):1215–6.
24. Kajimoto H, Kai H, Aoki H, Yasuoka S, Anegawa T, Aoki Y, et al. Inhibition of eNOS phosphorylation mediates endothelial dysfunction in renal failure: new effect of asymmetric dimethylarginine. Kidney Int. 2012;81(8):762–8.
25. Del Vecchio L, Locatelli F, Carini M. What we know about oxidative stress in patients with chronic kidney disease on dialysis--clinical effects, potential treatment, and prevention. Semin Dial. 2011;24(1):56–64.
26. Amann K, Breitbach M, Ritz E, Mall G. Myocyte/capillary mismatch in the heart of uremic patients. J Am Soc Nephrol. 1998;9(6):1018–22.
27. Lowbeer C, Stenvinkel P, Pecoits-Filho R, Heimburger O, Lindholm B, Gustafsson SA, et al. Elevated cardiac troponin T in predialysis patients is associated with inflammation and predicts mortality. J Intern Med. 2003;253(2):153–60.
28. Sezer S, Karakan S, Ozdemir N. Increased cardiac troponin T levels are related to inflammatory markers and various indices of renal function in chronic renal disease patients. Ren Fail. 2012;34(4):454–9.
29. London GM. Left ventricular alterations and end-stage renal disease. Nephrol Dial Transplant. 2002;17 Suppl 1:29–36.
30. Ooi DS, Veinot JP, Wells GA, House AA. Increased mortality in hemodialyzed patients with elevated serum troponin T: a one-year outcome study. Clin Biochem. 1999;32(8):647–52.
31. Omland T, de Lemos JA, Sabatine MS, Christophi CA, Rice MM, Jablonski KA, et al. A sensitive cardiac troponin T assay in stable coronary artery disease. N Engl J Med. 2009;361(26):2538–47.
32. McQueen MJ, Kavsak PA, Xu L, Shestakovska O, Yusuf S. Predicting myocardial infarction and other serious cardiac outcomes using high-sensitivity cardiac troponin T in a high-risk stable population. Clin Biochem. 2013;46(1–2):5–9.
33. Beatty AL, Ku IA, Christenson RH, DeFilippi CR, Schiller NB, Whooley MA. High-sensitivity cardiac troponin T levels and secondary events in outpatients with coronary heart disease from the Heart and Soul Study. JAMA Intern Med. 2013;173(9):763–9.
34. Omland T, Pfeffer MA, Solomon SD, de Lemos JA, Røsjø H, Šaltytė Benth J, et al. Prognostic value of cardiac troponin I measured with a highly sensitive assay in patients with stable coronary artery disease. J Am Coll Cardiol. 2013;61(12):1240–9.
35. Wang TJ, Evans JC, Benjamin EJ, Levy D, LeRoy EC, Vasan RS. Natural history of asymptomatic left ventricular systolic dysfunction in the community. Circulation. 2003;108(8):977–82.
36. Goldberg LR, Jessup M. Stage B heart failure: management of asymptomatic left ventricular systolic dysfunction. Circulation. 2006;113(24):2851–60.
37. Jessup M, Brozena S. Heart failure. N Engl J Med. 2003;348(20):2007–18.
38. Lieb W, Xanthakis V, Sullivan LM, Aragam J, Pencina MJ, Larson MG, et al. Longitudinal tracking of left ventricular mass over the adult life course: clinical correlates of short- and long-term change in the Framingham offspring study. Circulation. 2009;119(24):3085–92.

39. Drazner MH, Rame JE, Marino EK, Gottdiener JS, Kitzman DW, Gardin JM, et al. Increased left ventricular mass is a risk factor for the development of a depressed left ventricular ejection fraction within five years: the Cardiovascular Health Study. J Am Coll Cardiol. 2004;43(12):2207–15.
40. Neeland IJ, Drazner MH, Berry JD, Ayers CR, deFilippi C, Seliger SL, et al. Biomarkers of chronic cardiac injury and hemodynamic stress identify a malignant phenotype of left ventricular hypertrophy in the general population. J Am Coll Cardiol. 2013;61(2):187–95.
41. Seliger SL, de Lemos JA, Neeland IJ, Christenson R, Gottdiener J, Drazner MH, et al. Older adults, "malignant" left ventricular hypertrophy and associated cardiac specific biomarker phenotypes to identify the differential risk of new-onset reduced versus preserved ejection fraction heart failure – the Cardiovascular Health Study. JACC Heart Fail. 2015;3(6):445–55.
42. Glick D, DeFilippi CR, Christenson R, Gottdiener JS, Seliger SL. Long-term trajectory of two unique cardiac biomarkers and subsequent left ventricular structural pathology and risk of incident heart failure in community-dwelling older adults at low baseline risk. JACC Heart Fail. 2013;1(4):353–60.
43. Huelsmann M, Neuhold S, Resl M, Strunk G, Brath H, Francesconi C, et al. PONTIAC (NT-proBNP selected prevention of cardiac events in a population of diabetic patients without a history of cardiac disease): a prospective randomized controlled trial. J Am Coll Cardiol. 2013;62(15):1365–72.
44. Ledwidge M, Gallagher J, Conlon C, Tallon E, O'Connell E, Dawkins I, et al. Natriuretic peptide-based screening and collaborative care for heart failure: the STOP-HF randomized trial. JAMA. 2013;310(1):66–74.
45. Nishimura RA, Otto CM, Bonow RO, Carabello BA, Erwin 3rd JP, Guyton RA, et al. 2014 AHA/ACC guideline for the management of patients with valvular heart disease: a report of the American College of Cardiology/American Heart Association Task Force on Practice Guidelines. Circulation. 2014;129(23):e521–643.
46. Kupari M, Eriksson S, Turto H, Lommi J, Pettersson K. Leakage of cardiac troponin I in aortic valve stenosis. J Intern Med. 2005;258(3):231–7.
47. Rosjo H, Andreassen J, Edvardsen T, Omland T. Prognostic usefulness of circulating high-sensitivity troponin T in aortic stenosis and relation to echocardiographic indexes of cardiac function and anatomy. Am J Cardiol. 2011;108(1):88–91.
48. Chin CW, Shah AS, McAllister DA, Joanna Cowell S, Alam S, Langrish JP, et al. High-sensitivity troponin I concentrations are a marker of an advanced hypertrophic response and adverse outcomes in patients with aortic stenosis. Eur Heart J. 2014;35:2312–21.

Chapter 10
Use of High-Sensitive cTn Assays for the Evaluation of Patients Potentially at Risk for Cardiovascular Disease

Kai M. Eggers and Per Venge

Abstract There is increasing interest in measurement of cardiac troponin (cTn) levels for assessment of subjects from the community. Given the low prevalence of cardiovascular (CV) disease, the utility of cTn as a screening tool in the general population however, is debated. Measurement of cTn levels might instead be clinically useful in selected at-risk cohorts. In fact, several studies have consistently demonstrated that cTn levels in these cohorts are strong predictors of adverse outcome, mainly with respect to mortality and the development of heart failure. cTn levels also provide prognostic value beyond that obtained from standard risk assessment including measurement of other circulating biomarkers and might thus, serve as an important component in primary prevention.

In this chapter, we review the evidence on this topic including results from studies in selected at-risk cohorts, i.e. subjects with prevalent CV risk factors, diabetics and the elderly. The summarized notion from these investigations is that cTn measurements likely might serve as a 'gatekeeper' in the future, in particular to facilitate the identification of subjects with at-risk features in whom additional testing is needed to detect the particular source of cardiac injury and to design appropriate clinical responses.

Keywords Cardiac troponin • Primary prevention • Cardiovascular disease • Population studies • Diabetes mellitus • Elderly subjects

K.M. Eggers, MD, PhD (✉)
Departments of Medical Sciences, Cardiology, Uppsala University Hospital and Uppsala University, Uppsala, Sweden
e-mail: kai.eggers@ucr.uu.se

P. Venge, MD, PhD
Departments of Medical Sciences, Cardiology and Clinical Chemistry, Uppsala University Hospital and Uppsala University, Uppsala, Sweden
e-mail: per.venge@medsci.uu.se

© Springer International Publishing Switzerland 2016
A.S. Maisel, A.S. Jaffe (eds.), *Cardiac Biomarkers*,
DOI 10.1007/978-3-319-42982-3_10

The burden of cardiovascular disease (CV) is increasing worldwide. This has generated interest in strategies to estimate the risk of developing CV disease in community-dwelling subjects, and to detect and monitor CV disease at stages that might be modifiable by lifestyle interventions or pharmacotherapies.

Traditional risk factors (e.g. hypertension, hyperlipidemia, diabetes, smoking) do not fully explain the interindividual variation of risk. Standard clinical assessment (e.g. physical examination, ECG recordings) is moreover, not always sensitive enough to detect the subtle alterations associated with evolving CV disease. Because of the considerable need to improve risk detection, measurement of circulating CV biomarkers has been suggested as an important complement. However up until now, biomarker measurements are not considered in European guidelines for primary prevention [1] and U.S. guidelines only suggest measurement of C-reactive protein levels in subjects in whom standard risk assessment remains uncertain [2]. The reluctance regarding the broader application of biomarker measurements depends on concerns regarding cost-effectiveness and the lack of prospective studies documenting clinical benefit. From a conceptual perspective however, at-risk cohorts from general populations could be particularly suitable for biomarker-guided management as the (assumed) higher prevalence of CV disease in these cohorts would increase the utility of such an approach.

The cardiac troponins (cTn) are one of the most promising biomarkers in this regard. cTn is mainly bound to the thin filament of the contractile apparatus of cardiomyocytes, and its physiologic role is to control and regulate cardiac muscle contraction. In situations associated with acute myocardial damage, a considerable amount of cTn is released into the circulation. cTn levels may however, also be detectable in clinically stable subjects from the general population. The first reports on this issue have been published about 10 years ago [3]. These studies however, were based on results obtained using assays with, from todays perspective, suboptimal sensitivity. This hampered in-depth analyses regarding the mechanisms associated with cTn release. During recent years, high-sensitivity cTn assays with a 10- to 100-fold lower limit of detection compared with conventional methods have been developed. Latest-generation prototype assays yield measurable cTn concentrations in almost all healthy individuals [4]. With the use of these assays, it has become clear that cTn levels are associated with several aspects of chronic heart disease, entities portending to its development and the complications thereof in the years that follow.

In this chapter, we will present cases illustrating the implications of cTn levels in subjects at risk for developing CV disease. We will summarize the conditions contributing to cTn release in these cohorts with special emphasis on the elderly and diabetics. The role of cTn for the detection of chronic CV disease states is dealt with elsewhere in this book. We will moreover discuss issues that need to be considered if cTn measurement should be taken forward into clinical practice in at-risk subjects. As high-sensitivity assays soon will be standard, we will limit our review of the literature to studies using such assays.

Case 1: cTn Levels in a Patient with Prevalent CV Risk Factors

This case is a male with hypertension and dyslipidemia who has been smoking since age 20. His body mass index is 28 kg/m^2 and his LDL-cholesterol level is 170 mg/dL. He has a history of prostate cancer which had been treated with radiation therapy. At age 67, this patient participated in a routine health control. At that time, he was on continuous medication with betablockers and ACE-inhibitors. His blood pressure was 160/80 mmHg. The standard 12-lead ECG demonstrated surprisingly lateral ST-segment changes although the patient was free from exertional angina. Blood tests showed CRP 1.0 mg/L, NT-proBNP 1815 ng/L and creatinine 78 μmol/L. The cTnI level (Abbott Architect) was 12 ng/L (99th percentile 26 ng/L). Because of the ECG findings and the elevated NT-proBNP levels, the patient was referred for an echocardiography which was without evidence of left-ventricular (LV) hypertrophy, diastolic or systolic dysfunction. A treadmill test was not performed.

Three years later, the patient developed rapidly accelerating exertional chest pain for which he was hospitalized. A coronary angiography revealed a severe stenosis of the proximal segment of the right coronary artery which was treated by placement of a drug-eluting stent. At this time point, the patient started a medication with anti-platelets, atorvastatin and stopped smoking.

Two years after the coronary intervention, the patient had again developed mild and stable angina. His LDL-cholesterol level had decreased to 108 mg/dL but the NT-proBNP level had increased to 2199 ng/L with a concomitant increase in cTnI levels to 35 ng/L. For this reason, a new echocardiography was performed which demonstrated an impaired LV systolic function (LVEF 0.45). Consequently, the ACE-inhibitor dosage was increased to the maximally tolerated dose and the patient is since then followed with regular check-ups by his cardiologist.

Discussion

This case illustrates how results from combined testing of cTnI and NT-proBNP might signal the need for further cardiac evaluation, in this case with respect to LV abnormalities and possibly, coronary artery disease. It also highlights that higher cTn levels may be found when CV risk factors are present, e.g. hypertension, dyslipidemia, smoking but also diabetes and chronic kidney disease [5–8]. Higher cTn levels are moreover associated with increased LV mass, subnormal LVEF and diastolic dysfunction, entities that may be asymptomatic precursors of heart failure. cTn release in these conditions is mediated by increased LV filling pressures resulting in myocardial wall stress, inflammatory processes and/or oxidative stress [9]. A higher prevalence of LV abnormalities in combination with decreased subendocardial perfusion is also likely the cause of higher cTn levels seen in subjects with coronary artery disease [10].

There is thus, convincing evidence that cTn levels are elevated early on in the process of evolving CV disease, and intimately related to the progression towards adverse events. Measurement of cTn levels might therefore, be particularly useful in subjects with CV risk factors or those who already have developed CV disease. This is supported by data from the ULSAM study demonstrating stronger associations of cTnT with adverse outcome in subjects with prevalent CV disease compared to those without [7].

The prognostic implications of cTn levels in subjects at risk for cardiac disease has been confirmed in the HOPE study which enrolled subjects with either prevalent vascular disease or diabetes in combination with at least one additional CV risk factor. Over 4.5 years of follow-up, both cTnT and cTnI (Beckman-Coulter) exhibited independent and graded associations with CV death or myocardial infarction and improved metrics of prognostic discrimination [11, 12].

Case 2: cTn Levels in a Subject with Diabetes

The next case is an elderly, slightly overweight male smoker with non-insulin dependent diabetes type 2 since 23 years. His diabetes was reasonably well-controlled although admittedly he did not care very much about keeping strict diet. He had also pharmacologically treated hypertension and dyslipidemia with essentially normal blood pressure and lipid profile. Otherwise, this patient had no history of CV disease. At age 81 and 86, he underwent extended medical check-ups. His BMI at the first visit was 31 kg/m^2 and at the second visit 5 years later 25 kg/m^2. His blood pressure at the first visit was 154/78 mmHg and 118/60 mmHg at the second visit. The blood tests from the first visit showed LDL-cholesterol 77 mg/dL, CRP 2.7 mg/L and creatinine 81 μmol/L. At the second visit, blood tests showed LDL-cholesterol 109 mg/dL and creatinine 100 μmol/L. The cTnI level (Abbott Architect) was 36 ng/L at the first visit and 58 ng/L at the second visit.

While the CRP and creatinine results were non-alarming at the first visit, the creatinine level at the second visit showed a tendency towards elevation especially when the patients decreasing muscle mass was considered, thus suggesting a microvascular disease process in the kidney. At his first visit, the level of cTnI was at the level of the 99th percentile for males (34 ng/L) whereas the second result was clearly elevated and suggested ongoing myocardial damage. At the second visit, he had no obvious symptoms and signs of myocardial infarction or heart failure and the elevated cTnI levels were interpreted to be the consequences of microvascular disease in the myocardium caused by his diabetes, but a poor prognostic sign. Five weeks after this visit, the patient suffered from a myocardial infarction complicated by an ischemic stroke and passed away.

Discussion

Approximately 6% of the middle-aged population in the United States have diabetes, and twice as many have prediabetes. Diabetes significantly increases the risk for atherosclerotic disease depending on an overrepresentation of CV risk factors, e.g. hypertension, obesity, dyslipidemia with elevated triglycerides and reduced HDL-cholesterol, and renal dysfunction. Hyperglycemia and insulin resistance are probably also direct culprits at the cellular level. Patients with diabetes are at considerable risk for vascular complications and have a high prevalence of often asymptomatic CV disease.

The association between diabetes type 2 and the risk of premature death in CV disease is common knowledge [13, 14]. It has also been well documented that levels of cardiac markers such as cTn are elevated in blood in patients with diabetes but also in those with diabetes and no clinical CV disease [15]. Whether such elevations only reflect advanced arteriosclerosis in the coronary arteries or are direct consequences of glycation of myocardial structures resulting in microvascular and myocardial cell injuries is uncertain [16, 17]. Interestingly, an association between elevated cTnT levels and the development of microvascular complications, i.e. in the kidney, in diabetes was also recently shown and enhanced the prediction of end-stage renal disease beyond established risk factors [18, 19]. Thus, in any cohort studies on the predictive value of new biomarkers, the presence of diabetes has to be adjusted for to know the true predictive value of such biomarkers.

The clinical usefulness and utility of cTn for the prediction of adverse outcomes in CV disease in diabetes type 2 and whether these assays may be used to modify treatment has remained uncertain. However, with the recent introduction of the high-sensitivity cTn assays, results are emerging that indicate that this might be the case. Thus, in the Women's Health Study [20] and in the larger ADVANCE study [21], cTnT independently predicted major CV events and was clearly more powerful in this regard than conventional predictors. In a recent multicenter study in Europe, cTnT was one of six biomarkers that added to the prediction of CV disease over the Framingham score [22]. One limitation, though, of these studies was the fact that levels of cTnT were found undetectable in more than 35% of the participants, a fact which might underestimate the predictive power of cTnT, especially in women. A second limitation might be the fact that the ADVANCE study included a somewhat selected group of patients with diabetes type 2. Thus, before we can conclude the clinical utility of high-sensitivity cTn, these studies should be confirmed by community-based studies of unselected participants and also by assays of higher sensitivities that are able to measure cTn in blood of the vast majority (i.e. >95%) of such populations.

Case 3: cTn Levels in an Elderly Subject

This case is an elderly male without previous manifestations of CV disease. His body mass index is 27 kg/m^2 and he is a non-smoker. At age 70, he underwent a medical check-up. The standard 12-lead ECG and routine blood tests were normal apart from LDL-cholesterol 116 mg/dL. Levels of CRP and NT-proBNP were 3.9 mg/L and 143 ng/L, respectively. The cTnI level (Abbott Architect) was 29 ng/L which is above the assays 99th percentile (26 ng/L) but below the sex-specific 99th percentile of 34 ng/L. The patient was well-being and physically active.

A routine ECG control 5 years later revealed a left bundle branch block which was not known since before. The patient denied any cardiac complaints at that time. However, subsequent blood tests showed an increase in the NT-proBNP level to 1341 ng/L and in the cTnI level to 45 ng/L. For this reason, he was referred for an echocardiography which showed a slightly depressed LV ejection fraction of 0.50. No medical action was undertaken.

Seven months later, the patient was admitted to the hospital because of congestive heart failure associated with increasing fatigue and exertional shortness of breath. Anginal complaints were denied. The echocardiography showed mildly dilated chambers and the LV ejection fraction had further decreased to 0.40. The coronary angiography showed only mild stenoses. The patient started a medication with diuretics including spironolactone, betablockers, angiotensin-II receptor blockers, antiplatelets and a statin.

Since then, the patient's condition has improved. The last echocardiography 5 years after the hospitalization showed a partial reconstitution of the LVEF to 0.50. NT-proBNP levels have decreased to 300–500 ng/L upon further outpatient-controls. The patient has at present no cardiac symptoms and participates regularly in a physical training program.

Discussion

Ageing is associated with extensive alterations in CV anatomy and biochemistry [23]. With higher age, there is an increasing degree of tissue fibrosis due to increased collagen deposition and cross-linking, resulting in myocardial and vascular stiffness. Arterial stiffening results in a progressive rise in systolic blood pressure which increases impedance to LV ejection and consequently myocardial work and oxygen demand. Coronary oxygen supply may at the same time be reduced due to epicardial coronary artery disease depending on the life-time accumulated impact of CV risk factors. Myocardial fibrosis moreover, contributes to elevated LV enddiastolic filling pressures. The added effect of these alterations is a progressive rise in the prevalence of diastolic and systolic heart failure with increasing age. In fact, more than 50 % of hospitalizations for congestive heart failure occur in patients above age 75. Because of higher enddiastolic filling pressures, the proportion of LV filling during atrial contraction also increases which results in a subsequent dilatation of the left atrium. This predisposes to the development of atrial fibrillation, the most common arrhythmia in the geriatric population.

Many of these conditions may contribute to cTn release from the myocardium. This has been closer studied in three large studies investigating elderly community-dwelling subjects. In the Cardiovascular Health Study, higher cTnT levels were associated with lower LVEF, increased LV mass and coronary artery disease [5]. These findings were confirmed in the PREDICTOR study [24]. Similar as for NT-proBNP, the diagnostic accuracy of cTnT regarding the detection of elevated LV mass and impaired LV systolic function however, was only limited in that study emphasizing the need to specify subgroups in whom cTn measurement would be particularly useful. Data from the PIVUS study demonstrated that also levels of cTnI (Abbott Architect) were associated with increased LV mass, lower LVEF and indicators of coronary artery disease, even after multivariable adjustment [6].

Given these data, it is not surprising that outcome studies consistently demonstrated a strong prognostic value of cTn levels over and above standard CV risk assessment in the elderly, in particular with respect to mortality and heart failure hospitalizations (Table 10.1) [5–7]. While the association with ischemic cardiac events usually is less impressive in these studies, data from the ULSAM Study revealed an independent association between cTnT levels and the risk for future stroke [7]. This may reflect the association between cTn and atherosclerosis [5, 6] but also atrial fibrillation, a major cause of ischemic stroke in the elderly. In this setting, cTn levels correlate with the presence of spontaneous echocardiographic contrast and thrombi in the atria [25] which might represent a mechanistic link.

With the projected doubling in the size of the geriatric population between 2010 and 2030, elderly patients with CV disease will consume a considerable proportion of clinicians' time and health care resources. Clinicians may thus,

Table 10.1 Associations of cardiac troponin levels with adverse outcome in populations at risk for cardiovascular disease

Reference	n	Analyte	All-cause mortality	CV mortality	Coronary events	Incident HF	MACE
Diabetics							
Hillis (2014) [21]	3862	cTnT (Roche)	1.5 (1.4-1.7)	–	–	–	1.5 (1.4-1.7)
Looker (2015) [22]	2310	cTnT (Roche)	–	–	–	–	1.6 (1.4-1.8)
Elderly subjects							
deFilippi (2010) [5]	4221	cTnT (Roche)	–	1.5 (1.4-1.7)	–	1.4 (1.3-1.6)	–
Eggers (2013) [6]	1004	cTnI (Abbott)	1.4 (1.2-1.8)	1.7 (1.2-2.3)	–	–	–
Eggers (2013) [6]	940	cTnT (Roche)	1.3 (1.1-1.5)	1.5 (1.3-1.9)	1.4 (1.2-1.6)	–	1.4 (1.2-1.6)
Dallmeier (2015) [7]	1422	cTnT (Roche)	2.2 (1.6-2.9)	–	–	–	–
Dallmeier (2015) [7]	1422	cTnI (Abbott)	1.9 (1.6-2.4)	–	–	–	–

Data are given as hazard ratios with 95 % confidence intervals from Cox regressions using continuous cTn levels as dependent variable with adjustment for age, sex and cardiovascular risk factors.
CV cardiovascular, *HF* heart failure, *MACE* major cardiovascular events

appreciate cTn measurements as a tool to identify elderly subjects in particular need for preventive interventions, e.g. improving blood pressure and glycemic control. On the other hand, low cTn levels might support clinicians in their decisions about not starting or stopping medications with potential harmful side-effects.

This raises the question from which level a cTn result should raise attention. Notably, age is one of the strongest contributors to higher cTn levels with a breakpoint around age 60–65 from which cTn levels progressively start to rise [26]. This makes it difficult to define any prognostically useful cTn threshold. The commonly used cut-off in acute settings, i.e. the 99th percentile derived from healthy populations, does not fully cover the wealth of clinical and prognostic information provided by cTn levels as the prevalence of cardiac abnormalities and CV risk starts to rise at levels well below. This is illustrated by data from the CHS study, demonstrating an almost constant increase of risk starting at cTnT levels below the 99th percentile of 14 ng/L (Fig. 10.1) [6]. Optimal prognostic cut-offs usually have been described as 6–8 ng/L for cTnT [12] and tend to be even lower for cTnI [11, 27]. However, any single cut-off is problematic since it renders a continuous variable into a binary one. This is even more important in the elderly where a significant overlap of cTn levels in subjects with and without the condition of interest is common. A suitable approach to circumvene this dilemma might be the use of dual thresholds: one low cut-off to maximize sensitivity and one high cut-off to maximize specificity, leaving a subset of subjects with indeterminate test results warranting further evaluation.

Is Measurement of cTn Levels Justified? In Whom, Why and When?

Measurement of cTn levels for the assessment of at-risk cohorts requires the consideration of some important issues. Most importantly, there is a need to define such cohorts. Widespread cTn screening in the general population can at present not be recommended. However, screening may be justified in subjects with pathologic ECG findings or known CV or coronary artery disease. The higher prevalence of cardiac abnormalities in these subjects will improve the predictive accuracy of cTn, i.e. lower the number of subjects needed to be referred for further evaluation in case of an elevated level. This would improve the cost-benefit of such an approach to an acceptable level, similar as shown for B-type natriuretic peptide [28].

Second, the interpretation of cTn results is not straightforward and several caveats need to be considered. An understanding of the performance characteristics of the used cTn assay is essential as available methods differ in many aspects, see Chap. 2 in this book. This relates to the problems regarding the definition of appropriate decision thresholds. Age and sex strongly influence cTn levels why the use of sex-adjusted 99th percentiles has been recommended in acute settings.

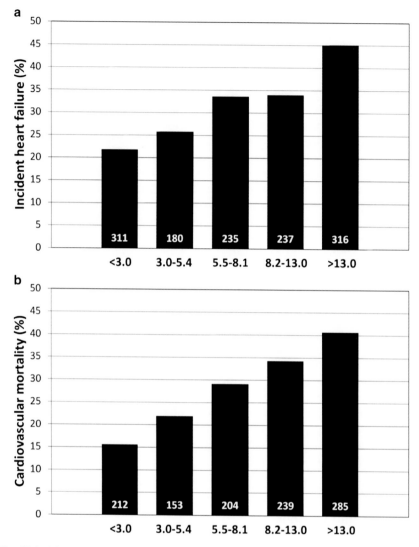

Fig. 10.1 Adverse events in relation to cTnT levels (ng/L) in participants from the CHS study (n = 3707; median follow-up 11.8 years). (**a**) Incident heart failure; (**b**) cardiovascular death (Data adapted from Ref. [5]). Study participants had been divided into cohorts with undetectable cTnT levels (<3.0 ng/L; n = 1427) and into quartiles in case of detectable cTnT levels. The numbers of events within each stratum are given at the bottom of the columns

It is however, not clear whether sex-adjustment will be needed at lower thresholds, i.e. prognostically useful cut-offs in community populations, as the relative contribution of sex likely will become less important at these low levels. However, the flipside of any lowered cut-off will inevitably be a larger number of false-positive test results and an increased relative importance of the biological variability of cTn.

Third, measurement of cTn levels will only be meaningful if this significantly improves clinical information beyond that obtained from standard risk assessment. As outlined above, data from several studies convincingly demonstrate that cTn levels carry prognostic information in at-risk cohorts that is incremental to traditional CV risk factors and even C-reactive protein or the B-type natriuretic peptides [5–8, 11, 15, 20, 21]. Changes in serially measured cTn levels augment the prognostic information obtained from single results. Data from the Cardiovascular Health Study suggest that increases in cTnT levels over a 3-year period predict CV death and heart failure, independent of traditional risk predictors and the baseline cTnT value [5]. The PIVUS study provided similar information when cTnI levels (Abbott Architect) were measured at age 70 and 75 [6]. In both studies, increases in cTn levels were associated with a greater burden of CV risk indicators, e.g. higher age, male sex, hypertension, coronary artery disease, poorer kidney function and impaired LVEF. Even new onset of atrial fibrillation appears to contribute to increasing levels. However, optimized time intervals for repeat testing of cTn still need to be defined.

Finally, measurement of cTn levels is only warranted if a positive finding has a clinical consequence, e.g. referral for echocardiography, lifestyle interventions or pharmacological treatment. This in turn requires that the beneficial effects of such measures would go hand in hand with a reduction of cTn levels. This still is the holy grail of any biomarker research. However up until now, we are lacking randomized trials to determine whether cTn-based interventions will improve CV outcomes. Observational data from available studies have so far provided mixed results. In PIVUS, no effect of the initiation of antihypertensive or lipid-lowering treatment, or coronary revascularization was seen on changes in cTnI levels between age 70 and 75 [6]. Contrasting to this, data from WOSCOPS showed a reduction in cTnI levels (Abbott Architect) 1 year after randomization of subjects with a previous myocardial infarction to treatment with Pravastatin [29]. Even lifestyle interventions in terms of regular physical exercise might lower cTn levels as shown by data from the Cardiovascular Health study [5].

Summary and Outlook

cTn levels measured with high-sensitivity assays provide important clinical information in at-risk cohorts, both regarding the detection of preclinical or mild CV disease and the prediction of subsequent complications. This information is incremental to that obtained from standard clinical assessment including measurement of other biomarkers. While the utility of cTn measurement in the general population is debated, it could serve as a tool to optimize management in at-risk cohorts. It is likely that cTn will have a 'gatekeeper' function in this setting, in particular to facilitate the identification of subjects in whom additional testing is needed to detect the particular source of cardiac injury and to design appropriate clinical responses. However, appropriate diagnostic and therapeutic responses to cTn results still remain to be defined by studies that include assessments of both clinical outcomes and costs.

References

1. Perk J, De Backer G, Gohlke H, et al. European Guidelines on cardiovascular disease prevention in clinical practice (version 2012). The Fifth Joint Task Force of the European Society of Cardiology and Other Societies on Cardiovascular Disease Prevention in Clinical Practice (constituted by representatives of nine societies and by invited experts). Eur Heart J. 2012;33:1635–701. Erratum in: Eur Heart J. 33:2126.
2. Goff DC Jr., Lloyd-Jones DM, Bennett G, et al. 2013 ACC/AHA guideline on the assessment of cardiovascular risk: a report of the American College of Cardiology/American Heart Association Task Force on Practice Guidelines. J Am Coll Cardiol. 2013;63:2935–59. Erratum in: J Am Coll Cardiol. 63:3026.
3. Wallace TW, Abdullah SM, Drazner MH, et al. Prevalence and determinants of troponin T elevation in the general population. Circulation. 2006;113:1958–65.
4. Apple FS, Ler R, Murakami MA. Determination of 19 cardiac troponin I and T assay 99th percentile values from a common presumably healthy population. Clin Chem. 2012;58:1574–81.
5. deFilippi CR, de Lemos JA, Christenson RH, et al. Association of serial measures of cardiac troponin T using a sensitive assay with incident heart failure and cardiovascular mortality in older adults. JAMA. 2010;304:2494–502.
6. Eggers KM, Venge P, Lindahl B, et al. Cardiac troponin I levels measured with a high-sensitive assay increase over time and are strong predictors of mortality in an elderly population. J Am Coll Cardiol. 2013;61:1906–13.
7. Eggers KM, Al-Shakarchi J, Berglund L, et al. High-sensitive troponin T and its relations to cardiovascular risk factors, morbidity and mortality in elderly men. Am Heart J. 2013;166:541–8.
8. Dallmeier D, Denkinger M, Peter R, et al. Sex-specific associations of established and emerging cardiac biomarkers with all-cause mortality in older adults: the ActiFE study. Clin Chem. 2015;61:389–99.
9. Kociol RD, Pang PS, Gheorghiade M, et al. Troponin elevation in heart failure prevalence, mechanisms, and clinical implications. J Am Coll Cardiol. 2010;56:1071–8.
10. Laufer EM, Mingels AM, Winkens MH, et al. The extent of coronary atherosclerosis is associated with increasing circulating levels of high sensitive cardiac troponin T. Arterioscler Thromb Vasc Biol. 2010;30:1269–75.
11. Kavsak PA, Xu L, Yusuf S, et al. High-sensitivity cardiac troponin I measurement for risk stratification in a stable high-risk population. Clin Chem. 2011;57:1146–53.
12. McQueen MJ, Kavsak PA, Xu L, et al. Predicting myocardial infarction and other serious cardiac outcomes using high-sensitivity cardiac troponin T in a high-risk stable population. Clin Biochem. 2013;46:5–9.
13. Sarwar N, Gao P, Seshasai SR, et al. Diabetes mellitus, fasting blood glucose concentration, and risk of vascular disease: a collaborative meta-analysis of 102 prospective studies. Lancet. 2010;375:2215–22.
14. Seshasai SR, Kaptoge S, Thompson A, et al. Diabetes mellitus, fasting glucose, and risk of cause-specific death. N Engl J Med. 2011;364:829–41.
15. Selvin E, Lazo M, Chen Y, et al. Diabetes mellitus, prediabetes, and incidence of subclinical myocardial damage. Circulation. 2014;130:1374–82.
16. Rubin J, Matsushita K, Ballantyne CM, et al. Chronic hyperglycemia and subclinical myocardial injury. J Am Coll Cardiol. 2012;59:484–9.
17. Zheng J, Ye P, Luo L, et al. Association between blood glucose levels and high-sensitivity cardiac troponin T in an overt cardiovascular disease-free community-based study. Diabetes Res Clin Pract. 2012;97:139–45.
18. Desai AS, Toto R, Jarolim P, et al. Association between cardiac biomarkers and the development of ESRD in patients with type 2 diabetes mellitus, anemia, and CKD. Am J Kidney Dis. 2011;58:717–28.

19. Welsh P, Woodward M, Hillis GS, et al. Do cardiac biomarkers NT-proBNP and hsTnT predict microvascular events in patients with type 2 diabetes? Results from the ADVANCE trial. Diabetes Care. 2014;37:2202–10.
20. Everett BM, Cook NR, Magnone MC, et al. Sensitive cardiac troponin T assay and the risk of incident cardiovascular disease in women with and without diabetes mellitus: the Women's Health Study. Circulation. 2011;123:2811–8.
21. Hillis GS, Welsh P, Chalmers J, et al. The relative and combined ability of high-sensitivity cardiac troponin T and N-terminal pro-B-type natriuretic peptide to predict cardiovascular events and death in patients with type 2 diabetes. Diabetes Care. 2014;37:295–303.
22. Looker HC, Colombo M, Agakov F, et al. Protein biomarkers for the prediction of cardiovascular disease in type 2 diabetes. Diabetologia. 2015;58:1363–71.
23. Stolker JM, Rich MW. Aging and geriatric heart disease. In: Crawford MH, DiMarco JP, Paulus WJ, editors. Cardiology. 3rd ed. Philadelphia: Mosby Elsevier; 2010. p. 1775–90.
24. Masson S, Latini R, Mureddu GF, et al. High-sensitivity cardiac troponin T for detection of subtle abnormalities of cardiac phenotype in a general population of elderly individuals. J Intern Med. 2013;273:306–17.
25. Providência R, Paiva L, Faustino A, et al. Cardiac troponin I: Prothrombotic risk marker in non-valvular atrial fibrillation. Int J Cardiol. 2013;167:877–82.
26. Hammarsten O, Fu ML, Sigurjonsdottir R, et al. Troponin T percentiles from a random population sample, emergency room patients and patients with myocardial infarction. Clin Chem. 2012;58:628–37.
27. Zeller T, Tunstall-Pedoe H, Saarela O, et al. High population prevalence of cardiac troponin I measured by a high-sensitivity assay and cardiovascular risk estimation: the MORGAM Biomarker Project Scottish Cohort. Eur Heart J. 2014;35:271–81.
28. Nielsen OW, McDonagh TA, Robb SD, et al. Retrospective analysis of the cost-effectiveness of using plasma brain natriuretic peptide in screening for left ventricular systolic dysfunction in the general population. J Am Coll Cardiol. 2003;41:113–20.
29. Mills NL, Shah AS, Mcallister DA, et al. High-sensitivity cardiac troponin I predicts long-term cardiovascular outcome in the west of Scotland coronary prevention study. Eur Heart J. 2014;35(Abstract Supplement):205.

Chapter 11
Other Biomarkers in Acute Coronary Syndrome

Roxana Ghashghaei and Nicholas Marston

Abstract Biomarkers play an important role in the early detection and diagnosis of acute coronary syndrome (ACS). While troponin is essential to the diagnosis of acute myocardial infarction, other markers have demonstrated utility in the setting of acute chest pain and ACS. CK-MB and myoglobin are two traditional markers that are frequently used in combination with troponin. More recently, novel markers such as pro-ADP, copeptin, and pro-ANP have shown promise in chest pain and may add to the clinical picture. This chapter will discuss the strengths, weaknesses, and supporting data for each of these traditional and novel chest pain biomarkers.

Keywords Biomarkers in acute coronary syndrome • Acute coronary syndrome biomarkers • Troponin in coronary syndromes • Pro-ADP • Copeptin • Pro-ANP • CK-MB biomarker

Biomarkers play an important role in the early detection and diagnosis of acute coronary syndrome (ACS). While troponin is essential to the diagnosis of acute myocardial infarction, other markers have demonstrated utility in the setting of acute chest pain and ACS. CK-MB and myoglobin are two traditional markers that are frequently used in combination with troponin. More recently, novel markers such as pro-ADP, copeptin, and pro-ANP have shown promise in chest pain and may add to the clinical picture. This chapter will discuss the strengths, weaknesses, and supporting data for each of these traditional and novel chest pain biomarkers.

R. Ghashghaei, MD
Department of Internal Medicine, University of California San Diego Health System, San Diego, CA, USA
e-mail: rghashgh@ucsd.edu

N. Marston, MD (✉)
Department of Internal Medicine, UCSD Medical Center, San Diego, CA, USA
e-mail: nmarston@ucsd.edu

© Springer International Publishing Switzerland 2016
A.S. Maisel, A.S. Jaffe (eds.), *Cardiac Biomarkers*,
DOI 10.1007/978-3-319-42982-3_11

Traditional Markers

CK-MB

Creatinine kinase-myocardial band (CK-MB) is the cardiac specific isoform of creatinine kinase (CK) and is found in high concentrations in the myocardium. After an acute myocardial injury, CK-MB levels peak within 4–6 h. This delayed rise of CK-MB limits its early diagnostic utility for ACS [1]. However, after approximately 8 h the negative predictive value of CK-MB reaches 95 % [2], providing valuable information for clinicians attempting to rule out myocardial infarction with serial sampling.

CK-MB is especially useful when assessing a patient for possible re-infarction. Its shorter half-life leads to normal values within 24–48 h after an event [1]. Troponin, on the other hand, is often elevated up to 2 weeks following an acute myocardial infarction [3] and will not be as reliable. In these situations CK-MB is the biomarker of choice and can aid in diagnosis of re-infarction.

Consecutive CK-MB measurements have also been shown to correlate with infarct size. This could be clinically useful and may provide insight into the extent of myocardial damage. Conversely, one study found that CK-MB rises later in smaller infarcts, resulting in lower sensitivity and specificity within the first 8 h of symptom onset. This effect is less evident in other biomarkers such as myoglobin [2].

CK-MB can be found in many organs other than the heart, contributing to its lack of specificity. Minor quantities are found in skeletal muscles including the diaphragm, intestine, uterus, and prostate. Thus an injury to any of these organs or in patients undergoing invasive surgical procedures can cause CK-MB levels to rise, effectively reducing its specificity for myocardial injury. The combination of decreased specificity and delayed rise on presentation brings to question the utility of CK-MB as an initial diagnostic biomarker for chest pain [1].

Prognostic Value

In addition to its utility in diagnosing re-infarction, CK-MB appears to have prognostic value in ACS. In one study, plasma levels of CK-MB were measured in 8654 patients presenting with non-ST segment elevation ACS (NSTE-ACS). CK-MB positivity was found to be predictive of increased all-cause mortality in patients presenting with NSTE-ACS regardless of their troponin status. This study validated the prognostic role of the CK-MB biomarker in patients presenting with NSTE-ACS [4].

Myoglobin

Similar to CKMB, myoglobin has traditionally been used alongside troponin in the assessment of chest pain. High concentrations can be found in both cardiac and skeletal muscle. The distinct advantage of myoglobin is its ability to detect myocardial injury soon after chest pain onset, with plasma concentrations rising rapidly 1 h after the onset of myocardial necrosis. This is in contrast to cardiac troponin and CK-MB which often take more than 4 h to become detectable. This early rise of myoglobin provides high sensitivity and high negative predictive value early in the chest pain presentation [3].

The clinical usefulness of myoglobin decreases over time due to its accelerated clearance. Within 7 h blood levels often return to near normal and the negative predictive value is greatly reduced. Additionally, myoglobin has low specificity in patients with trauma (i.e. damage to skeletal muscles) or in patients with renal failure (i.e. reduced clearance of myoglobin). Therefore levels can be falsely elevated in these populations and the ability to assess ACS is significantly limited [4].

Prognostic Value

Myoglobin not only has a role in early diagnosis of myocardial infarction, but can also be used for prognostic value. Two large studies (Thrombolysis in Myocardial Ischemia/ Infarction (TIMI) study and Treat Angina with Aggrastat and Determine Cost of Therapy with an Invasive or Conservative Therapy-Thrombolysis In Myocardial Ischemia/Infarction (TACTICS-TIMI)) assessed myoglobin's ability to risk stratify patients with non-ST elevation acute coronary syndrome (NSTE-ACS). Blood levels measured in over 2000 patients demonstrated an association between elevated myoglobin and increased 6 month mortality in both populations. Notably, no significant correlation was noted between elevated myoglobin levels and nonfatal myocardial infarction. After accounting for other factors including electrocardiographic changes, troponin, and CK-MB, the study concluded that elevated levels of myoglobin are independently associated with an increased risk of 6 month mortality [5].

Novel Markers

Copeptin

Copeptin, or C-terminal pro-vasopressin, is a pre-cursor of the neurohormone arginine vasopressin. Copeptin is co-released from the pituitary gland along with vasopressin during significant stressors such as an acute myocardial infarction [6]. Due to vasopressin's short half life in plasma, the more stable copeptin is an ideal

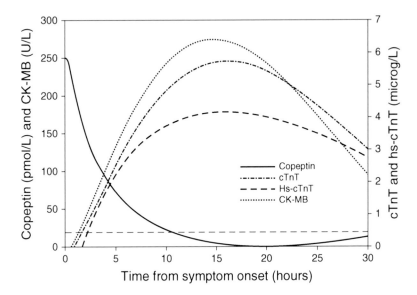

Fig. 11.1 Temporal release pattern of copeptin versus CK-MB, cTnT, and hs-cTnT. The dashed horizontal line represents the upper reference limit (99th percentile) for copeptin. *CK-MB* creatine kinase isoenzyme, *cTnT* cardiac troponin T, *hs-cTnT* high-sensitivity cardiac troponin T (From Ref. [8], with permission)

surrogate marker [7]. Similar to myoglobin, copeptin rises rapidly upon release and peaks within hours [6]. This can be useful in early chest pain presentations when the troponin is still negative. On the other hand, the similarly rapid fall of copeptin can make the test less useful in later presentations (Fig. 11.1 [8]).

This early rise and fall of copeptin led to interest in its diagnostic utility for AMI. It was hypothesized that normal levels of copeptin provided strong evidence against AMI. The CHOPIN trial (Copeptin Helps in the Early Detection of Patients with Acute Myocardial Infarction) [9] confirmed this hypothesis by enrolling over 2,000 patients with chest pain and found that if the initial troponin and copeptin were both negative then acute myocardial infarction could be ruled out with >99 % negative predictive value. The first randomized control trial soon followed and confirmed that patients with a negative baseline troponin and copeptin could be safely discharged from the ED with low risk for 30 day events [10].

Prognostic Value

While the diagnostic utility of copeptin is gaining strength, the prognostic value is a bit more established. The LAMP study was the first large study to address the utility of copeptin in ACS [11]. It showed that an elevated copeptin correlated with worse outcomes including death and heart failure at 60 days. Further studies have gone on to show that the prognostic value holds true as early as 30 days and beyond

1 year (Fig. 11.2a [12]). Its predictive ability extends to patients with a range of disease severity including ST-elevation myocardial infarction (STEMI), non-STEMI, and non-ACS etiologies of chest pain [13].

PRO-ADM and PRO-ANP

Midregional proadrenomedullin (pro-ADM) and midregional proatrial natriuretic peptide (pro-ANP) are two peptides released in response to hemodynamic stress and are emerging as novel biomarkers for risk stratification of patients with acute coronary syndrome (ACS). MR-proADM is a segment of the prohormone adreno-medullin, which is secreted from the adrenal medulla, vascular endothelial cells, and the myocardium in response to physical stretch in the context of volume and pressure overload. It acts as a strong vasodilator which also impacts cardiac contrac-tility, diuresis, and natriuresis. Meanwhile, pro-ANP is a vasodilator and a natri-uretic that is produced in the myocardium as a result of elevated intraatrial pressure [14]. Pro-ADM and pro-ANP have both been studied as biomarkers that offer the potential for more refined risk assessment of ACS and have been prognostically associated with adverse cardiovascular outcomes.

Prognostic Value

In a prospective observational multi center cohort study, 1386 patients with chest pain had plasma levels of pro-ADM and pro-ANP measured. Patients were followed for adverse outcomes including death, myocardial infarction, stroke and the need for revascularization. Those patients who experienced an adverse outcome had sig-nificantly higher pro-ANP and pro-ADM levels. These biomarker elevations were typically present on admission and increased rapidly during the event [15]. In con-trast, pro-ADM and pro-ANP were stable in patients with non-ACS chest pain.

The MERLIN TIMI (Metabolic Efficiency With Ranolazine for Less Ischemia in Non ST-Elevation Acute Coronary Syndromes–Thrombolysis In Myocardial Infarction 36) trial also supported the prognostic role of pro-ADM and pro-ANP. It demonstrated that each marker was independently associated with increased risk of cardiovascular death and heart failure (Fig. 11.2b, c [12]). This predictive value held true for STEMI patients where one study revealed pro-ADM levels at initial presen-tation were strongly predictive of short and long term mortality [16], and another showed pro-ANP's ability to independently predict all-cause mortality and major adverse cardiovascular events in STEMI patients undergoing percutaneous inter-vention [17].

In addition to prognostication, Pro-ADM and pro-ANP may be useful in guiding therapy. As part of the PEACE (Prevention of Events with Angiotensin Converting Enzyme) trial, plasma levels of pro-ADM and pro-ANP were measured in 3717 patients with stable coronary artery disease. Patients were randomly assigned to

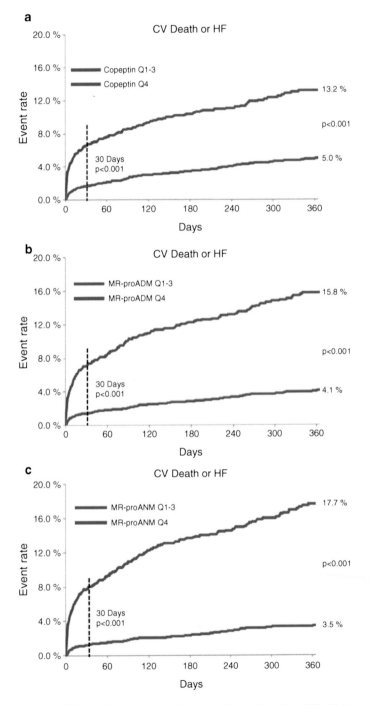

Fig. 11.2 Unadjusted Kaplan-Meier estimated 1-year incidence of death or HF with (**a**) copeptin, (**b**) MR-proADM, and (**c**) MR-proANP. *Copeptin* C-terminal provasopressin, *CV* cardiovascular, *HF* heart failure, *MR-proADM* midregional proadrenomedullin, *MR-proANP* midregional proatrial natriuretic peptide, *Q* quartile (From Ref. [12], with permission.)

receive either trandolapril or placebo. Not only were elevated levels independently associated with the risk of cardiovascular death and heart failure, but the results implied that elevated levels of pro-ADM and pro-ANP may also be used to select patients who might benefit from treatment with angiotensin converting enzyme inhibitors [14].

Conclusion

Cardiac biomarkers can be a useful tool in the evaluation of chest pain when used appropriately. Traditional markers such as CKMB and myoglobin have unique strengths distinct from troponin, providing additional clinical value. Specifically, CKMB is useful in cases of re-infarction when troponin remains elevated. Myoglobin on the other hand peaks earlier than troponin, making it useful in early presenters. Novel markers such as copeptin, pro-ADM, and pro-ANP also have distinct characteristics distinguishing them from troponin. They appear to aid in diagnosis, prognosis, and may even guide therapeutic interventions. More research is needed on these novel biomarkers to fully understand their clinical utility.

Case 1: Using Myoglobin to Detect Early Myocardial Ischemia

A 75-year old male presents to the emergency department with acute chest pain. The pain is substernal, 7 out of 10 in severity, and radiates to his left arm. It came on suddenly one hour ago while walking and has persisted to presentation. He denies diaphoresis, shortness of breath, nausea/vomiting and abdominal pain. He has a history of hypertension, diabetes mellitus, and hyperlipidemia with no known coronary artery disease. Social history is significant for a 30 pack years of smoking but no alcohol and illicit drug use. On admission, the patient's vital signs are notable for systolic blood pressures in the 130 s, HRs 60-65s and otherwise normal respiratory rate, and oxygen saturation. On physical exam he has clear lungs and normal S1 and S2 with no murmurs. Jugular venous distension is approximated 8 cm and there is no pedal edema. EKG is obtained and notable for non-specific t-wave flattening in lateral leads V5 and V6. In the ED he is given sublingual nitroglycerin which provides temporary relief. The first set of cardiac troponin I and CK-MB are within normal limits but myoglobin is elevated to 14 ng/ml. Given his risk factors and clinical presentation, he is admitted for rule out of acute coronary syndrome. Once admitted, repeat troponins 6 and 12 h later uptrended from 0.059 to 0.169 ng/ml, respectively. Concurrent CK-MB levels were mildly elevated at 10 and 13 ng/ml, and myoglobin levels rose to 189 and 299, respectively. Given the typical chest pain, EKG findings, and uptrending cardiac biomarkers, the patient was diagnosed with a Non-ST segment Elevation Myocardial Infarction (NSTEMI) and he was started on a heparin drip.

Case 2: Using CKMB to Assess Possible Re-Infarction

The same 75-year old man is taken for cardiac catheterization the following morning. A drug-eluding stent is placed in the left circumflex artery and the patient is started on clopidogrel. That night after dinner he develops some burning chest discomfort while lying flat in bed. His cardiac exam is unremarkable and EKG unchanged from admission. Cardiac enzymes were repeated and show persistently elevated troponins at 0.281 and normal CKMB. The patient reports a history of GERD and ranitidine was given with significant relief. The troponins were trended overnight and gradually downtrended. His CKMB remained negative. The following day he was discharged home with aspirin, clopidogrel, statin, lisinopril, and metoprolol.

References

1. Moe KT, Wong P. Current trends in diagnostic biomarkers of acute coronary syndrome. Ann Acad Med Singapore. 2010;39:210–5.
2. Winter R, Koster R, Sturk A, Sanders G. Value of myoglobin, troponin T, and CK-MBmass in ruling out an acute myocardial infarction in the emergency room. Circulation. 1995;92:3401–7.
3. Morrow D, Cannon C, Jesse R, Newby K, Ravkilde J, Storrow A, Wu A, Christenson R. National Academy of Clinical Biochemistry Laboratory Medicine Practice Guidelines: clinical characteristics and utilization of biochemical markers in acute coronary syndromes. Circulation. 2007;115:e356–75.
4. Kalayeh N, Yarkoni A, Kahn Y, Gonzalez F, Loli A, Halligan R, Cardello F, Gerkin R, Desser K. Creatine kinase-MB enzyme elevation is a powerful independent predictor of all cause mortality in non-ST segment elevation acute coronary syndrome. Circulation. 2007;116:II_364.
5. Lemos J, Morrow D, Gibson M, Murphy S, Sabatine M, Rifai N, McCabe C, Antman E, Cannon C, Braunwald E. J Am Coll Cardiol. 2002;40(2):238–44.
6. Elshafei A, Abdalla G, El-Motaal OA, Salman T. Copeptin: a neuroendocrine biomarker in acute myocardial infarction. Ann Rev Res Biol. 2013;3(4):1040–54.
7. Morgenthaler NG, Struck J, Alonso C, Bergmann A. Assay for the measurement of copeptin, a stable peptide derived from the precursor of vasopressin. Clin Chem. 2006;52:112–9.
8. Gu YL, Voors AA, Zijlstra F, Hillege HL, Struck J, Masson S, et al. Comparison of the temporal release pattern of copeptin with conventional biomarkers in acute myocardial infarction. Clin Res Cardiol. 2011;100:1069–76.
9. Maisel A, Mueller C, Neath S, et al. Copeptin helps in the early detection of patients with acute myocardial infarction: primary results from the CHOPIN trial. J Am Coll Cardiol. 2013;62:150–60.
10. Möckel M, Searle J, Hamm C, et al. Early discharge using single cardiac troponin and copeptin testing in patients with suspected acute coronary syndrome (ACS): a randomized, controlled clinical process study. Eur Heart J. 2014;36:369–76.
11. Khan SQ, Dhillon OS, O'Brien RJ, et al. C-terminal provasopressin (copeptin) as a novel and prognostic marker in acute myocardial infarction: Leicester Acute Myocardial Infarction Peptide (LAMP) study. Circulation. 2007;115:2103–10.
12. O'Malley R, Bonaca M, Scircia B, Murphy S, Jarolim P, Sabatine M, Braunwald E, Morrow D. Prognostic performance of multiple biomarkers in patients with non-ST segment elevation acute coronary syndrome. J Am Coll Cardiol. 2014;63:1644–53.

13. Marston N, Maisel A. The prognostic value of copeptin in patients with acute chest pain. Expert Rev Cardiovasc Ther. 2014;12(10):1237–42.
14. Tzikas S, Keller T, Ojeda FM, Zeller T, Wild PS, Lubos E, Kunde J, Baldus S, Bickel C, Lackner KJ, Munzel TF, Blankenberg S. MR-proANP and MR-proADM for risk stratification of patients with acute chest pain. Heart. 2013;99(6):388–95.
15. Omland T, Aakvaag A, Bonarjee V, et al. Plasma brain natriuretic peptide as an indicator of left ventricular systolic function and long- term survival after acute myocardial infarction: comparison with plasma atrial natriuretic peptide and N-terminal proatrial natriuretic peptide. Circulation. 1996;93:1963–9.
16. Silvain J, Beygui F, Bernard M, Cayla G, O'Conner S, Bellemain-Appaix A, Barthelemy O, Brugier D, Collet JP, Montalescot G. Pro-adrenomedullin (Mr-ProADM) can predict short and long term mortality in STEMI patients. Circulation. 2011;124:A15899.
17. Lindberg S, Jensen JS, Pedersen SH, Galatius S, Goetze JP, Mogelvang R. MR-ProANP improves prediction of mortality and cardiovascular events in patients with STEMI. Eur J Prev Cardiol. 2014;22:693–700.

Chapter 12
Newer Lipid Markers: Apolipoprotein B, LDL Particle Concentration, and Triglyceride-Rich Lipoproteins – When Are They Needed?

Renato Quispe, Seth S. Martin, and Steven R. Jones

Abstract Lowering low-density lipoprotein cholesterol (LDL-C) is a well-established strategy for cardiovascular risk reduction. Inherently, the focus is on LDL's cholesterol content rather than its particle concentration. However, a number of studies have demonstrated that measures of particles burden, such as apolipoprotein B (apoB) and LDL particle concentration (LDL-P) can be discordant with LDL-C. When discordant, they appear to more strongly predict cardiovascular events, compared with LDL-C. Triglyceride-rich lipoproteins (TRL) play a key role in generating small dense LDL particles and are now causally implicated in atherosclerosis. This book chapter reviews the most important information about TRL, apoB, and LDL-P, and discusses relevant scenarios for the clinician where discordance between lipoprotein cholesterol content and lipoprotein particle concentration measurements should be considered.

Keywords Lipid markers • Triglycerides • Apolipoprotein B • Low-density lipoprotein cholesterol • Low-density lipoprotein particle number • Remnant lipoprotein particles cholesterol • Discordance

A wealth of evidence from over two decades of clinical trials has shown that lowering low-density lipoprotein cholesterol (LDL-C), by means of medications such as statins, reduces the risk of atherosclerotic cardiovascular diseases (ASCVD) events

R. Quispe, MD • S.S. Martin, MD, MHS
The Johns Hopkins Ciccarone Center for the Prevention of Heart Disease,
Baltimore, MD, USA

S.R. Jones, MD (✉)
Division of Cardiology, Johns Hopkins Hospital, The Johns Hopkins Ciccarone Center for the Prevention of Heart Disease, Baltimore, MD, USA
e-mail: sjones64@jhmi.edu

© Springer International Publishing Switzerland 2016
A.S. Maisel, A.S. Jaffe (eds.), *Cardiac Biomarkers*,
DOI 10.1007/978-3-319-42982-3_12

[1]. However, the observation that substantial residual cardiovascular risk still exists even at seemingly "optimal" LDL-C levels has motivated greater exploration of other cardiovascular markers – beyond LDL-C – that may provide more comprehensive management of dyslipidemia-related cardiovascular risk.

This chapter presents updated information on lipid biomarkers beyond LDL-C, such as apolipoprotein B (apoB), LDL particle concentration (LDL-P) and triglyceride-rich lipoproteins, with an emphasis on clinical settings where relevant discordance may exist.

Lipid Metabolism and Fundamental Aspects of Dyslipidemia

Five major lipoprotein classes exist: chylomicrons, very low-density lipoprotein (VLDL), intermediate-density lipoprotein (IDL), LDL and high-density lipoprotein (HDL). Triglyceride-rich lipoproteins (TRL) include VLDL – secreted by the liver – and IDL in the fasting and nonfasting state, with the addition of chylomicrons – secreted by the gut – and their resulting remnant particles in the nonfasting state.

Triglyceride-rich VLDL particles are hydrolyzed by lipoprotein lipase (LPL) – activated by its cofactor apoC-II – to produce VLDL remnants and IDL, the smallest remnant. As a consequence of LPL action, IDLs have a higher concentration of cholesteryl esters (CE) but lower concentration of triglycerides, compared with VLDL. Although some IDL particles are taken up by remnant receptors on the liver, other IDL particles are then hydrolyzed by hepatic lipase (HL) to produce LDL. CE is transferred from the core of HDL and LDL to TG-rich lipoproteins (VLDL, IDL and chylomicrons) by action of cholesteryl ester transfer protein (CETP), which exchanges CE from HDL and LDL, for TG from TG-rich lipoproteins.

In the setting of hypertriglyceridemia, CETP action has important implications for HDL and LDL metabolism. First, triglyceride-enriched HDL particles are hydrolyzed by HL, producing a smaller HDL particle that is more easily removed from plasma. Second, triglyceride-enriched LDL particles undergo hydrolysis via lipoprotein lipase or hepatic lipase, reducing LDL particle size.

Dyslipidemia in individuals with obesity, metabolic syndrome or diabetes mellitus is driven by hypertriglyceridemia. Increased visceral (intra-abdominal) adiposity promotes insulin resistance, generating high levels of circulating free fatty acids that ultimately promote hepatic oversecretion of larger triglyceride-enriched VLDL particles. Patients with type 2 diabetes mellitus in particular can have a marked increase in small dense LDL particles, but do not necessarily have a higher LDL-C concentration when compared with non-diabetic individuals. Since, at a given LDL-C concentration, diabetic patients may have a greater number of LDL particles, discordance can be generated between LDL-C and estimates of atherogenic lipoprotein particles, such as LDL-P and apoB.

Triglyceride-Rich Lipoproteins (TRL)

TRL as Causal in Atherosclerosis and Cardiovascular Diseases

A singular, independent effect of hypertriglyceridemia on cardiovascular risk is difficult to assess given the coexistent modifications in HDL and LDL. However, recent Mendelian randomization data are consistent with TRL playing a causal role in ASCVD [2].

Potentially atherogenic features inherent in TRL include: TRL enhance expression of endothelial adhesion molecules and stimulate macrophage chemotaxis; and TRL enter the arterial wall when they are ingested by macrophages. Elevated fasting and especially non-fasting plasma triglyceride levels are significant predictors of CVD [3, 4]. For instance, the Copenhagen City Heart Study – a prospective Danish population based cohort – showed that increasing levels of nonfasting triglycerides were associated with an increased risk of ischemic stroke [5], and in a longer follow-up, that higher levels of nonfasting cholesterol and nonfasting triglycerides were similarly associated with a higher risk of myocardial infarction [6].

Relevance of TRL Remnants in Cardiovascular Risk

Previously, triglycerides per se were considered questionable as a causal factor for atherosclerosis and coronary heart disease (CHD). However, remnant cholesterol – the cholesterol content of TRL – has been shown to be a causal factor. Remnant particles have been associated with development of atherosclerosis by smooth cell proliferation, macrophage-derived foam cell formation, modulation of monocyte-endothelial interactions, inhibition of endothelial progenitor cell development, and endothelial dysfunction. Normally, these potentially atherogenic remnants are rapidly cleared from blood circulation postprandially. However, non-fasting triglyceride and remnant cholesterol levels are strongly correlated [4].

Two Mendelian randomization studies of TRL have been performed in the Copenhagen General Population Study. One showed that nonfasting remnant cholesterol (estimated as TG/5 in mg/dL) is a causal risk factor for ischemic heart disease (IHD), independent of reduced HDL-C [7]. The other revealed that elevated nonfasting remnant cholesterol is causally associated with low-grade inflammation and IHD whereas high LDL-C was only associated with IHD [8].

Among high TRL dyslipidemia phenotypes, type III dyslipidemia (familial dysbetalipoproteinemia) conveys about a five- to eightfold higher risk for CAD [9]. Type III dyslipidemia is caused by TRL remnant accumulation due to impaired removal or processing of TRL remnants, often together with excess TRL production. Although patients with this disorder have increased concentrations of TRL remnants in general, the excess of β-VLDL is considered diagnostic. Unfortunately, this disorder remains underdiagnosed, because the standard lipid profile cannot identify this lipoprotein excess. In order to distinguish type III dyslipidemia from other dyslipidemias with similar levels of hypertriglyceridemia, other methods such as ultracentrifugation [10], direct measurement of remnant VLDL [11] or diagnostic schemes concurrently using apoB measurement [12] are effective.

Hypertriglyceridemia and Small Dense LDL Particles

A significant proportion of hypertriglyceridemia-related atherogenicity is attributable to the production of small dense LDL particles. Small dense LDL particles have been associated with high atherogenicity [13]. Compared with their larger, normal-size counterparts, some evidence suggests that small dense LDL particles are more easily oxidized, have a higher affinity for the extracellular matrix, more readily migrate through arterial walls, and are highly retained in the subendothelial space. Their affinity for uptake by hepatic LDL receptor may be reduced, leading to lower rates of degradation and longer residence time in the circulation.

Apolipoprotein B

Concept and Pathophysiology

Apolipoprotein B is a structural surface protein of non-HDL lipoprotein particles. One molecule of apoB is embedded within the phospholipid monolayer of each lipoprotein particle secreted by the liver or the intestine, remaining with each particle for its lifetime. Two types of apoB coexist in plasma: [1] apoB-100, which is synthesized by the liver and incorporated into VLDL, and resulting IDL, LDL, and Lipoprotein(a) [Lp(a)]; and [2] apoB-48, which is synthesized in the gut and incorporated into chylomicrons, and present in resulting chylomicron remnant particles. Total circulating apoB levels are mostly represented by apoB-100, given that under normal circumstances apoB-48 containing particles contribute minimally to the total number of apoB containing particles in plasma, even postprandially. ApoB concentration in plasma is proportional to the concentration or "number" of apoB containing lipoprotein particles since there is a 1:1 stoichiometric relationship between apoB and lipoprotein particles; that is, one molecule of apoB per particle. Thus, apoB is proportional to the sum of all atherogenic plasma lipoprotein particles: LDL, IDL, VLDL and Lp(a) and chylomicron derived particles. Typically, LDL-P is the major determinant of apoB: about 90 % of total circulating apoB is associated with LDL particles (Fig. 12.1).

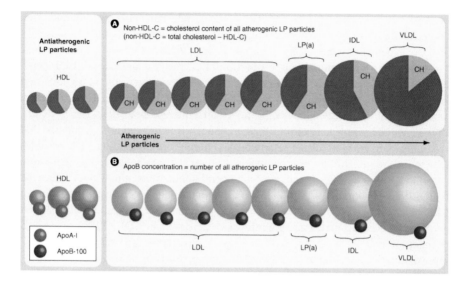

Fig. 12.1 Composition of lipoprotein particles varies widely across the range of lipoprotein classes resulting in varying relationship between lipoprotein cholesterol and particle concentration (From Ref. [34], with permission)

Table 12.1 Estimated percentiles of LDL-C, non-HDL-C, apoB and LDL-P

	Percentile						
	5th	10th	25th	50th	75th	90th	95th
LDL-C (mg/dL)	80	90	110	130	160	180	200
Non-HDL-C (mg/dL)	110	120	140	160	190	210	230
ApoB (mg/dL)	60	70	80	100	120	140	150
LDL-P (nmol/L)	800	900	1100	1400	1800	2000	2100

Estimates were derived from the Framingham Heart Study. Men and women are combined

Evidence of apoB and Cardiovascular Risk

The concept of discordance between lipid markers has been increasingly described over the last few years. Lipid discordance is defined as a disproportional level of one lipid measure compared with another, either disproportionally high or disproportionally low, deviating from bulk correlation. Since lipid measures are not all on the same scale, assignment of population percentiles allows direct comparison of one parameter with another on a standard scale. For instance, within a given population, a diabetic patient may have an LDL-C level at the 50th percentile but a disproportionally high apoB level at the 90th percentile. Table 12.1 shows population percentiles estimated from the Framingham Heart Study.

If the cholesterol content of LDL particles were constant, then LDL-C would closely reflect LDL particle concentration, and LDL-C and apoB would always be concordant. However, LDL particles are extremely heterogeneous with respect to cholesterol concentration contained in LDL particle core [14]. Additionally, the cholesterol content of LDL particles may vary more than twofold between individuals [15], especially in the setting of elevated triglycerides or insulin-resistant states. For example, when composition (proportion of cholesterol and size) of LDL particles is normal, LDL-C is a reasonably accurate approximation of LDL-P, and LDL-C is concordant with apoB levels. On the other hand, if LDL particles are small and cholesterol-depleted, LDL-C would underestimate LDL-P, and hence, LDL-C will be discordant with LDL-P and apoB. It is important to recognize that risk appears to be more closely correlated to number of circulating LDL particles than to their aggregate cholesterol content, LDL-C [13]. Although LDL-C generally correlates well with LDL-P and apoB in general populations, it may not capture the risk attributable to LDL in the individual patient when the cholesterol content of LDL particles is perturbed. In this context, a number of studies have demonstrated apoB to be a better predictor of cardiovascular risk than LDL-C [16–19]. ApoB concentration and LDL-P tend to track very closely, rarely discordant, with LDL-P representing the vast majority of apoB containing non-HDL lipoprotein particles.

Non-HDL-C as an Alternative to apoB

Non-HDL-C concentration, defined as total cholesterol minus HDL-C, reflects the aggregate cholesterol carried by apoB-containing particles. Non-HDL-C can also be discordant with LDL-C and may predict risk better than LDL-C in both normotriglyceridemic and hypertriglyceridemic individuals [20] because it includes cholesterol content in triglyceride-rich VLDL and chylomicron derived apoB48 containing particles, and also because it does not suffer from downfalls of the Friedewald equation. Recent evidence indicates that both non-HDL-C and apoB are more accurate indices of cardiovascular risk than LDL-C, but there are no conclusive results for comparing apoB and non-HDL-C as risk markers. Some studies suggest they are equivalent, but others suggest apoB is superior. Results from the Emerging Risk Factors Collaboration (ERFC) showed that hazard ratios for CHD for non-HDL-C (1.73 [95 % CI 1.52–1.96]) and apoB (1.71 [95 % CI 1.51–1.95]) were statistically equivalent [21]. A more recent meta-analysis based on all previously published epidemiologic studies that contained estimates of relative risks of non-HDL-C, LDL-C and apoB, suggested that apoB was the most potent cardiovascular risk marker though confidence intervals were overlapping (RRR: 1.43; 95 % CI 1.35–1.51), followed by non-HDL-C (RRR: 1.34; 95 % CI 1.24–1.44) and lastly, LDL-C (RRR: 1.25; 95 % CI 1.18–1.33) [22].

Several experts consider non-HDL-C preferable to apoB [23], as a replacement for LDL-C as a risk marker citing two main reasons: [1] non-HDL-C and apoB are similarly effective in predicting cardiovascular events; and [2] non-HDL-C is easily calculated from the existing standard lipid profile, whereas apoB measurement would result in additional complexity and expense. Despite these concerns, apoB is non-proprietary, commonly available in most clinical laboratories, relatively inexpensive and makes use of internationally standardized assays.

In clinical practice, discordance between apoB and non-HDL-C tends to exist in 3 particular settings: [1] apoB levels are disproportionately higher than corresponding non-HDL-C levels due to small dense LDL; in this case, apoB is generally considered a more reliable risk marker; [2] non-HDL-C levels are higher than corresponding apoB levels, which may occur in circumstances where there is an accumulation of cholesterol-enriched VLDL remnant particles, such as in type III dyslipidemia (familial dysbetalipoproteinemia); in this case, non-HDL-C may more accurately reveal risk [24]; or [3] non-HDL-C is disproportionately higher than apoB due to cholesterol-enriched LDL particles in the setting of very low triglycerides. In this case, a relatively lower concentration of atherogenic particles is present than would be expected on the basis of non-HDL-C, suggesting that apoB may better predict risk compared with non-HDL-C.

Therapeutic Implications

While much of the research cited above has focused on using baseline levels of lipids to predict risk, the reality is that current risk models around the world use total cholesterol and HDL-C as individual variables for risk prediction. At present, the question of discordance may be of greatest interest for on-treatment surveillance to guide further management. Compared with LDL-C, on-treatment apoB, as well as non-HDL-C levels, showed a more significant relation with residual risk of vascular disease, which endorses their use – instead of LDL-C – as potential targets of statin therapy [25]. However, statins produce a greater reduction in LDL-C and non-HDL-C than apoB levels, exaggerating discordance between LDL-C and apoB. Basing LDL-lowering therapy only on cholesterol based measures could result in a treatment gap and lost opportunity to achieve optimal reductions in atherogenic lipoprotein concentration and resulting risk reduction [26]. However, the most aggressive guideline recommended an apoB target of 80 mg/dL, which is at the 25th population percentile by Framingham data compared to LDL-C and non-HDL-C goals set at <5th percentile for high-risk patients. Limited by such a liberal apoB target, a change in intensity of lipid lowering therapy is infrequent once LDL-C and non-HDL-C targets are already met. It is arguable that apoB targets representing equivalent population percentiles to existing LDL-C and non-HDL-C goals may be more appropriate, although this approach is not widely accepted. An apoB level of 60 mg/dL represents approximately equivalent population percentile as the high risk LDL-C goal.

In summary, available evidence supports the conclusion that apoB is a generally one of the strongest indicators of risk and treatment adequacy. However, routine apoB measurement may carry additional costs – as opposed to LDL-C and non-HDL-C derived from the standard lipid panel. Moreover, given current guidelines set the apoB target at a high population percentile, apoB is unlikely to lead to more aggressive management in someone who has reached LDL-C and non-HDL-C targets unless these measures are discordant. There is still debate about how to best incorporate apoB into routine clinical practice. ApoB is expected to be of greatest clinical relevance when it differs in information content from other measures, as in discordant individuals or type III dyslipidemia, something that cannot be reliably known a priori. At the baseline patient evaluation, considering apoB levels would enable an accurate diagnosis of all apoB dyslipoproteinemias. Indeed, a diagnostic algorithm has been developed and is available for mobile devices (iOS application) [12].

LDL Particle Number

Cholesterol assays have been available for many years, for which LDL concentrations in clinical practice – for risk assessment and management – are routinely expressed in terms of its cholesterol concentration. LDL-C has been most commonly estimated via the Friedewald equation from the standard lipid panel. However, we showed that Friedewald-estimated LDL-C is a poor estimate at low LDL-C and high triglycerides levels [27]. A new estimation formula that takes into account the variability in the TG:VLDL-C relationship represents a better estimate compared with Friedewald method [28, 29]. Although direct measures of LDL-C exist, there is inconsistency between assays.

For many patients, levels of LDL-C and LDL-P – as well as apoB – are concordant. However, data from the Multi-Ethnic Study of Atherosclerosis showed that half of the study population had difference of ≥12 percentile units between LDL-C and LDL-P [30]. The presence of small dense LDL in individuals with elevated triglycerides or low HDL-C, diabetes mellitus or metabolic syndrome leads to high levels of LDL-P despite normal LDL-C levels [31]. LDL-lowering therapy causes a higher reduction in LDL-C and non-HDL-C levels compared with LDL-P – generating discordance as well – for which LDL-P may provide a better assessment of on-treatment residual risk (Fig. 12.2). Consequently, LDL-P has been found to be a better predictor of cardiovascular risk than LDL-C [30, 32].

In clinically relevant discordant scenarios, such as individuals with diabetes or CHD and optimal LDL-C and non-HDL-C, LDL-P might provide additional information with therapeutic implications. For instance, LDL lowering therapy could be addressed more aggressively if LDL-P is discordantly high; similarly, if LDL-P is discordantly decreased compared with LDL-C or non-HDL-C, LDL lowering therapy may be more conservative. However, it has not been established what an appropriate on-treatment LDL-P target would be. In clinical trials, post-hoc analysis showed that on-treatment levels of LDL-P better predicted residual risk than discordant LDL-C [33].

A significantly high proportion of total circulating apoB is associated with LDL particles, independently of triglycerides levels. It is expected that LDL-P and apoB are highly concordant, which frequently occurs. However, patients with type III

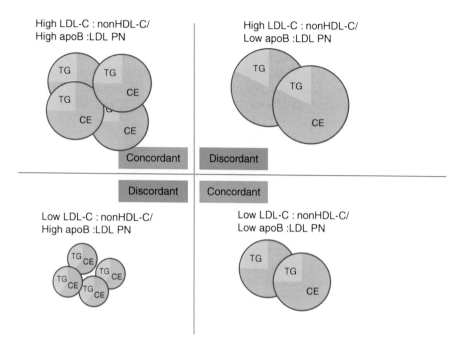

Fig. 12.2 Discordance between low density lipoprotein particle number and aggregate particle cholesterol concentration results from variation in relative particle cholesterol content and particle size (From Ref. [36], with permission)

hyperlipidemia have a large amount of apoB-48 in remnant lipoprotein, for which apoB-100 represents only about 50 % of total apoB particles [24].

Compared with LDL-P, apoB is analytically superior as it is non-proprietary, inexpensive, widely available and uses internationally standardized assays. On the other hand, LDL-P is available by several methodologies, most commonly Nuclear Magnetic Resonance (NMR) spectroscopy; nonetheless, it does not have as wide degree of availability as it is a proprietary assay. Unlike apoB, it without internationally standardization. Further, evidence is needed to assess the cost-effectiveness of LDL-P by comparison to the standard lipid profile or apoB.

Clinical Cases

Clinical Case 1

Consider a 55-year-old woman with a body mass index of 37 kg/m², diabetes mellitus and hypertension, who is admitted with an acute coronary syndrome. On admission, she had a lipid profile of Friedewald-estimated LDL-C of 90 mg/dL, non-HDL-C of 130 mg/dL, triglycerides of 200 mg/dL and HDL-C of 30 mg/

dL. This scenario illustrates some discordance concepts discussed in this chapter. In these individuals, cardiovascular risk may be underestimated if only LDL-C is considered, especially if LDL-C is determined by Friedewald estimation. Given her obesity and high triglyceride/low HDL-C profile, her LDL-C levels are probably represented mostly by cholesterol-depleted, small dense LDL particles. Therefore, discordance will probably exist between LDL-C and non-HDL-C and measurements of particle burden, such as LDL-P or apoB.

She was discharged on high-intensity statin therapy and at 1 month follow-up, her standard lipid profile showed a Friedewald-estimated LDL-C of 60 mg/dL, non-HDL-C of 90 mg/dL, triglycerides of 150 mg/dL and HDL-C of 35 mg/dL. This patient's Friedewald-estimated LDL-C level is now 60 mg/dL, but not optimized at closer to 50 mg/dL as shown recently in the IMPROVE-IT trial, where there was a particular benefit in diabetic patients. Measurement of apoB would detect the concentration of all atherogenic particles and, thus, may help better determine residual risk and monitor therapeutic adequacy. It is also important to note that statin therapy reduces LDL-C levels by a greater percentage than it does apoB levels, altering the association of LDL-C to LDL-P. In other words, this patient probably reached her LDL-C (<70) and non-HDL-C (<100) goals but may continue to have a high number of LDL particles.

Since there are not well-established clinical targets for LDL-P, it is difficult to know how their measurement would impact treatment decisions. The American Diabetes Association/American College of Cardiology (ADA/ACC) recommends, in addition to an LDL-C and non-HDL-C goals of 70 and 100 mg/dL, respectively, an apoB goal of 80 mg/dL for patients with prior cardiovascular events or diabetes with one risk factor. This apoB goal, set relatively high on a population percentile basis, is also recommended by other guidelines such as the European dyslipidemia guidelines. The PROVE-IT trial showed that patients with high-intensity statin therapy (atorvastatin 80 mg/day) reached a median apoB level of 67 mg/dL and 16 % reduction in the hazard ratio for death or a major cardiovascular event compared with moderate statin therapy (pravastatin 40 mg/day), which reached a median apoB level of 90 mg/dL [34]. Since LDL-C is not optimized – although non-HDL-C is lower than 100 mg/dL – it may be reasonable to increase the intensity of statin therapy and/or add ezetimibe on this basis alone. An apoB test would provide additional information for patients on statin therapy about their real cardiovascular risk attributed to atherogenic lipid particles, and could support further intensification of therapy if the clinician and patient select an apoB goal that is lower than recommended in guidelines (e.g., <70 mg/dL based on PROVE-IT).

Clinical Case 2

A 27 year-old obese man presents with palmar xanthomas and tubero-eruptive exanthomas of both elbows. His family history is significant for dyslipidemia and premature coronary disease. His father and two of his siblings had significant hypercholesterolemia. His clinical signs raised suspicion of type III dyslipidemia, which is defined by an increase in levels of chylomicron and VLDL remnants. The excess remnant particles characteristic of this disorder contribute substantial cholesterol and triglyceride leading to both hypercholesterolemia and hypertriglyceridemia.

His standard lipid profile shows levels of triglycerides of 5.0 mmol/L (442 mg/dL) and total cholesterol of 13 mmol/L (502 mg/dL). An apoB measurement was 0.70 g/L. His triglycerides/apoB ratio is <10, and total cholesterol/apoB is ≥6.2, which using diagnostic algorithm developed by Sniderman et al. [12] along with clinical findings and family history confirms diagnosis of familial dysbetalipoproteinemia. Further genotyping assays showed classic apoE2 homozygosity, which is typical of this disorder.

Classical dyslipidemias are characterized by changes in the number and/or composition of apoB lipoprotein particles, and can be identified using a diagnostic algorithm that integrates standard lipid measurements, such as total cholesterol and triglycerides, as well as apoB levels. It is important to note that type III dyslipidemia is the exception to the rule that total plasma apoB is the best measurement of atherogenic lipoproteins.

Summary

The routine use of apoB for initial diagnosis, especially in the setting of hypertriglyceridemia, would improve accuracy of diagnosis and subsequent selection of treatment. For therapeutic purposes, it may be reasonable to measure LDL-P, or preferably apoB, in high-risk patients at risk for discordance, such as those with hypertriglyceridemia or diabetes mellitus once non-HDL-C is at goal on initial treatment. However, LDL-P goals have not been established and apoB goals are probably too high to have any significant impact on clinical management. TRL, especially RLP-C, has emerged as an important cardiovascular risk marker that warrants further studies in order to be included in a more comprehensive assessment of cardiovascular risk. These new lipid biomarkers are continuously explored, but much still needs to be done in order to optimize patient care and better approach the use of these lipid measures in clinical practice.

References

1. Cholesterol Treatment Trialists C, Baigent C, Blackwell L, Emberson J, Holland LE, Reith C, Bhala N, Peto R, Barnes EH, Keech A, Simes J, Collins R. Efficacy and safety of more intensive lowering of LDL cholesterol: a meta-analysis of data from 170,000 participants in 26 randomised trials. Lancet. 2010;376(9753):1670–81.
2. Do R, Willer CJ, Schmidt EM, et al. Common variants associated with plasma triglycerides and risk for coronary artery disease. Nat Genet. 2013;45(11):1345–52.

3. Triglyceride Coronary Disease Genetics Consortium, Emerging Risk Factors Collaboration, Sarwar N, Sandhu MS, Ricketts SL, Butterworth AS, Di Angelantonio E, Boekholdt SM, Ouwehand W, Watkins H, Samani NJ, Saleheen D, Lawlor D, Reilly MP, Hingorani AD, Talmud PJ, Danesh J. Triglyceride-mediated pathways and coronary disease: collaborative analysis of 101 studies. Lancet. 2010;375(9726):1634–9.

4. Nordestgaard BG, Benn M, Schnohr P, Tybjaerg-Hansen A. Nonfasting triglycerides and risk of myocardial infarction, ischemic heart disease, and death in men and women. JAMA. 2007;298(3):299–308.

5. Freiberg JJ, Tybjaerg-Hansen A, Jensen JS, Nordestgaard BG. Nonfasting triglycerides and risk of ischemic stroke in the general population. JAMA. 2008;300(18):2142–52.

6. Langsted A, Freiberg JJ, Tybjaerg-Hansen A, Schnohr P, Jensen GB, Nordestgaard BG. Nonfasting cholesterol and triglycerides and association with risk of myocardial infarction and total mortality: the Copenhagen City Heart Study with 31 years of follow-up. J Intern Med. 2011;270(1):65–75.

7. Varbo A, Benn M, Tybjaerg-Hansen A, Jorgensen AB, Frikke-Schmidt R, Nordestgaard BG. Remnant cholesterol as a causal risk factor for ischemic heart disease. J Am Coll Cardiol. 2013;61(4):427–36.

8. Varbo A, Benn M, Tybjaerg-Hansen A, Nordestgaard BG. Elevated remnant cholesterol causes both low-grade inflammation and ischemic heart disease, whereas elevated low-density lipoprotein cholesterol causes ischemic heart disease without inflammation. Circulation. 2013;128(12):1298–309.

9. Hopkins PN, Nanjee MN, Wu LL, McGinty MG, Brinton EA, Hunt SC, Anderson JL. Altered composition of triglyceride-rich lipoproteins and coronary artery disease in a large case–control study. Atherosclerosis. 2009;207(2):559–66.

10. Kulkarni KR, Garber DW, Marcovina SM, Segrest JP. Quantification of cholesterol in all lipoprotein classes by the VAP-II method. J Lipid Res. 1994;35(1):159–68.

11. Wang T, Nakajima K, Leary ET, Warnick GR, Cohn JS, Hopkins PN, Wu LL, Cilla DD, Zhong J, Havel RJ. Ratio of remnant-like particle-cholesterol to serum total triglycerides is an effective alternative to ultracentrifugal and electrophoretic methods in the diagnosis of familial type III hyperlipoproteinemia. Clin Chem. 1999;45(11):1981–7.

12. Sniderman A, Couture P, de Graaf J. Diagnosis and treatment of apolipoprotein B dyslipoproteinemias. Nat Rev Endocrinol. 2010;6(6):335–46.

13. St-Pierre AC, Cantin B, Dagenais GR, Mauriege P, Bernard PM, Despres JP, Lamarche B. Low-density lipoprotein subfractions and the long-term risk of ischemic heart disease in men: 13-year follow-up data from the Quebec Cardiovascular Study. Arterioscler Thromb Vasc Biol. 2005;25(3):553–9.

14. Chapman MJ, Laplaud PM, Luc G, Forgez P, Bruckert E, Goulinet S, Lagrange D. Further resolution of the low density lipoprotein spectrum in normal human plasma: physicochemical characteristics of discrete subspecies separated by density gradient ultracentrifugation. J Lipid Res. 1988;29(4):442–58.

15. Otvos JD, Jeyarajah EJ, Cromwell WC. Measurement issues related to lipoprotein heterogeneity. Am J Cardiol. 2002;90(8A):22i–9.

16. Benn M, Nordestgaard BG, Jensen GB, Tybjaerg-Hansen A. Improving prediction of ischemic cardiovascular disease in the general population using apolipoprotein B: the Copenhagen City Heart Study. Arterioscler Thromb Vasc Biol. 2007;27(3):661–70.

17. McQueen MJ, Hawken S, Wang X, Ounpuu S, Sniderman A, Probstfield J, Steyn K, Sanderson JE, Hasani M, Volkova E, Kazmi K, Yusuf S, Investigators Is. Lipids, lipoproteins, and apolipoproteins as risk markers of myocardial infarction in 52 countries (the INTERHEART study): a case–control study. Lancet. 2008;372(9634):224–33.

18. Ingelsson E, Schaefer EJ, Contois JH, McNamara JR, Sullivan L, Keyes MJ, Pencina MJ, Schoonmaker C, Wilson PW, D'Agostino RB, Vasan RS. Clinical utility of different lipid measures for prediction of coronary heart disease in men and women. JAMA. 2007;298(7):776–85.

19. Mora S, Otvos JD, Rifai N, Rosenson RS, Buring JE, Ridker PM. Lipoprotein particle profiles by nuclear magnetic resonance compared with standard lipids and apolipoproteins in predicting incident cardiovascular disease in women. Circulation. 2009;119(7):931–9.

20. Pischon T, Girman CJ, Sacks FM, Rifai N, Stampfer MJ, Rimm EB. Non-high-density lipoprotein cholesterol and apolipoprotein B in the prediction of coronary heart disease in men. Circulation. 2005;112(22):3375–83.

21. Emerging Risk Factors C, Di Angelantonio E, Sarwar N, Perry P, Kaptoge S, Ray KK, Thompson A, Wood AM, Lewington S, Sattar N, Packard CJ, Collins R, Thompson SG, Danesh J. Major lipids, apolipoproteins, and risk of vascular disease. JAMA. 2009;302(18):1993–2000.

22. Sniderman AD, Williams K, Contois JH, Monroe HM, McQueen MJ, de Graaf J, Furberg CD. A meta-analysis of low-density lipoprotein cholesterol, non-high-density lipoprotein cholesterol, and apolipoprotein B as markers of cardiovascular risk. Circ Cardiovasc Qual Outcomes. 2011;4(3):337–45.

23. Ramjee V, Sperling LS, Jacobson TA. Non-high-density lipoprotein cholesterol versus apolipoprotein B in cardiovascular risk stratification: do the math. J Am Coll Cardiol. 2011;58(5):457–63.

24. Sniderman A, Tremblay A, Bergeron J, Gagne C, Couture P. Diagnosis of type III hyperlipoproteinemia from plasma total cholesterol, triglyceride, and apolipoprotein B. J Clin Lipidol. 2007;1(4):256–63.

25. Boekholdt SM, Arsenault BJ, Mora S, Pedersen TR, LaRosa JC, Nestel PJ, Simes RJ, Durrington P, Hitman GA, Welch KM, DeMicco DA, Zwinderman AH, Clearfield MB, Downs JR, Tonkin AM, Colhoun HM, Gotto Jr AM, Ridker PM, Kastelein JJ. Association of LDL cholesterol, non-HDL cholesterol, and apolipoprotein B levels with risk of cardiovascular events among patients treated with statins: a meta-analysis. JAMA. 2012;307(12):1302–9.

26. Sniderman AD. Differential response of cholesterol and particle measures of atherogenic lipoproteins to LDL-lowering therapy: implications for clinical practice. J Clin Lipidol. 2008;2(1):36–42.

27. Martin SS, Blaha MJ, Elshazly MB, Brinton EA, Toth PP, McEvoy JW, Joshi PH, Kulkarni KR, Mize PD, Kwiterovich PO, Defilippis AP, Blumenthal RS, Jones SR. Friedewald-estimated versus directly measured low-density lipoprotein cholesterol and treatment implications. J Am Coll Cardiol. 2013;62(8):732–9.

28. Martin SS, Blaha MJ, Elshazly MB, Toth PP, Kwiterovich PO, Blumenthal RS, Jones SR. Comparison of a novel method vs the Friedewald equation for estimating low-density lipoprotein cholesterol levels from the standard lipid profile. JAMA. 2013;310(19):2061–8.

29. Meeusen JW, Lueke AJ, Jaffe AS, Saenger AK. Validation of a proposed novel equation for estimating LDL cholesterol. Clin Chem. 2014;60(12):1519–23.

30. Otvos JD, Mora S, Shalaurova I, Greenland P, Mackey RH, Goff Jr DC. Clinical implications of discordance between low-density lipoprotein cholesterol and particle number. J Clin Lipidol. 2011;5(2):105–13.

31. Garvey WT, Kwon S, Zheng D, Shaughnessy S, Wallace P, Hutto A, Pugh K, Jenkins AJ, Klein RL, Liao Y. Effects of insulin resistance and type 2 diabetes on lipoprotein subclass particle size and concentration determined by nuclear magnetic resonance. Diabetes. 2003;52(2):453–62.

32. Cromwell WC, Otvos JD, Keyes MJ, Pencina MJ, Sullivan L, Vasan RS, Wilson PW, D'Agostino RB. LDL Particle Number and Risk of Future Cardiovascular Disease in the Framingham Offspring Study – Implications for LDL Management. J Clin Lipidol. 2007;1(6):583–92.

33. Rosenson RS, Otvos JD, Freedman DS. Relations of lipoprotein subclass levels and low-density lipoprotein size to progression of coronary artery disease in the Pravastatin Limitation of Atherosclerosis in the Coronary Arteries (PLAC-I) trial. Am J Cardiol. 2002;90(2):89–94.

34. Ray KK, Cannon CP, Cairns R, Morrow DA, Ridker PM, Braunwald E. Prognostic utility of apoB/AI, total cholesterol/HDL, non-HDL cholesterol, or hs-CRP as predictors of clinical risk

in patients receiving statin therapy after acute coronary syndromes: results from PROVE IT-TIMI 22. Arterioscler Thromb Vasc Biol. 2009;29(3):424–30.

35. Vaverkova H. LDL-C or apoB as the best target for reducing coronary heart disease: should apoB be implemented into clinical practice? Clin Lipidol. 2011;6(1):35–48.

36. Sniderman A, Lamarche B, Contois J, et al. Discordance analysis and the Gordian knot of LDL and non-HDL cholesterol versus apoB. Curr Opin Lipidol. 2014;25(6):461–7.

Part II
Heart Failure

Chapter 13
Natriuretic Peptides: Physiology for the Clinician

Siu-Hin Wan and Horng H. Chen

Abstract Natriuretic peptides (NPs) are a family of hormones that have significant cardiorenal properties. As an important component of blood pressure homeostasis in humans, NPs are potent vasodilatory hormones that mediate diuresis, natriuresis and cardiac remodeling (Levin et al., N Engl J Med 339(5):321–328, 1998). Neurohormonal signaling plays an essential role in cardiovascular disease. Whereas antagonism of the renin-angiotensin-aldosterone pathway, a mediator of pro-vascocontriction, leads to improved outcomes in heart failure, the potentiation of the NPs leads to vasodilation and improved cardiac remodeling. Therefore, NPs have been investigated both as a biomarker for cardiovascular disease as well as a potential treatment agent.

Keywords Natriuretic peptides • Cardiovascular properties of natriuretic peptides • Therapeutic modalities for heart failure • Atrial natriuretic peptide (ANP) • B-type natriuretic peptide (BNP) • C-type natriuretic peptide

Background

Natriuretic peptides (NPs) are a family of hormones that have significant cardiorenal properties. As an important component of blood pressure homeostasis in humans, NPs are potent vasodilatory hormones that mediate diuresis, natriuresis and cardiac remodeling [1]. Neurohormonal signaling plays an essential role in cardiovascular disease. Whereas antagonism of the renin-angiotensin-aldosterone pathway, a mediator of pro-vascocontriction, leads to improved outcomes in heart failure, the potentiation of the NPs leads to vasodilation and improved cardiac remodeling. Therefore, NPs have been investigated both as a biomarker for cardiovascular disease as well as a potential treatment agent.

S.-H. Wan, MD (✉) • H.H. Chen, MB, BCh (✉)
Department of Cardiovascular Diseases, Mayo Clinic and Foundation,
Rochester, MN, USA
e-mail: wan.siuhin@mayo.edu; chen.horng@mayo.edu

© Springer International Publishing Switzerland 2016
A.S. Maisel, A.S. Jaffe (eds.), *Cardiac Biomarkers*,
DOI 10.1007/978-3-319-42982-3_13

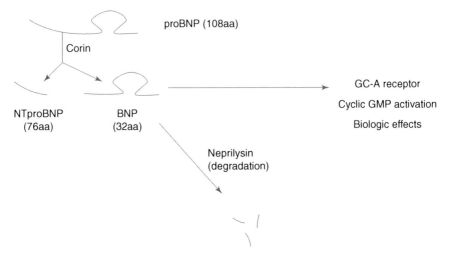

Fig. 13.1 Processing and molecular forms of BNP

The natriuretic peptide family consists of atrial natriuretic peptide (ANP), B-type natriuretic peptide (BNP), and C-type natriuretic peptide (CNP). ANP is found mainly in the cardiomyocytes of the atria and is released with increased intravascular volume and atrial stretch. Urodilatin, a peptide derived from the ANP precursor, is found in the kidneys; similar to ANP, it is also a mediator of natriuresis and diuresis.

BNP, also known as brain natriuretic peptide because of its original location of discovery, is perhaps the most well-known of the natriuretic peptide family, and has a prominent role in the diagnosis and management of heart failure as well as other cardiovascular diseases. It is released primarily in the cardiac ventricles and contains multiple molecular forms. The precursor 108 amino acid pro-BNP is processed to the 32 amino acid BNP as well as an NT-proBNP fragment. Pro-BNP, BNP and NT-proBNP are found in the circulating plasma, and their levels increased with heart failure (Fig. 13.1).

CNP is of endothelial cell origin and has low plasma concentrations, but has potent cardiovascular properties. While CNP does not have direct natriuretic properties, it does have important vasodilatory properties. The unique physiological actions of ANP, BNP, and CNP are mediated by different affinities of each peptide for the different NP receptors.

Three natriuretic peptide receptors have been identified. Natriuretic peptide receptor A (NPRA) and natriuretic peptide receptor B (NPRB) are both linked to the cyclic GMP (cGMP) signaling pathway [2, 3]. NPRA is activated by both ANP and BNP. Northern blot studies have demonstrated that NPRAs are predominantly found in the heart, lungs, kidneys, adrenals, and adipose tissue [2]. NPRB is activated by CNP, and NPRBs are predominantly found in the heart, lungs, kidneys, and the brain [2]. Natriuretic peptide receptor C (NPRC) is unique in that it does not possess a guanylyl cyclase domain. NPRC is activated by ANP, BNP, and CNP, and is important in the clearance of the NPs through peptide binding and internalization [3]. NPRCs are predominantly expressed in the lungs, kidneys, placenta, and the heart. While the principal function of NPRC is its role as a clearance receptor for the NPs, it has also been reported that NPRC may be responsible for the antiproliferative and beneficial remodeling effects of natriuretic peptides [4, 5].

Physiology of Natriuretic Peptides

The natriuretic peptides have important cardiovascular properties. The effects of ANP result in a reduction in blood pressure via multiple mechanisms [1]. ANP causes reduction of vascular tone in the peripheral vascular system. It also reduces preload via intravascular fluid shifts. ANP and BNP also result in suppression of sympathetic activity and antagonize the renin-angiotensin-aldosterone system, which contributes to reduction in blood pressure. CNP, compared to ANP and BNP, has more venodilatation effects. In addition to blood pressure reduction effects, the NPs also have anti-proliferative properties, which are important in cardiac remodeling. In studies with knockout NPRA mice, arterial blood pressure rose dramatically with subsequent cardiac fibrosis and hypertrophy as the animal aged, compared to wild type [6]. Similarly, knockout mice for ANP and BNP genes led to hypertension, cardiac hypertrophy and fibrosis, obesity, and heart failure [7].

In the renal system, natriuretic peptides promote diuresis and natriuresis by their neurohormonal and hemodynamic actions. By antagonizing the renin-angiotensin-aldosterone system as well as the vasopressin system, the neurohormonal effects of natriuretic peptides antagonize water and salt retention. By dilating the afferent renal arterioles and constricting the efferent renal arterioles, natriuretic peptides result in increased glomerular pressure and glomerular filtration rate. By relaxing mesangial cells, the surface area for filtration in the glomerulus is also increased [1]. Urodilatin, via its local renal actions, has potent effects on diuresis and natriuresis [1].

Other important natriuretic peptide actions include anti-proliferation, anti-inflammation, and lipolysis. Natriuretic peptides inhibit cell division, and thus, are important, not only in cardiac remodeling and ventricular hypertrophy, but also vascular wall remodeling in hypertension and atherosclerosis. In rat models with disruption of BNP, there was a significant increase in fibrosis via increased activation of TGF-beta as well as collagen activation [8]. NPs also have important anti-inflammatory properties. In rat models with ANP infusion, there was a reduction in TNF-alpha, interleukin-1, and nitric oxide synthase, reflecting ANP's anti-inflammatory properties [9]. ANP also has lipolytic properties in adipose tissue [10].

Natriuretic Peptide Synthesis and Release

Natriuretic peptide release is stimulated by cardiac stretch, such as from intravascular volume overload and heart failure. In congestive heart failure, development of ventricular hypertrophy results in increased recruitment of ventricular cardiomyocytes in synthesizing BNP, which is subsequently released with increased transmural wall stress [11]. ANP is predominantly found in the cardiac atria, BNP is predominantly synthesized in the cardiac ventricles, and CNP is found mostly in the peripheral vasculature. CNP mRNA expression and secretion were augmented with shear stress in cell culture studies [12]. Thus, NPs are released in response to an acute volume load. The inactivation and degradation of natriuretic peptides is carried out by neutral endopeptidases or neprilysin.

Processing and Molecular Forms of Natriuretic Peptides

Natriuretic peptides are synthesized as inactive molecules prior to their conversion to biologically active proteins. Through studies utilizing human embryonic kidney (HEK) cells, the processing and molecular forms of the natriuretic peptides have been able to be better elucidated.

Understanding the different molecular forms of natriuretic peptides is important. While the high-molecular weight form of BNP is elevated in heart failure as a response to cardiac stretch, there may be a state of deficiency of and resistance to the low-molecular weight and biologically active form of 32 amino acid BNP in heart failure [13].

For BNP, the removal of the signaling peptide, via a signal peptidase, from the 134 amino acid preproBNP results in conversion to proBNP. This propeptide is subsequently converted into an inactive N terminal peptide as well as the active C terminal natriuretic peptide via convertases. Corin and furin are largely responsible for the conversion of proBNP, a 108 amino acid peptide, to physiologically active 32 amino acid BNP and inactive 76 amino acid NTproBNP [14, 15]. Certain molecular changes, such as glycosylation of the threonine 71 residue, have been shown to inhibit propeptide conversion. ProBNP and NTproBNP have little activity on the NP receptors and therefore, have minimal cGMP activation [16].

ANP is synthesized in cardiac myocytes as a 126 amino acid preproANP. Removal of the signaling peptide from preproANP results in proANP, which is stored in granules [17]. ProANP is subsequently cleaved to an N-terminal propeptide, as well as the biologically active 26 amino acid ANP. Corin is a cardiac serine protease responsible for cleaving proANP to the biologically active ANP [18].

Those that have genetic defects in the natural processing of the natriuretic peptide system may have decreased active natriuretic peptide levels and subsequent increased cardiovascular risk. A genetic defect in corin has been associated with increased adverse outcomes in blacks with systolic heart failure [19]. A dysfunction in the relative proportions of different molecular forms is associated with cardiovascular disease. In early hypertension, there is impaired response of the natriuretic peptide system, with poor BNP activity and reduced NTproBNP levels. In later stages of hypertension, there are compensatory increases in both BNP and NTproBNP.

B-Type Natriuretic Peptide Assays

In a clinical setting, there are currently a variety of assays available for measurement of serum BNP or serum NTproBNP. Furthermore, both rapid point-of-care assays as well as central laboratory assays are available. In normal subjects, the levels of BNP and NTproBNP are comparable, approximately 10 pmol/mL. Among those with heart failure, the levels of NTproBNP tend to rise more rapidly than that of BNP. While there is not a simple equation for conversion from a BNP measurement to NTproBNP value and vice versa, in heart failure, the NTproBNP level may be approximately four times that of BNP. Additionally, concurrent renal dysfunction with heart failure may cause greater elevations in NTproBNP than BNP. Plasma BNP assays detect BNP as well as proBNP and BNP degradation products. NTproBNP assays also detect proBNP. However, the exact proportion of cross-reactivity highly depends on the specific type and brand of assay used. Previous comparisons have demonstrated that BNP assays vary but some have up to 40 % cross-reactivity with proBNP detection [20]. NTproBNP assays are generally more specific, with little cross-reactivity to BNP, but up to over 200 % cross-reactivity to proBNP [20].

The Breathing Not Properly study evaluated over 1500 patients with acute dyspnea presenting to the emergency department, and found that plasma BNP levels were significantly higher in those with clinical heart failure compared to those without. Furthermore, it was found that the sensitivity and specificity for heart failure was 90 % and 76 %, respectively, when a cutoff BNP of greater than 100 pg/mL was used. Of note, the specificity greatly declined among those that had concurrent atrial fibrillation.

Case 1

A 70 year old man with history of myocardial infarction 5 years ago and hypertensive chronic kidney disease presented to an outside institution with complaint of progressively worsening exertional dyspnea. He had bilateral crackles on lung auscultation and positive jugular venous distention. The outside hospital obtained an NTproBNP level of 1050 pg/mL. Despite initiation of aggressive diuretic agents, the patient had persistent dyspnea. The use of advanced therapy was considered. The patient was subsequently transferred to your hospital and a BNP level was obtained and showed a level of 450 pg/mL. What are the laboratory interpretation, diagnostic and management implications of these findings?

Heart failure is first and foremost a clinical diagnosis. The patient's history of a prior myocardial infarction should increase clinical suspicion for heart failure, as ischemic cardiomyopathy is the leading cause of heart failure in developed countries. The history of progressively worsening exertional dyspnea as well as the findings of fluid overload should further raise the suspicion of the diagnosis of heart failure. The use of BNP assays should, therefore, aid in the narrowing of possible diagnoses. At the outside institution, the patient had a significantly elevated NTproBNP level. An NTproBNP level of greater than 900 pg/mL has a high sensitivity and specificity for the diagnosis of heart failure, especially in the right clinical context. However, upon hospital transfer, a measurement of BNP levels yielded a lower 450 pg/mL. While the absolute value is smaller, the findings are still consistent with heart failure, as a cutoff of 100 pg/mL for BNP is roughly equivalent to 900 pg/mL for NTproBNP. Furthermore, given that the patient has renal dysfunction, the NTproBNP assay may yield an even higher value than that of BNP. While the half-life of NTproBNP is greater than that of BNP, the ratio of the assay values cannot be used to determine timing of fluid overload onset, as the available commercial assays for both BNP and NTproBNP likely measure a mixture of BNP, NTproBNP, and proBNP.

Factors Affecting Endogenous BNP Levels

Age and Gender

There are multiple factors that affect BNP levels. BNP levels tend to be higher among the elderly population, as well as the female gender. Redfield et al, in determining the discriminatory value of BNP in heart failure, emphasized the importance of taking into account age and gender in the interpretation of BNP levels. The likely mechanism of female gender's association with increased BNP levels is estrogen, as levels were particularly elevated in those taking hormone replacement therapy [21, 22]. While age may be associated with increased ventricular hypertrophy, there appears to be an association of age with increased BNP levels independent of left ventricular dimensions and mass, which argues for alterations in cardiac biology that are undetectable by standard imaging techniques [22].

Redfield et al found that the average BNP levels for normal men for the age categories of 45–54, 55–64, 65–74, and 75–83 years are 7–17, 11–31, 18–28, and 21–38 pg/mL respectively. The average BNP levels for normal women for the age categories of 45–54, 55–64, 65–74, and 75–83 years are 18–28, 27–32, 29–45, and 58–67 pg/mL respectively. For age adjusted cut-off values for BNP and NTproBNP in the diagnosis of congestive heart failure, please refer to Table 13.1.

Table 13.1 Age-adjusted cut-off values for BNP and NTproBNP in those with normal renal function in the diagnosis of congestive heart failure

Age (years)	BNP		NTproBNP	
	Exclude HF (pg/mL)	Diagnose HF (pg/mL)	Exclude HF (pg/mL)	Diagnose HF (pg/mL)
<50	<35	>400	<300	>450
50–75	<40	>400	<300	>900
>75	<76	>400	<300	>1800

Data from Refs. [23, 24]

Obesity

Individuals with heart failure and obesity have suppressed BNP levels. There have been several proposed mechanisms for the findings of relatively lower BNP levels in those with obesity. Those with obesity, prior to development of heart failure, may already have increased intravascular volume, and therefore, a blunted BNP increase upon development of heart failure. The association of lower levels of BNP with obesity may also relate to the increased risk of hypertension development among the obese. There may be reduction in production and release of BNP in obesity. Also, the release and degradation of BNP may be higher in those with obesity, given the increase in natriuretic peptide clearance receptors in adipose tissue.

Different Pathophysiological States

Given that ANP and BNP are released with atrial and ventricular stretch, different cardiomyopathies will result in different levels of natriuretic peptide increase. With concentric left ventricular hypertrophy, even though there is increased myocardial mass, there is less wall stretch given the parallel arrangement of sarcomeres. Therefore, there is often less of an increase in natriuretic peptide levels in pure left ventricular concentric hypertrophy compared to dilated cardiomyopathy or eccentric hypertrophy, where there is greater myocardial stretch from sarcomeres in series. Given the pathophysiological dependence on stretch for natriuretic peptide release, in constrictive pericarditis, there is often lower levels of NPs than what would be expected, given that the pericardium is preventing the myocytes from appropriately stretching.

With ANP being released by atrial stretch, there are also interesting pathophysiological correlations with atrial fibrillation development. In addition, there appears to be an inverse correlation of BNP levels with heart rate. The effects of heart rate and atrial fibrillation on NP levels remain to be further investigated.

Renal Function

Decreased renal function and decreased kidney clearance results in increased circulating BNP levels. Given that in cardiorenal syndrome, renal dysfunction is a common comorbid condition of heart failure, BNP interpretation must be made with caution. Clinically, when the glomerular filtration rate falls below 60 mL/min, the traditional BNP cutoff of 100 pg/mL used for supporting a heart failure diagnosis should be used with caution.

Neprilysin Inhibitors

Neprilysin degrades biologically active BNP into inactive fragments, and the use of neprilysin inhibitors as a therapeutic modality will be further discussed in the therapy section. Administration of a neprilysin inhibitor will increase the levels of biologically active BNP, but will not affect NT-pro BNP.

Case 2

A 45 year old woman with body mass index (BMI) of 48 presents to clinic with acute dyspnea. Examination was notable for a parasternal heave as well as bilateral crackles of the lungs. Chest XR demonstrates pulmonary vascular congestion. A plasma BNP was obtained, which showed a value of 60 pg/mL. She appears to be uncomfortable and remains dyspneic. How should her BNP level be interpreted in this setting?

This obese patient presents with acute dyspnea in the setting of heart failure. The BNP level is in the indeterminate range, and not greater than the 100 pg/mL cutoff for heart failure diagnosis. However, given the patient's elevated BMI, there may be increased degradation of BNP with adipose tissue and reduced production and release of natriuretic peptides. Therefore, despite the relatively lower BNP finding in this case than expected, the suspicion for dilated cardiomyopathy remains high, and the patient should have prompt further evaluation such as an echocardiogram and appropriate management.

Case 3

A 78 year old woman on hormone replacement therapy and history of diabetes and chronic kidney disease stage 3 presents to clinic for a routine checkup. She is asymptomatic. Examination demonstrated clear lung fields bilaterally with no evidence of jugular venous distension or lower extremity edema. An NTproBNP level was obtained, which showed a level of 900 pg/mL. An NTproBNP level obtained last year during her routine physical examination was 850 pg/mL. How should this value be interpreted?

This patient has multiple reasons to have an elevated BNP and NTproBNP levels. She is elderly and on hormone replacement therapy. Age, female gender and estrogen all contribute to elevated natriuretic peptide levels. Furthermore, she has a history of chronic kidney disease, and reduction in renal function will lead to elevated levels of BNP. In the absence of heart failure signs and symptoms, even though the NTproBNP level is at or greater than the 900 pg/mL cutoff, the patient should not be diagnosed with heart failure. Furthermore, a comparison of NTproBNP levels from previous measurements, which is often useful, does not demonstrate a significant elevation in NTproBNP levels.

Natriuretic Peptide Therapeutics

Given the vasodilatory and renal natriuretic and diuretic effects, as well as the cardiovascular pleotropic and antifibrotic effects of natriuretic peptides, there has been increasing interest in the use of natriuretic peptides as a therapeutic modality. Nesiritide, or human recombinant BNP, has been extensively studied in patients hospitalized with acute heart failure. While there was mild improvement of dyspnea symptoms, there was no improvement in mortality or rehospitalization, and there was an association with increased hypotension [25]. For those with acute heart failure and renal dysfunction, low dose nesiritide also did not provide any benefit in decongestion or renal function [26]. Additionally, the addition of serial outpatient infusions of nesiritide to standard therapy also failed to demonstrate a significant outcomes benefit in those with chronic heart failure [27]. Given the challenges of nesiritide infusion and the side effect of hypotension, there has been investigation into different delivery methods of BNP, such as subcutaneous administration, which has demonstrated improvement in cardiorenal parameters [28].

Caperitide, or alpha-human atrial natriuretic peptide, has demonstrated promise in use in those with acute heart failure, and is approved in Japan. Acute low dose infusion of caperitide was found to result in improved long term prognosis in those with acute heart failure [29]. Given the efficacy in vasodilatation and diuresis, caperitide has also been studied as a first line therapy for those with acute heart failure, pulmonary congestion, and preserved blood pressure [30]. Furthermore, urodilatin, a renally synthesized ANP, was found to reduce filling pressures and improve symptoms in those with acute heart failure [31]. Ularitide, pharmacologic urodilatin, is currently undergoing phase III study in the TRUE-AHF clinical trial.

The approval of LCZ696, an angiotensin-neprilysin inhibitor, in 2015 heralded a new age in the treatment of heart failure. Neprilysin, which degrades many peptides including natriuretic peptides, has long been seen as a potential target for drug therapy. Previous studies have been complicated by angioedema side effects. However, the approval of LCZ696 for chronic heart failure patients reinforced the important pleotropic effects of natriuretic peptides. Angiotensin-neprilysin inhibition was found to be better than ACE inhibition alone at reducing mortality and rehospitalization for heart failure [32].

Case 4

A 72 year old man with NYHA class III heart failure with reduced ejection fraction and multiple rehospitalizations presents to clinic for an additional opinion. He has been placed on guideline directed therapy including optimal doses of beta blockers, ACE inhibitors, and aldosterone antagonists, and has a heart rate of 65 beats per minute. His quality of life is significantly limited to the point where he has difficulty with activities of daily living. He asks if there are any additional options for his chronic heart failure.

LCZ696 is a newly approved agent for chronic heart failure, NYHA class II to IV. The patient is currently already on optimal guideline directed therapy with an ACE inhibitor, but continues to do poorly functionally. LCZ696 has been shown to reduce mortality as well as rehospitalization compared to ACE inhibition alone, and this agent should be offered to the patient both for quality of life improvement as well as for mortality reduction. In transitioning from ACE inhibition, a washout period of 36 h should be used, and the patient should be warned about the potential risks of the medication, including angioedema, hyperkalemia, and hypotension.

Future studies are necessary to develop therapeutic modalities for heart failure with preserved ejection fraction, as well as additional therapies for chronic heart failure. Given the success of dual angiotensin-neprilysin inhibition, chimeric peptides have also been increasingly studied. The natriuretic peptide system remains an exciting opportunity for growth and development in the treatment of heart failure as well as other cardiovascular diseases.

References

1. Levin ER, Gardner DG, Samson WK. Natriuretic peptides. N Engl J Med. 1998;339(5):321–8. doi:10.1056/NEJM199807303390507.
2. Nakao K, Ogawa Y, Suga S, Imura H. Molecular biology and biochemistry of the natriuretic peptide system. II: Natriuretic peptide receptors. J Hypertens. 1992;10(10):1111–4.
3. Potter LR, Hunter T. Guanylyl cyclase-linked natriuretic peptide receptors: structure and regulation. J Biol Chem. 2001;276(9):6057–60. doi:10.1074/jbc.R000033200.
4. Rubattu S, Sciarretta S, Morriello A, Calvieri C, Battistoni A, Volpe M. NPR-C: a component of the natriuretic peptide family with implications in human diseases. J Mol Med (Berl). 2010;88(9):889–97. doi:10.1007/s00109-010-0641-2.
5. Hutchinson HG, Trindade PT, Cunanan DB, Wu CF, Pratt RE. Mechanisms of natriuretic-peptide-induced growth inhibition of vascular smooth muscle cells. Cardiovasc Res. 1997;35(1):158–67.

6. Pandey KN. Biology of natriuretic peptides and their receptors. Peptides. 2005;26(6):901–32. doi:10.1016/j.peptides.2004.09.024.

7. Gupta DK, Wang TJ. Natriuretic peptides and cardiometabolic health. Circ J. 2015;79(8):1647–55. doi:10.1253/circj.CJ-15-0589.

8. Ogawa Y, Tamura N, Chusho H, Nakao K. Brain natriuretic peptide appears to act locally as an antifibrotic factor in the heart. Can J Physiol Pharmacol. 2001;79(8):723–9.

9. Mori M, Yamanashi Y, Kobayashi K, Sakamoto A. Atrial natriuretic peptide alleviates cardiovascular and metabolic disorders in a rat endotoxemia model: a possible role for its anti-inflammatory properties. J Nippon Med Sch. 2010;77(6):296–305.

10. Sengenes C, Zakaroff-Girard A, Moulin A, Berlan M, Bouloumie A, Lafontan M, et al. Natriuretic peptide-dependent lipolysis in fat cells is a primate specificity. Am J Physiol Regul Integr Comp Physiol. 2002;283(1):R257–65. doi:10.1152/ajpregu.00453.2001.

11. Belluardo P, Cataliotti A, Bonaiuto L, Giuffre E, Maugeri E, Noto P, et al. Lack of activation of molecular forms of the BNP system in human grade 1 hypertension and relationship to cardiac hypertrophy. Am J Physiol Heart Circ Physiol. 2006;291(4):H1529–35. doi:10.1152/ajpheart.00107.2006.

12. Chun TH, Itoh H, Ogawa Y, Tamura N, Takaya K, Igaki T, et al. Shear stress augments expression of C-type natriuretic peptide and adrenomedullin. Hypertension. 1997;29(6):1296–302.

13. Chen HH. Heart failure: a state of brain natriuretic peptide deficiency or resistance or both! J Am Coll Cardiol. 2007;49(10):1089–91. doi:10.1016/j.jacc.2006.12.013.

14. Semenov AG, Tamm NN, Seferian KR, Postnikov AB, Karpova NS, Serebryanaya DV, et al. Processing of pro-B-type natriuretic peptide: furin and corin as candidate convertases. Clin Chem. 2010;56(7):1166–76. doi:10.1373/clinchem.2010.143883.

15. Ichiki T, Huntley BK, Burnett Jr JC. BNP molecular forms and processing by the cardiac serine protease corin. Adv Clin Chem. 2013;61:1–31.

16. Heublein DM, Huntley BK, Boerrigter G, Cataliotti A, Sandberg SM, Redfield MM, et al. Immunoreactivity and guanosine 3′,5′-cyclic monophosphate activating actions of various molecular forms of human B-type natriuretic peptide. Hypertension. 2007;49(5):1114–9. doi:10.1161/HYPERTENSIONAHA.106.081083.

17. Wu F, Yan W, Pan J, Morser J, Wu Q. Processing of pro-atrial natriuretic peptide by corin in cardiac myocytes. J Biol Chem. 2002;277(19):16900–5. doi:10.1074/jbc.M201503200.

18. Wu Q, Xu-Cai YO, Chen S, Wang W. Corin: new insights into the natriuretic peptide system. Kidney Int. 2009;75(2):142–6. doi:10.1038/ki.2008.418.

19. Rame JE, Tam SW, McNamara D, Worcel M, Sabolinski ML, Wu AH, et al. Dysfunctional corin i555(p568) allele is associated with impaired brain natriuretic peptide processing and adverse outcomes in blacks with systolic heart failure: results from the Genetic Risk Assessment in Heart Failure substudy. Circ Heart Fail. 2009;2(6):541–8. doi:10.1161/CIRCHEARTFAILURE.109.866822.

20. Luckenbill KN, Christenson RH, Jaffe AS, Mair J, Ordonez-Llanos J, Pagani F, et al. Cross-reactivity of BNP, NT-proBNP, and proBNP in commercial BNP and NT-proBNP assays: preliminary observations from the IFCC Committee for Standardization of Markers of Cardiac Damage. Clin Chem. 2008;54(3):619–21. doi:10.1373/clinchem.2007.097998.

21. Loke I, Squire IB, Davies JE, Ng LL. Reference ranges for natriuretic peptides for diagnostic use are dependent on age, gender and heart rate. Eur J Heart Fail. 2003;5(5):599–606.

22. Redfield MM, Rodeheffer RJ, Jacobsen SJ, Mahoney DW, Bailey KR, Burnett Jr JC. Plasma brain natriuretic peptide concentration: impact of age and gender. J Am Coll Cardiol. 2002;40(5):976–82.

23. McCullough PA, Nowak RM, McCord J, Hollander JE, Herrmann HC, Steg PG, et al. B-type natriuretic peptide and clinical judgment in emergency diagnosis of heart failure: analysis from Breathing Not Properly (BNP) Multinational Study. Circulation. 2002;106(4):416–22.

24. Januzzi JL, van Kimmenade R, Lainchbury J, Bayes-Genis A, Ordonez-Llanos J, Santalo-Bel M, et al. NT-proBNP testing for diagnosis and short-term prognosis in acute destabilized heart failure: an international pooled analysis of 1256 patients: the International Collaborative of NT-proBNP Study. Eur Heart J. 2006;27(3):330–7. doi:10.1093/eurheartj/ehi631.

25. O'Connor CM, Starling RC, Hernandez AF, Armstrong PW, Dickstein K, Hasselblad V, et al. Effect of nesiritide in patients with acute decompensated heart failure. N Engl J Med. 2011;365(1):32–43. doi:10.1056/NEJMoa1100171.
26. Chen HH, Anstrom KJ, Givertz MM, Stevenson LW, Semigran MJ, Goldsmith SR, et al. Low-dose dopamine or low-dose nesiritide in acute heart failure with renal dysfunction: the ROSE acute heart failure randomized trial. JAMA. 2013;310(23):2533–43. doi:10.1001/jama.2013.282190.
27. Yancy CW, Krum H, Massie BM, Silver MA, Stevenson LW, Cheng M, et al. Safety and efficacy of outpatient nesiritide in patients with advanced heart failure: results of the Second Follow-Up Serial Infusions of Nesiritide (FUSION II) trial. Circ Heart Fail. 2008;1(1):9–16. doi:10.1161/CIRCHEARTFAILURE.108.767483.
28. Chen HH, Redfield MM, Nordstrom LJ, Horton DP, Burnett Jr JC. Subcutaneous administration of the cardiac hormone BNP in symptomatic human heart failure. J Card Fail. 2004;10(2):115–9.
29. Hata N, Seino Y, Tsutamoto T, Hiramitsu S, Kaneko N, Yoshikawa T, et al. Effects of carperitide on the long-term prognosis of patients with acute decompensated chronic heart failure: the PROTECT multicenter randomized controlled study. Circ J. 2008;72(11):1787–93.
30. Nomura F, Kurobe N, Mori Y, Hikita A, Kawai M, Suwa M, et al. Multicenter prospective investigation on efficacy and safety of carperitide as a first-line drug for acute heart failure syndrome with preserved blood pressure: COMPASS: Carperitide Effects Observed Through Monitoring Dyspnea in Acute Decompensated Heart Failure Study. Circ J. 2008;72(11):1777–86.
31. Mitrovic V, Seferovic PM, Simeunovic D, Ristic AD, Miric M, Moiseyev VS, et al. Haemodynamic and clinical effects of ularitide in decompensated heart failure. Eur Heart J. 2006;27(23):2823–32. doi:10.1093/eurheartj/ehl337.
32. McMurray JJ, Packer M, Desai AS, Gong J, Lefkowitz MP, Rizkala AR, et al. Angiotensin-neprilysin inhibition versus enalapril in heart failure. N Engl J Med. 2014;371(11):993–1004. doi:10.1056/NEJMoa1409077.

Chapter 14
Natriuretic Peptides: Basic Analytic Considerations

Alan H.B. Wu

Abstract The analysis of natriuretic peptides in blood is important and widely used for clinical practice for the diagnosis and management of patients with heart failure. As with the analysis of any biomarker, the analytical attributes of the assay for B-type natriuretic peptide and NT-proBNP can influence the interpretation of results. Point-of-care testing is an attractive alternative to sending samples to a central laboratory. The advantage of getting results sooner must be weighed into the additional costs and sacrifice in analytical performance.

Keywords Natriuretic peptide • Analytical precision in natriuretic peptides • Pro-BNP • Commercial immunoassays for BNP • Natriuretic peptide testing in heart failure • NT-proBNP

Case Report

A 57-year old male is admitted to the emergency department with acute dyspnea. He has a history of asthma and suffered an acute myocardial infarction (AMI) three years earlier. He has no prior history of heart failure. The patient has normal temperature and blood pressure, and has an increase pulse and respiratory rate. The patient is overweight (BMI = 30 kg/m^2) and is a smoker. Given his history, the patient was place under the hospital's protocol for diagnosis and rule out of AMI. Table 14.1 shows the results of some of his laboratory results upon ED presentation. All test results were conducted from a central laboratory. The patient had mild renal insufficiency (eGFR > 50 mL/min). The cardiac troponin I

A.H.B. Wu, PhD
Department of Laboratory Medicine, University of California, San Francisco/San Francisco General Hospital, San Francisco, CA, USA
e-mail: Alan.Wu@ucsf.edu; wualan@labmed2.ucsf.edu

© Springer International Publishing Switzerland 2016
A.S. Maisel, A.S. Jaffe (eds.), *Cardiac Biomarkers*,
DOI 10.1007/978-3-319-42982-3_14

Table 14.1 Selected laboratory results of case report

ED admission		
Test	Result	Reference range
Creatinine	2.1	0.7–1.4 mg/dL
eGFR	50 mL/min	>60 mL/min
hs-CRP	4.1 mg/dL	high risk: >3 mg/dL
Cardiac troponin I	0.58 ng/mL	<0.04 ng/mL
B-type natriuretic peptide	825 pg/mL	<100 pg/mL
Three hours after ED presentation		
3-h cardiac troponin I	0.62 ng/mL	<0.04 ng/mL
6-h cardiac troponin	0.59 ng/mL	<0.04 ng/mL
Day 1 hospitalization		
B-type natriuretic peptide	235 pg/mL	<100 pg/mL
Discharge (day 7 after hospitalization)		
B-type natriuretic peptide	146 pg/mL	<100 pg/mL
Two-month followup		
B-type natriuretic peptide	323 pg/mL	<100 pg/mL

concentration was above the 99th percentile cutoff. A repeat test troponin test conducted 3 and 6 h later showed no significant change in cTnI relative to baseline levels, and the patient was ruled out for AMI. The B-type natriuretic peptide (BNP) level was abnormally increased. Based on the result of the BNP, the patient was diagnosed as having decompensated heart failure, and was admitted for further treatment and diagnostic workup. The patient was treated with diuretics which was effective in reducing his shortness-of-breath symptoms.

On the first hospital day, nurses noted a large volume of fluid that was excreted into the patient's urine. The doctors ordered a repeat BNP on the next day. The BNP level declined from 825 to 235 ng/mL. The substantial decline in BNP results suggested to his doctors that the patient had compensated for his heart failure through the removal of fluids. Physicians needed to determine if his current increased BNP concentration was due to his mild renal insufficiency or pulmonary disease so an echocardiogram was ordered. The patient had a normal ejection fraction and was diagnosed as having preserved diastolic function heart failure. He was treated with a β-blocker and an angiotensin converting enzyme (ACE) inhibitor. After 4 hospitalized days, the patient was discharged. His repeat BNP produced a result of 146 pg/mL. As an outpatient, he underwent regular checkups for his heart failure. At two months for his discharge, his BNP increased to 323 pg/mL. Based on this result, the patient's physician increased the ACE inhibitor dosage.

Analytical Considerations for Natriuretic Peptides

Biochemistry and Commercial Assays

Pro-BNP is a 108 amino acid precursor peptide found in cardiac myocyte that metabolizes by the enzyme corin to BNP, 32-amino acid hormone, and NT-proBNP, an inactive76 amino acid peptide [1]. BNP and NT-proBNP are release into the circulation following volume overload and cardiac wall stress and vasoconstriction and the loss of electrolytes. BNP counters the action of renin and aldosterone which are vasodilators and retention of salt and water. Once released, BNP binds to natriuretic peptide receptors at the site of action and is degraded by peptidases. BNP has a short half-life of about 20 min, while the half-life of NT-proBNP is longer at 2 h [2]. In patients with heart failure, proBNP also circulates in blood as the native form and glycosylated [3].

There are four major manufacturers of commercial BNP assays, Abbott Laboratories, Alere Inc., Beckman Coulter, and Siemens (Centaur). Due to the instability of the analyte, Blood must be collected into tubes containing EDTA and tested for BNP within a few hours of collection. Major manufacturers for NT-proBNP include Roche, Siemens (Dimension), and Ortho Vitros. NT-proBNP is more stable than BNP and can be tested in serum or plasma. In addition to Alere, there are also a number of point-of-care (POC) assays for BNP and NT-proBNP have been FDA cleared (Response Biomedical, Biomerieux, and Mitsubishi) while many others are in development. POC testing devices operate on whole blood and provide natriuretic test results within 20 min of collection. However, individual test cartridges are more expensive and assays are less precise than those obtained from the central laboratory.

The use of BNP and NT-proBNP are protected by patents, and licenses are required to implement commercial assays for clinical practice. There is no clinical utility of providing both set of results on a given patient. The choice of the biomarker is dependent on the laboratory's choice of clinical laboratory instrumentation. Although antibodies can be raised against proBNP that have no cross reactivity towards the metabolites (BNP and NT-proBNP) [4], there are no commercial assays for proBNP.

The reference range for BNP and NT-proBNP increase with each decade of age, with women having higher values than men. Despite these differences in these populations, the manufacturers have received approval by the FDA for a single cutoff for BNP the cutoff (100 pg/mL) and two cutoffs for NT-proBNP (125 pg/mL for individuals less than 75 years and 450 for individuals ≥75 years. In the absence of heart failure, BNP and NT-proBNP are lower for both men and women who are obese [5] and are higher for those with renal insufficiency [6]. In order to provide more clarity, some investigators have suggested use of other cutoff concentrations

Table 14.2 Proposed cutoff concentrations for BNP and NT-proBNP

	Cutoff	
	BNP, pg/mL	NT-proBNP, pg/mL
Acute decompensated HF	100 rule out	450 for <50 years,
	100–400 gray zone	900 for 50–75 years
	400 rule in	1800 for >75 years
Renal dysfunction (eGFR <60 mL/min)	200	1200
Obesity	170, for BMI <25 kg/m^2	900
	110, for BMI 25–25 kg/m^2	
	54, for BMI ≥35 kg/m^2	

Data from Kim and Januzzi [2]

for BNP and NT/proBNP when incorporates a "gray zone" between diagnosis and rule out, BMI and glomerular filtration rate (Table 14.2) [2]. This strategy of selecting a cutoff concentration that optimizes clinical sensitivity and specificity for heart failure is unlike the approached used in determining the cutoff concentration for cardiac troponin. In the latter case, any increase of cardiac troponin above the 99th percentile of a healthy population is used as the cutoff concentration to indicate myocardial injury, irrespective to ischemic or non-ischemic etiologies.

In this case report, the assay used for BNP was not specified as would be the typical in routine practice today. BNP results at presentation greatly exceeded the cutoff concentrations shown in Table 14.2 and decompensated heart failure is established as the diagnosis. An increase would have been evident irrespective to the BNP assay used. A decline in BNP value to 235 pg/mL on the next day, and then a further decline to 146 pg/mL at the patient's discharge from the hospital suggest compensation. A subsequent increase to 323 pg/mL suggests heart failure disease progression.

Imprecision, Bias and Total Allowable Error

Analytical attributes of a clinical laboratory test can have a significant influence on how a biomarker is interpreted in clinical practice. Through the use of quality control materials, the analytical imprecision of an assay is tracked by the clinical laboratory daily. For the natriuretic peptides, testing conducted from the centration laboratory typically has imprecision between 5 and 10%. BNP and/or NT-proBNP testing performed through the use of point-of-care devices can produce higher analytical imprecision (e.g., 10–20%). While this is higher than for results obtained from the central laboratory, there is no clinical consequence [7]. This is because the interpretation of BNP/NT-proBNP is made relative to large increases or decreases in results. This is in contrast to troponin, where small changes in troponin results may indicate myocardial necrosis, and high analytical precision is needed. The

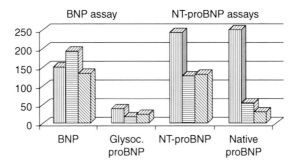

Fig. 14.1 Differences in cross reactivities among commercial immunoassays for BNP and NT-proBNP. *1st group*: recombinant BNP (aa 77–108). *2nd group*: glycosylated proBNP (aa: 1–108). *3rd group*: recombinant NT-proBNP (aa 1–76). 4th group: native recombinant proBNP (aa: 1–108). *Left pair*: BNP assays (*vertical* bar: Abbott Architect, *horizontal bar*: Siemens Centaur, diagonal bar: Alere Triage). *Right pair*: NT-proBNP assays (*vertical bar*: Siemens Dimension, *horizontal bar*: Ortho Vitros, *diagonal bar*: Roche Elecsys) (Data from Luckenbill et al. [8])

biological variation for the natriuretic peptides is high relative to other clinical laboratory tests. In this case report, differences in BNP results from one sample to the next change by large fractions, i.e., they greatly exceed the assay's imprecision. Therefore the medical decisions that are needed for this patient are not influenced by the assay's imprecision when point-of-care testing devices are used.

Bias refers to differences in laboratory results between the one used in a clinical laboratory and a reference standard. For BNP/NT-proBNP, neither a reference standard nor a reference method exists. Therefore *absolute* bias of a particular assay cannot be determined. For routine clinical practice, *relative* bias is important. This relates to differences in test results between different analytical testing platforms. There are several manufacturers of BNP and NT-proBNP reagents. Biases exist between assays for the same biomarker. While there is a common cutoff concentration, BNP results are not commutable, i.e., the result by one assay cannot be recalculated through the use of a correction factor, with any degree of confidence, to the other assay. There are also non-commutable differences in NT-proBNP results, despite the fact that one company (Roche Diagnostics) owns the patent on the clinical use of this peptide and has licensed their antibodies to other manufactures and requires use of their standards. A major cause of lack of assay harmony refers to the differential sensitivity of antibodies used in BNP assays against the targeted peptides, post-translational modifications, and reactivity towards the precursor protein (proBNP) [8]. Figure 14.1, group 1 and 3 shows that among BNP and NT-proBNP assays, there are different degrees of cross-reactivities towards the targeted protein. Figure 14.1, group 2 and 4 shows different cross-reactivities towards the precursor protein (glycosylated and native proBNP), known to circulate in blood of heart failure patients. These differences will produce different BNP and NT-proBNP results, even if they are calibrated to the same standard. In this case report, all serial BNP results were produced from the same manufacturer of reagents. This is the most appropriate manner to interpret results. Conclusions cannot be so readily rendered if tests were conducted from different platforms. Clinical laboratories do not indicate the manufacturer or instruments on clinical laboratory reports. Physicians must inquire about how testing is performed if a patient is seen at different institutions. It is extremely difficult to interpret results when results of BNP vs. NT-proBNP are interchanged from the same patient.

The total allowable error is the sum of the bias (absolute value) and imprecision. This concept is used by clinical laboratories to establish goals for quality control for their laboratories. Several regulatory agencies such as the Center for Medicare and Medicaid (CMS) have established minimum performance by laboratories for commonly tested analytes. Neither CMS nor any other regulatory agency have established total allowable error goals for the natriuretic peptides.

Biological Variation

The biological variation of a laboratory test refers to the variances within an individual over time and among a group of individuals. Biological variation studies are conducted on healthy subjects. The within-individual variances, calculated as the coefficient of variance (CV_I), is computed by serial collection of blood from the same individual over a period of time. The time interval of blood collection is determined by the intended utility of the test and range from hours, to days, weeks, and months. Typically 4–6 samples are required for each individual. The group variances are calculated as the CV_G and is the experimental variability across all subjects tested. Usually, only a dozen or more different individuals are needed. These two measured attributes along with the analytical imprecision (CV_A) are used to determine various attributes of a test such as the index of individuality and the reference change value. The RCV is a means to establish a cutoff value between the results of serial biomarker results [9].

Compared to other cardiac risk assessment markers, e.g., cholesterol, the natriuretic peptides have a relatively high biological variation when measured over days, weeks, and months. Table 14.3 lists the biological variation for the natriuretic peptides, results broken down according to the interval of blood collections [10]. The longer the duration of observation the higher the biological variation and the corresponding RCV value. Table 14.3 also shows that the biological variation for BNP is higher than for NT-proBNP, making it slightly less useful for long-term monitoring of disease [11].

Table 14.3 Biological variation for BNP and NT-proBNP[1]

	Within-day	Day-to-day	Week-to-week
B-type natriuretic peptide	±32 %	±74 %	±113 %
NT-proBNP	±25 %	±55 %	±98 %
Cholesterol	NA	NA	±15 %

NA not applicable

In the case report, the BNP result dropped from 825 to 235 pg/mL, a decline of 350 %. This greatly exceeds the within-day RCV cutoff of 32 %, indicating that this decline in result exceeds the variation that is expected during health. One might conclude that diuretic therapy was effective in treating this patient's decompensation. A further decline to 146 pg/mL also exceeds the day-to-day RCV. Since this result was obtained on the day of discharge, it serves as a baseline for any outpatient monitoring. At six months, a repeat BNP result was 323 pg/mL, a 220 % increase over baseline. This exceeds the week-to-week RCV of 112 % indicating a situation of worsening of heart failure. Depending on the symptoms, this patient may benefit from a more aggressive treatment of his heart failure.

Summary

The analytical attributes of a biomarker can be critically important in assessing the performance of the test in clinical practice. Ideally, the biomarker should be stable and assays should be precise, standardized across testing platforms, and exhibit low biological variation. Assays for the natriuretic peptides fulfil many but not all of these desirable attributes. For example, the high biological variation makes room for the use of other heart failure markers such as soluble ST-2 and galectin-3, which have lower reference change values [12]. For these biomarkers, it may be possible that a smaller degree of change in results over time may indicate a significant change in the clinical status of the heart failure patient, thereby warranting a change in their management. Recently, sacubitrol has FDA cleared for treating heart failure patients. This drug inhibits neprilysin, an enzyme that breaks down BNP and other vasoactive peptides. The levels of BNP are decreased following sacubitrol treatment, whereas NT-proBNP levels are increased.

References

1. Hall C. Essential biochemistry and physiology of (NT-pro)BNP. Eur J Heart Fail. 2004;6:257–60.
2. Kim HA, Januzzi JL. Natriuretic peptide testing in heart failure. Circulation. 2011;123:2015–9.
3. Dries DL, Ky B, Wu AH, Rame JE, Putt ME, Cappola TP. Simultaneous assessment of unprocessed ProBNP1-108 in addition to processed BNP32 improves identification of high-risk ambulatory patients with heart failure. Circ Heart Fail. 2010;3:220–7.
4. Giuliani I, Rieunier F, Larue C, Delagneau JF, Granier C, Pau B, Ferriere M, et al. Assay for measurement of intact B-type natriutretic peptide prohormone in blood. Clin Chem. 2006;52:1054–61.
5. Clerico A, Giannoni A, Vittorini S, Emdin M. The paradox of low BNP levels in obesity. Heart Fail Rev. 2012;17:81–96.

6. McCullough PA, Sandberg KR. B-type natriuretic peptide and renal disease. Heart Fail Rev. 2003;8:355–8.
7. Kupchak P, Wu AHB, Ghani F, Newby LK, Ohman EH, Christenson RH. The influence of imprecision on receiver-operating characteristic curve analysis for cardiac markers. Clin Chem. 2006;52:752–3.
8. Luckenbill KN, Christenson RH, Jaffe AS, Mair J, Ordonez-Llanos J, Pagani F, Tate JR, Wu AHB, Ler R, Apple FS. Cross-reactivity of BNP, NT-proBNP and proBNP in commercial BNP and NT-proBNP assays: preliminary observations. Clin Chem. 2008;54:619–21.
9. Fraser CG. Biological variation: from principles to practice. Washington DC: AACC Press; 2002.
10. Fokkema MR, Herrmann Z, Muskiet FAJ, Moecks J. Reference change values for brain natriuretic peptide revisted. Clin Chem. 2006;52:1602–3.
11. Wu AHB. Serial testing of B-type natriuretic peptide and NTpro-BNP for monitoring therapy of heart failure: the role of biological variation in interpretation of results. Am Heart J. 2006;152:828–34.
12. Wu AHB, Wians Jr F, Jaffe AS. Biological variation of galectin-3 and soluble ST2 for chronic heart failure: implication on interpretation of test results. Am Heart J. 2013;165:995–9.

Chapter 15
Natriuretic Peptide Use in Screening in the Community

Noel S. Lee and Lori B. Daniels

Abstract Congestive heart failure is a widely prevalent chronic condition affecting over 23 million people worldwide. The heart failure spectrum spans from asymptomatic individuals at risk to those suffering symptoms even at rest. In between are patients with silent left ventricular dysfunction, which is often only diagnosed after an abnormal electrocardiogram or chest imaging is obtained during workup for other medical conditions. One in 10 of such individuals will develop symptoms annually. The 2013 American College of Cardiology Foundation and the American Heart Association practice guideline for the management of heart failure recommends screening particularly high risk individuals with echocardiography, as studies indicate pharmacologic treatment of asymptomatic left ventricular dysfunction improves outcomes. One area of interest is the role of natriuretic peptides – such as B-type natriuretic peptide, or BNP, and its N-terminal fragment, NT-proBNP – in screening. Although investigators have debated their cost effectiveness, studies have found that these biomarkers are useful not only in evaluating for current left ventricular dysfunction, but also in predicting future dysfunction, incident heart failure, and all-cause mortality. Accurate risk stratification, diagnosis, and prompt initiation of treatment in these individuals are important facets of heart failure care that natriuretic peptides may facilitate.

Keywords Biomarkers • Echocardiography • Heart failure • Natriuretic peptides • Primary prevention and natriuretic peptide • Risk stratification and natriuretic peptide • Screening with natriuretic peptide

N.S. Lee, MD
Department of Medicine, Division of Cardiovascular Medicine, Sulpizio Cardiovascular Center, University of California, San Diego, La Jolla, CA, USA
e-mail: nolee@ucsd.edu

L.B. Daniels (✉)
Division of Cardiovascular Medicine, University of California, San Diego, La Jolla, CA, USA
e-mail: lbdaniels@ucsd.edu

© Springer International Publishing Switzerland 2016
A.S. Maisel, A.S. Jaffe (eds.), *Cardiac Biomarkers*,
DOI 10.1007/978-3-319-42982-3_15

But I don't have heart failure! – American Heart Association infographic

A 2013 American Heart Association (AHA) policy statement [1] cautioned all Americans against nonchalantly brushing off congestive heart failure. The takeaway message was underscored emphatically in an accompanying infographic. Just below the heading "But I don't have heart failure!" read the stark truth: "By 2030 heart failure costs could reach $70 billion, meaning every U.S. taxpayer could owe $244 a year, whether they have it or not." Aside from emphasizing the more than doubling of present costs, the publication spotlighted several predictions for 2030, including that over 8 million people in the United States, or 1 in 33, will have this chronic condition. But the policy statement also clearly stated that the calculations assumed a steady rate of scientific advancement and unchanged clinical practices. Community-based prevention and treatment are keys to curtailing this escalation.

With an annual incidence of over 550,000 Americans and a 20 % lifetime risk for people over 40 years, the heart failure healthcare crisis is not limited to the United States [2]. The prevalence of heart failure worldwide is over 23 million [2]. Primary care physicians bear the majority of the weight not only in caring for this patient population but also for the population at risk. These providers generally already actively screen for heart failure risk factors by checking blood pressure, hemoglobin A1c and/or fasting glucose levels, and lipid panels. They look for signs of obesity and tobacco abuse. In these areas, they counsel and initiate medications where appropriate. Such interventions have a remarkable impact. For example, long-term antihypertensive therapy for both systolic and diastolic hypertension cuts the risk of heart failure by about half [3].

Controlling risk factors is not the only way to reduce the impending growth in heart failure, though. A subset of people with left ventricular (LV) dysfunction fall into Stage B heart failure: structural disease without symptoms. Many remain undiagnosed. One community study out of Olmsted County, Minnesota found that over half of the residents with moderate or severe diastolic dysfunction or systolic dysfunction with an LV ejection fraction no greater than 40 % either had not been evaluated for heart failure at all or were asymptomatic [4]. Of the 40 individuals with an ejection fraction of 40 % or less, only 47.5 % were taking angiotensin-converting enzyme [ACE] inhibitors, and only 22.5 % were taking beta-blockers [4]. Identifying this preclinical Stage B heart failure population is important, as randomized trials have demonstrated that medical therapy significantly reduces incident heart failure and heart failure-related hospitalizations in patients with asymptomatic LV dysfunction [5].

Thus, screening for heart failure may be beneficial: the condition is serious and prevalent, particularly among expanding older age groups, and treatment before onset of symptoms occur can improve outcomes. The AHA and American College of Cardiology (ACC) have produced evidence-based guidelines for the prevention and treatment of heart failure [3]. However, screening strategies are still under investigation. Should everyone in the community be checked? Or only the highest risk subgroup? And at what frequency? One screening modality has garnered much attention but equally as much controversy: the use of natriuretic peptides like B-type

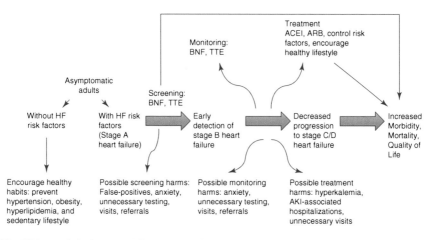

Fig. 15.1 Analytic framework for screening for heart failure

natriuretic peptide (BNP) and its N-terminal fragment (NT-proBNP). Both have been widely employed in diagnosing heart failure in acute dyspnea, guiding management, and evaluating prognosis but are not yet formally recommended for routine measurement in current screening guidelines [3].

Even over 15 years ago, BNP was postulated as a promising screening tool [6]. A simple blood test, it is easily obtained and causes minimal discomfort. Although much cheaper than the gold-stand echocardiogram, it still yields reliable and consistent results, and it already serves as an adjunct in distinguishing heart failure from non-heart failure related symptoms in various settings.

Like the AHA and ACC, the U.S. Preventive Services Task Force (USPSTF) advocates evidence-based approaches to clinical practice guidelines. In evaluating screening scenarios, the USPSTF has used analytic frameworks that ask whether high-risk groups can be identified; whether screening can accurately test for the condition, affect treatment decisions, and reduce morbidity and mortality; and whether screening or treatment results in adverse effects [7]. Figure 15.1 illustrates such an analytic framework for screening for heart failure.

Although the AHA/ACC guidelines assert that not enough data exist yet to recommend utilizing natriuretic peptides for routine screening, emerging research suggests these markers might be helpful. Specifically, the St Vincent's Screening TO Prevent Heart Failure (STOP-HF) study [8] was the first randomized, prospective investigation on this topic and was published after the guidelines were released.

In this investigation, 1374 subjects over age 40 at risk of heart failure (with one or more of the following risk factors: hypertension, hypercholesterolemia, obesity, vascular disease, diabetes, arrhythmias, moderate to serve valve disease) were randomly assigned to receive standard non-BNP-guided primary care or screening with BNP. Patients in the latter group with BNP levels of at least 50 pg/mL underwent echocardiography and were referred to multifaceted cardiology specialty care. Of the 697 patients randomized to BNP screening, 263 patients (41.6%) had elevated levels that placed them in this collaborative treatment plan. Analysis after a mean follow-up of 4.2 years demonstrated that BNP screening and targeted care significantly reduced rates of LV dysfunction with and without heart failure (5.3 % vs. 8.7 % in the intervention group and the control group, respectively; p=0.003) [8].

The STOP-HF study is just one of the studies advocating the value of natriuretic peptides as a screening tool for heart failure. Here we will examine clinical cases in which the natriuretic peptides BNP and NT-proBNP may be applied to screening for heart failure risk in the community.

Case 1

Mr. HF, a 65-year-old African-American man, presents to your primary care office to establish care. He reports a history of well-controlled hypertension, diabetes, and hyperlipidemia, but he recently lost his job and is concerned about being able to afford his medications. He was diagnosed with hypertension at age 47 and subsequently made several lifestyle modifications, including a 7-pound weight loss through exercising 30 min per day, 5 days per week, and reducing his fast-food intake. Medications include daily baby aspirin, metformin, lisinopril, hydrochlorothiazide, and simvastatin.

Despite these commitments to improving his lifestyle, Mr. HF has struggled with tobacco abuse. He has a 16-pack-year history and is currently smoking ½ a pack per day. He drinks a glass of wine occasionally with dinner. Family history is notable for obesity, diabetes, and coronary artery disease in his mother, who suffered a myocardial infarction at age 68. Review of systems is negative for shortness of breath, dyspnea with exertion, lower extremity edema, chest pain, palpitations, cough, and orthopnea. He sleeps with one pillow and denies paroxysmal nocturnal dyspnea.

His blood pressure is 129/85; pulse 79 beats per minute. BMI is 27.6 kg/m². His cardiovascular exam reveals a regular heart rate and rhythm with a fourth heart sound and a nondeviated point of maximum impulse. Jugular venous pressure is 7 cm. His lungs are clear to auscultation, and he has no lower extremity edema. Distal pulses are palpable bilaterally, and his extremities are warm to touch. Electrocardiogram shows normal sinus rhythm without abnormalities.

Discussion Points

1. What risk factors for heart failure does this patient have, and how should they be managed?

In order to understand the utility of natriuretic peptides and to potentially apply them to heart failure screening, practitioners must be able to identify patient risk factors.

This patient falls into the stage A category of heart failure: he is at risk but does not have known structural heart disease. Uncontrollable risk factors in this patient include male sex, older age, and black race. People who live to age 40 have a 20% lifetime risk of developing heart failure, and studies have found an incidence of up to 19.3 per 1000 person-years in people over 65 years of age [2]. Increased risk in black individuals is at least partially attributed to a higher prevalence of other risk factors, such as obesity, chronic kidney disease, diabetes, and hypertension [2].

Controllable risk factors in this patient include obesity, hypertension, diabetes, smoking, and dyslipidemia. He should be encouraged to continue his weight loss, diet control, and exercise. A BMI of 30 kg/m² or greater doubles the risk of heart failure; diabetes can double the risk in men and increase it by fivefold in women [2]. Smoking cessation strategies should be discussed, as this habit is independently associated with a 47% increased risk of heart failure [2]. Ex-smokers have been shown to have a 30% lower mortality rate than current smokers after 2 years of cessation [2].

Additionally, psychological stress may be a risk factor for heart failure, and his stressors are clearly affecting his health. Patients may benefit from learning stress, anger, and time management skills. He should be reminded to take his blood pressure medication, as this disease doubles his risk (it triples the risk in females) [2]. Treatment of hypertension can reduce the incidence of heart failure by nearly half [2]. Additionally, individuals with blood pressure greater than 160/90 are at double the risk of those with blood pressure less than 140/90 [2].

In other patients, providers should be mindful of a history of coronary artery disease, valvular heart disease, drug exposures (such as chemotherapy, cocaine, or non-steroidal anti-inflammatory drugs), alcohol use, and family history of heart failure or coronary artery disease [2, 3]. Patients should also be screened for sleep-disordered breathing, anemia, and chronic kidney disease.

The Health Aging and Body Composition (ABC) heart failure risk score [9] and the Framingham heart failure risk score (FHFRS) [10] are examples of proposed risk stratification tools. These scores take into account predictors of incident heart failure such as age, coronary artery disease, LV hypertrophy, systolic blood pressure, and heart rate.

2. **The patient is particularly concerned about congestive heart failure: his friend suffered from it until his death last year. He recalls that his friend had several ultrasounds of his heart over the course of a few years. He is strapped for cash but asks if any tests or an ultrasound can be done.**

According to the ACC/AHA guidelines, routine periodic population screening for asymptomatic reduced LV ejection fraction is not cost-effective and is not recommended [3]. This patient has numerous risk factors, though. Although routine use of natriuretic peptides is not yet justified, the guidelines acknowledge that screening with BNP prior to echocardiography may be a cost-effective approach to identifying high-risk patients [3].

Heidenreich et al. [11] studied the cost-effectiveness of utilizing BNP to screen for LV dysfunction by comparing four screening strategies:

- BNP with follow-up echocardiography for those with abnormal concentration and subsequent treatment with ACE inhibitors for those with LV ejection fraction under 40%
- BNP with treatment based on abnormal results

- Echocardiography with treatment based on abnormal results
- No screening

In populations with a 1 % prevalence of reduced LV ejection fraction, screening with BNP followed by echocardiography provided a cost-effective health benefit. Using the cost-effective standard threshold of $50,000 per quality-adjusted life year (QALY), this combined approach in men offered a $22,3000 incremental cost per QALY gained compared to no screening. Screening with echocardiography alone had an incremental cost of $123,500 per QALY gained. Using BNP alone was not only more expensive but led to a worse outcome. Due to a lower prevalence of disease (<1 %) in women, screening with BNP with follow-up echocardiography in this subset was less cost-effective at $77,700 per QALY gained. Both BNP alone and echocardiography alone, however, led to worse and more expensive outcomes [11].

Other data indicate NT-proBNP may be used as a "rule-out" tool for asymptomatic LV dysfunction in hypertensive or diabetic individuals, so could be considered in this patient's case. Betti et al. used NT-proBNP and echocardiography to screen 1,012 primary care patients on medications for type 2 diabetes and/or systemic hypertension for Stage B heart failure [12]. Diastolic dysfunction was present in 36.4 % of patients; systolic dysfunction was present in 1.1 %. Using an NT-proBNP cutoff value of 125 pg/mL was best for ruling out asymptomatic LV dysfunction, with a sensitivity and negative predictive value of 100 % in identifying pooled moderate-to-severe diastolic and systolic dysfunction in all subjects except males under 67 years, in whom the sensitivity was 87.5 %, and the negative predictive value was 99.5 % [12]. These results suggest low levels of natriuretic peptides basically exclude the presence of disease.

3. **The result return with NT-proBNP of 156 pg/ml. How should you interpret this result? What counseling is appropriate?**

Studies of BNP and NT-proBNP use various cutoffs. Currently, none have been validated for diagnosing or excluding heart failure in an outpatient setting, though several have been suggested. Betti et al. found that low NT-proBNP levels (<125 pg/mL) might rule-out LV dysfunction [12]; others have suggested utilizing a somewhat higher cut-point of 190 pg/mL [13], and still others have had successful screening strategies with even lower levels (i.e., 50 pg/mL in STOP-HF [8]).

How should this patient's result be interpreted? Betti et al. also discovered significant trends in NT-proBNP levels across different types of LV dysfunction. Levels were significantly higher in patients with asymptomatic LV dysfunction than in patients with normal echocardiograms. The highest values were observed in those with systolic dysfunction. They were also significantly different comparing mild, moderate, and severe diastolic dysfunction subgroups. Overall, however, the test was not useful for ruling in LV dysfunction: its specificity ranged from only 59.9 to 92.7 %, lowest for females over 67 years [12].

Though not diagnostic, natriuretic peptide testing provides incremental prognostic information. Choi et al. measured NT-proBNP in 5,597 multi-ethnic (non-Hispanic white, African-American, Hispanic, and Chinese) American men and women ages 45–84 years without a history of cardiovascular disease or heart failure [14]. During an average 5.5-year follow up, 111 experienced incident heart failure.

Of these cases, 77 % had NT-proBNP concentrations in the top quartile. NT-proBNP levels in the top quartile were significantly associated with incident heart failure in the total population (overall hazard ratio 10.52, 95 % CI 6.78–16.33, p<0.001) as well as in the non-Hispanic white, African-American, and Hispanic subsets [14]. (Incident heart failure in Chinese-Americans was lower than in the other ethnic groups, and the rate was deemed too low for statistical analysis.)

Thus, the patient in Case 1 should be counseled that although his NT-proBNP level is above the recommended cutoff of 125 pg/mL, it neither suggests nor diagnoses LV dysfunction; rather, it elevates the patient's risk level and provides grounds for a higher degree of vigilance including, perhaps, further investigation. Elevated natriuretic peptide concentrations can sometimes result from non-heart failure etiologies, such as obstructive sleep apnea, anemia, renal failure, or older age [3]. Nonetheless, since he is high-risk, further investigation should be considered.

4. When should this person be rescreened?

Analysis suggests that yearly screening with natriuretic peptides is not cost-effective [11]. Some studies suggest that serial NT-proBNP measurements, which can change substantially over 2–3 years, can reflect change in subclinical disease, though. In one study, apparently healthy individuals with an initially low NT-proBNP concentration who had an increase of 25 % (to a level of at least 190 pg/mL) had approximately twice the risk of incident heart failure and cardiovascular mortality over the next 10 or so years compared with those whose NT-proBNP level decreased or remained the same [13]. The same was true for subjects with initially high NT-proBNP whose levels increased by at least 25 % (approximately twice the risk compared to those with persistently high levels), whereas the opposite was true for those whose initially high levels decreased by at least 25 % to <190 pg/mL (approximately half the risk) [13].

As heart failure screening guidelines evolve, practitioners must realize that a single natriuretic peptide measurement may potentially rule-out LV dysfunction or contribute prognostic information at that time point, but trending levels may provide additional insight into a patient's cardiovascular health and whether it has changed. Although at present, natriuretic peptides are not routinely used for screening in clinical care, future screening guidelines may endorse not just one, but perhaps repeated natriuretic peptide measurements every 2–3 years.

5. When should echocardiography be considered?

As discussed, evidence suggests using BNP for screening prior to echocardiography is more cost-effective than echocardiography alone in ruling out heart failure [11]. Assessment of LV ejection fraction in asymptomatic individuals based on elevated natriuretic peptide levels should be considered but may not always lead to increased benefit. The Cardiovascular Health Study (CHS) was a multicenter, prospective observational cohort study of cardiovascular disease in 4,137 adults at least 65 years old without heart failure. Investigators measured baseline NT-proBNP and LV ejection fractions, a repeat NT-proBNP measurement after 2–3 years, and a repeat echocardiogram after 5 years. In this population with a 10.7 year median follow-up, the LV ejection fraction contributed minimally to the information provided by a single or repeat NT-proBNP level in evaluating risk for incident heart failure or cardiovascular mortality [15]. To detect one abnormal LV ejection fraction, 14 patients with a high baseline NT-proBNP concentration (>190 pg/mL) or 34 participants with initially normal (<190 pg/mL) but subsequently increased levels (with a >25 % increase to ≥190 pg/mL) would need to be screened [15].

Follow-up echocardiography in select patients could be useful, though. The same study demonstrated that individuals with either a high baseline or with an increasing NT-proBNP level were significantly more likely to develop a reduced LV ejection fraction compared to those with stably low NT-proBNP levels [15]. Since pharmacologic treatment of asymptomatic LV dysfunction has a proven benefit, a cost-effective approach might be screening the highest risk individuals for asymptomatic LV dysfunction with natriuretic peptides followed by echocardiography in those with either a high baseline value or an increasing value on repeat measurement a few years later.

6. He asks if he should see a cardiologist. How would you uptitrate care?

Physicians should be vigilant in patients with elevated natriuretic peptides levels. Individuals with Stage A or B heart failure and elevated BNP levels (≥100 pg/mL) carry as poor a prognosis as Stage C or D patients with BNP <100 pg/mL [16, 17]. Aside from LV dysfunction and incident heart failure, natriuretic peptide levels are predictive of stroke or transient ischemic attack, atrial fibrillation, and all-cause mortality [18]. Cognizant of this information, physicians should be motivated to enact more aggressive preventive treatment plans in certain patients.

The effectiveness of uptitration of care based on BNP was evident in STOP-HF. Patients in both the control and intervention groups significantly improved their hypertension control on follow-up (p < 0.001), but those in the latter group were prescribed significantly more renin-angiotensin-aldosterone-system agents (either aldosterone antagonists, angiotensin receptor blockers, or ACE inhibitors) (p < 0.01) [8]. In the intervention group, those with high BNP had a trend toward lower LDL-cholesterol (p = 0.07) and a significantly higher HDL-cholesterol (p = 0.004) level at the end of the study period, although both study arms had a similar increase in statin therapy [8]. Dedicated counseling may have led to increased awareness on both the parts of the primary care physician and the patient, and therefore improved adherence to therapy.

Summary of Case 1

This case highlights basics in screening for heart failure, which is still an area of investigation. Treatment of patients with asymptomatic LV dysfunction has a known benefit. In caring for patients, identifying risk factors is important. The ease of natriuretic peptide testing compared to echocardiography should be recognized and considered in clinical decision-making. Caveats in test interpretation, frequency of rescreening, and possible uptitration of care must be taken into consideration when ordering an initial BNP or NT-proBNP level. Patient and practioner awareness is crucial.

Special Populations

Heidenreich et al., among other investigators, noted that the utility and cost-effectiveness of natriuretic peptides as a screening modality depends on the prevalence of LV dysfunction in the subgroup being screened: the test may be more economical in higher risk patients, such as those with prior atherosclerotic events, rather than all-comers [11]. The next cases discuss special patient populations.

> **Case 2**
> Consider the scenario if the patient in Case 1 were female.

How Might Clinical Decision-Making Based on Natriuretic Peptide Levels Change?

The STOP-HF study used a non-gender-specific BNP cutoff of 50 pg/mL for further evaluation with echocardiography and referral to specialized cardiology care, but most data suggest that sex- and age-specific cut-points would strengthen the value of natriuretic peptides in screening [18–20]. This idea correlates with the increase in concentrations of natriuretic peptides observed in women and also with older age. The physiologic mechanism for higher natriuretic peptide concentrations in women compared with men is not fully established but is likely related to sex hormones [20].

Despite the fact that natriuretic peptide levels tend to run higher in women compared to men, most studies have shown that, with appropriate cut-points, their ability to predict heart failure risk is at least as strong in women as it is in men [14, 18, 21].

> **Case 3**
> Your patient is a 19-year-old college sophomore who currently runs 6 miles per day. She presents to your office for a required physical prior to joining the varsity cross-country team. She mentions occasional dizziness after her most strenuous runs but reports a quick recovery. She denies a history of syncope and has no significant past medical history. She takes no medications. She denies tobacco, alcohol, or recreational drug use. Her family history is negative for cardiovascular disease. Her pulse is 59, and her blood pressure is 103/68. Her BMI is 20 kg/m².

Would BNP Be Useful in Pre-participation Screening for Cardiac Abnormalities in This Patient?

Currently, data indicate that BNP is not useful as part of the pre-participation screening for cardiac abnormalities. One study of 457 college varsity athletes examined BNP and NT-proBNP levels at least 1 h after exercise [22]. Cardiac structure and function were evaluated by hand-held echocardiography in 200 of the subjects. Most athletes had low natriuretic peptide levels. Subjects with a history of exertional dizziness or passing out had significantly higher natriuretic peptide levels, which ultimately did not correlate with any structural abnormalities or exam indicator such as hypertension or cardiac murmur [22]. Further studies are needed prior to applying natriuretic peptides to clinical decision-making in this population.

> **Case 4**
> Your patient is a 45-year-old Caucasian woman with no significant past medical history. Her adoptive father had a heart attack last year, and since then, has developed heart failure that significantly limits his physical activities. Your patient recently read a newspaper article describing the benefits of treating patients with asymptomatic LV dysfunction, and she wonders if she falls into this category. She takes no medications and uses no substances. Her blood pressure is 116/76; pulse is 84.

Should You Consider Screening This Patient for LV Dysfunction with Natriuretic Peptides?

A study including 703 healthy individuals without traditional risk factors for heart failure found that NT-proBNP was not predictive of death, heart failure, cerebral vascular accident, or myocardial infarction, suggesting against the use of this biomarker in obtaining information regarding future cardiovascular events, including heart failure, in healthy normal subjects in the community [23].

Other Considerations: Natriuretic Peptides in Conjunction with Risk Scores and Other Biomarkers

Some studies advocate that natriuretic peptides can be helpful in screening for stage B heart failure when used in conjunction with risk scores such as the Health Aging and Body Composition heart failure risk score and the Framingham heart failure risk score [24]. In the future, BNP could also be used as part of a multi-marker approach to screening. Several studies have evaluated highly sensitive troponin in conjunction with natriuretic peptides to screen for heart failure risk, with incremental benefit found [21, 25]. Taking it even a step further, one study found that a panel of soluble ST2, growth differentiation factor-15, highly sensitive troponin I, high-sensitivity C-reactive protein, and BNP was useful in categorizing risk and prognosticating death, heart failure, and cardiovascular events [26]. Combining multiple biomarkers that reflect distinct pathophysiologic disturbances within the heart failure spectrum may be a way to improve both specificity and sensitivity when assessing risk. Ultimately, this approach may also be a way to tailor preventive therapy in a more individualized fashion, by identifying and targeting the particular pathways that show biomarker perturbations.

Although the use of panels of biomarkers for risk assessment is not yet validated, such combined approaches are a realistic possibility for heart failure screening in the future.

Conclusions

In considering the value of natriuretic peptides in screening for heart failure in the community, the analytic framework in Fig. 15.1 provides a useful and important foundation. High-risk groups are identifiable by clinical characteristics and can be further delineated by natriuretic peptide levels. Many studies have emphasized the potential of natriuretic peptides as an easy "rule-out" test, but positive results and change in results over time also yield important prognostic information. These levels can affect clinical decisions, as treating asymptomatic LV dysfunction improves outcomes. Still, whether natriuretic peptide-guided screening or treatment leads to significant adverse effects remains unknown. The 2013 AHA policy statement called for a change in community practices to avoid the impending growth in heart failure prevalence and healthcare expenditure, including increased prevention of hypertension, hyperlipidemia, smoking, and obesity; adherence to guideline-based therapies; and application of new heart failure therapies [1]. Perhaps application of natriuretic peptides is the crucial advancement that could spur a decrease in heart failure incidence. Future guidelines may include a screening algorithm as in Fig. 15.2 – one that relies on good clinical judgment and uses BNP or NT-proBNP as a stepping-stone to uptitration of care for screening and treatment of stage B heart failure.

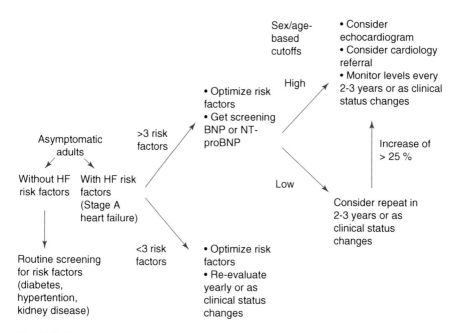

Fig. 15.2 Possible baseline algorithm for future natriuretic peptide use for screening for heart failure in the community

References

1. Heidenreich PA, Albert NM, Allen LA, Bluemke DA, Butler J, Fonarow GC, et al. Forecasting the impact of heart failure in the United States: a policy statement from the American Heart Association. Circ Heart Fail. 2013;6(3):606–19.
2. Bui AL, Horwich TB, Fonarow GC. Epidemiology and risk profile of heart failure. Nat Rev Cardiol. 2011;8(1):30–41.
3. Yancy CW, Jessup M, Bozkurt B, Butler J, Casey Jr DE, Drazner MH, et al. 2013 ACCF/AHA guideline for the management of heart failure: a report of the American College of Cardiology Foundation/American Heart Association Task Force on Practice Guidelines. J Am Coll Cardiol. 2013;62(16):e147–239.
4. Redfield MM, Jacobsen SJ, Burnett Jr JC, Mahoney DW, Bailey KR, Rodeheffer RJ. Burden of systolic and diastolic ventricular dysfunction in the community: appreciating the scope of the heart failure epidemic. JAMA. 2003;289(2):194–202.
5. Effect of enalapril on mortality and the development of heart failure in asymptomatic patients with reduced left ventricular ejection fractions. N Engl J Med. 1992;327(10):685–91.
6. McDonagh TA, Robb SD, Murdoch DR, Morton JJ, Ford I, Morrison CE, et al. Biochemical detection of left-ventricular systolic dysfunction. Lancet. 1998;351(9095):9–13.
7. Harris RP, Helfand M, Woolf SH, Lohr KN, Mulrow CD, Teutsch SM, et al. Current methods of the US Preventive Services Task Force: a review of the process. Am J Prev Med. 2001;20(3 Suppl):21–35.
8. Ledwidge M, Gallagher J, Conlon C, Tallon E, O'Connell E, Dawkins I, et al. Natriuretic peptide-based screening and collaborative care for heart failure: the STOP-HF randomized trial. JAMA. 2013;310(1):66–74.
9. Butler J, Kalogeropoulos A, Georgiopoulou V, Belue R, Rodondi N, Garcia M, et al. Incident heart failure prediction in the elderly: the health ABC heart failure score. Circ Heart Fail. 2008;1(2):125–33.
10. Kannel WB, D'Agostino RB, Silbershatz H, Belanger AJ, Wilson PW, Levy D. Profile for estimating risk of heart failure. Arch Intern Med. 1999;159(11):1197–204.
11. Heidenreich PA, Gubens MA, Fonarow GC, Konstam MA, Stevenson LW, Shekelle PG. Cost-effectiveness of screening with B-type natriuretic peptide to identify patients with reduced left ventricular ejection fraction. J Am Coll Cardiol. 2004;43(6):1019–26.
12. Betti I, Castelli G, Barchielli A, Beligni C, Boscherini V, De Luca L, et al. The role of N-terminal PRO-brain natriuretic peptide and echocardiography for screening asymptomatic left ventricular dysfunction in a population at high risk for heart failure. The PROBE-HF study. J Card Fail. 2009;15(5):377–84.
13. deFilippi CR, Christenson RH, Gottdiener JS, Kop WJ, Seliger SL. Dynamic cardiovascular risk assessment in elderly people. The role of repeated N-terminal pro-B-type natriuretic peptide testing. J Am Coll Cardiol. 2010;55(5):441–50.
14. Choi EY, Bahrami H, Wu CO, Greenland P, Cushman M, Daniels LB, et al. N-terminal pro-B-type natriuretic peptide, left ventricular mass, and incident heart failure: Multi-Ethnic Study of Atherosclerosis. Circ Heart Fail. 2012;5(6):727–34.
15. deFilippi CR, Christenson RH, Kop WJ, Gottdiener JS, Zhan M, Seliger SL. Left ventricular ejection fraction assessment in older adults: an adjunct to natriuretic peptide testing to identify risk of new-onset heart failure and cardiovascular death? J Am Coll Cardiol. 2011;58(14):1497–506.
16. Daniels LB. Natriuretic Peptides and Assessment of Cardiovascular Disease Risk in Asymptomatic Persons. Curr Cardiovasc Risk Rep. 2010;4(2):120–7.
17. Daniels LB, Clopton P, Jiang K, Greenberg B, Maisel AS. Prognosis of stage A or B heart failure patients with elevated B-type natriuretic peptide levels. J Card Fail. 2010;16(2):93–8.
18. Wang TJ, Larson MG, Levy D, Benjamin EJ, Leip EP, Omland T, et al. Plasma natriuretic peptide levels and the risk of cardiovascular events and death. N Engl J Med. 2004;350(7):655–63.

19. Vasan RS, Benjamin EJ, Larson MG, Leip EP, Wang TJ, Wilson PW, et al. Plasma natriuretic peptides for community screening for left ventricular hypertrophy and systolic dysfunction: the Framingham heart study. JAMA. 2002;288(10):1252–9.
20. Redfield MM, Rodeheffer RJ, Jacobsen SJ, Mahoney DW, Bailey KR, Burnett Jr JC. Plasma brain natriuretic peptide concentration: impact of age and gender. J Am Coll Cardiol. 2002;40(5):976–82.
21. Nambi V, Liu X, Chambless LE, de Lemos JA, Virani SS, Agarwal S, et al. Troponin T and N-terminal pro-B-type natriuretic peptide: a biomarker approach to predict heart failure risk-- the atherosclerosis risk in communities study. Clin Chem. 2013;59(12):1802–10.
22. Daniels LB, Allison MA, Clopton P, Redwine L, Siecke N, Taylor K, et al. Use of natriuretic peptides in pre-participation screening of college athletes. Int J Cardiol. 2008;124(3):411–4.
23. McKie PM, Cataliotti A, Lahr BD, Martin FL, Redfield MM, Bailey KR, et al. The prognostic value of N-terminal pro-B-type natriuretic peptide for death and cardiovascular events in healthy normal and stage A/B heart failure subjects. J Am Coll Cardiol. 2010;55(19):2140–7.
24. Gupta S, Rohatgi A, Ayers CR, Patel PC, Matulevicius SA, Peshock RM, et al. Risk scores versus natriuretic peptides for identifying prevalent stage B heart failure. Am Heart J. 2011;161(5):923–30. e2.
25. Glick D, DeFilippi CR, Christenson R, Gottdiener JS, Seliger SL. Long-term trajectory of two unique cardiac biomarkers and subsequent left ventricular structural pathology and risk of incident heart failure in community-dwelling older adults at low baseline risk. JACC Heart Fail. 2013;1(4):353–60.
26. Wang TJ, Wollert KC, Larson MG, Coglianese E, McCabe EL, Cheng S, et al. Prognostic utility of novel biomarkers of cardiovascular stress: the Framingham Heart Study. Circulation. 2012;126(13):1596–604.

Chapter 16
Natriuretic Peptide Use in the Emergency Department

W. Frank Peacock and Salvator DiSomma

Abstract Shortness of breath is a common emergency department presentation frequently requiring early treatment to realize optimal outcomes. The most rapidly performed diagnostics, that of taking a history and physical, or limited by their poor accuracy, and the most accurate determinates are not available in a fashion early enough for emergency medicine usage. Because they are available shortly after emergency department presentation, natriuretic peptides can improve diagnostic accuracy and thus guide the implementation of mortality reducing interventions.

The most frequent ED presenting symptom of acute decompensated heart failure is shortness of breath. Unfortunately, this extremely common presentation can be a diagnostic challenge as it can occur in a large number of conditions, an abbreviated list of which appears in Table 16.1.

Keywords Natriuretic peptides • B-type Natriuretic peptide • N-terminal pro-B type natriuretic peptide • Emergency Department • Heart Failure

The Case of Elbow Macaroni

Elbow Macaroni is a 77 year old morbidly obese female patient who presents by EMS to the ED after walking up the stairs to her church at 10 am Sunday morning. Well known to the hospital, she has suffered with a long history of COPD, and was hospitalized twice in the last year; once for pneumonia and once for a gastrointestinal bleeding event felt to be

W.F. Peacock, MD, FACEP (✉)
Department of Emergency Medicine, Baylor College of Medicine, Houston, TX, USA

Ben Taub General Hospital, Houston, TX, USA
e-mail: frankpeacock@gmail.com

S. DiSomma, MD, PhD
Department of Internal Medicine, Emergency Medicine, San Andrea Hospital,
San Andreas, CA, USA

Department of Medical-Surgery Sciences and Translational Medicine, University Rome
Sapienza, Rome, Italy

© Springer International Publishing Switzerland 2016
A.S. Maisel, A.S. Jaffe (eds.), *Cardiac Biomarkers*,
DOI 10.1007/978-3-319-42982-3_16

secondary to the anticoagulant she takes for her atrial fibrillation. Mrs. Macaroni has also suffered from diabetes for the last 28 years, during which despite being moderately compliant with her therapy, both her vision and renal function have markedly declined. Today's visit was predicated by increasing fatigue, and nausea, the latter of which caused her to miss her morning antihypertensive diuretic dose on the day of presentation. She also reports cough, which she states kept her up most of last night.

On arrival, the patient's vital signs demonstrate an irregularly irregular tachycardia of 122, a respiratory rate of 28, BP 165/99, and an oxygen saturation of 89%. She is dyspneic to the point of having difficulty speaking, diaphoretic, and sitting upright in the bed.

Because of the delays in therapy are associated with increased rates of adverse outcomes, early treatment is critical. But what treatment is immediately necessary is not always obvious. The importance of both early and correct treatment is supported by the following investigation by Wuerz [1], In a cohort of 499 patients transferred by ambulance and ultimately found to suffer heart failure, the probability of survival was 251% (95% CI 137–455, p<0.01) higher if treatment was performed before getting in the ambulance, rather than delayed until hospital arrival, which occurred average of 36 min later. However, patients who received early treatment, but for the wrong disease suffered even more. In patients with non-HF causes of dyspnea, their mortality increased >350% (p<0.05) if treated with HF therapy instead of bronchodilators. Ultimately, there is a clear premium on diagnostic accuracy (Table 16.1).

It would seem that Mrs. Macaroni would require immediate treatment, and oxygen supplementation should be started as soon as possible. Considering her level of distress, positive pressure ventilation would be a reasonable intervention. Careful and constant observation to detect any signs of respiratory fatigue should be implemented. If she appears to be tiring, preparations for endotracheal intubations should be readied. At this junction the differential includes too many therapeutic options, beyond airway stabilization. The history and physical may provide useful clues, and an initial approach to evaluating the severely dyspneic patient appears in Fig. 16.1.

Unfortunately, in the EMS environment and early after ED arrival, investigation beyond a simple history and physical exam are just not available. The history and physical should be done in phases, first as an initial survey, and then later when more stable a more complete investigation can be performed, all based on patient tolerance and the need to initiate immediate treatment.

It is helpful to know the extent to which the exam and clinical impression is useful. Table 16.2 shows the performance of various aspects of the history and physical. Even a finding such as the S3, which has excellent specificity, has such poor sensitivity that its value is minimized in a large portion of the HF population.

Physicians must be willing to constantly re-asses their initial impression in response to therapy, and as new data become available. Utilization of established criteria help in making a diagnosis. The Framingham criteria [2, 3], using history and physical findings, require at least 1 major and 2 minor criteria for diagnosis. (Table 16.3). The Boston criteria (Table 16.4) adds chest x-ray (CXR) to the history and exam [4]. More points give higher probabilities for HF. A score>4 correlates with a PAOP >12 mmHg, and has a sensitivity and specificity of 90% and 85%, respectively. These criteria are validated, but are limited when asymptomatic.

Table 16.1 Abbreviated list of causes of shortness of breath

1. Cardiac
(a) Heart Failure
(b) Myocardial Infarction
(c) Pericarditis
(d) Atrial fibrillation
2. Pulmonary
(a) Pneumonia
(b) Pneumothorax
(c) Pulmonary Embolus
(d) Asthma/COPD exacerbation
(e) Lung Cancer
(f) Pleural effusion/Empyema
(g) Pneumomediatstinum
(h) Aspiration/Foreign Body
3. Metabolic
(a) Anemia
(b) Compensation for metabolic acidosis (e.g., DKA)
(c) Poisoning (e.g., metHgb, cyanide)
(d) Anaphylaxis/Allergic reaction
4. Psychiatric
(a) Anxiety
(b) Panic Attack
5. Musculoskeletal
(a) Tietze's (costrochondritis)
(b) Mondor's syndrome (chest wall thrombophlebitis)
6. Miscellaneous
(a) Amniotic fluid embolus
(b) Subdiaphragmatic abscess
(c) Large volume ascities

The Importance of Obtaining a History

If a patient's dyspnea is not too extreme and they are able to provide a history, a number of parameters can suggest either new or exacerbated HF. While the ED HF patient commonly has shortness of breath, other complaints supporting a diagnosis of HF include dyspnea on exertion, orthopnea, peripheral edema, weight gain, paroxysmal nocturnal dyspnea, cough and fatigue. As HF commonly occurs in elderly patients with multiple comorbidities, conditions that worsen or precipitate HF should be considered. These include acute anemia, infection, worsening comorbidities, selected over-the-counter medication use, and iatrogenic electrolyte abnormalities. Dietary and medication non-compliance commonly account for HF decompensation, and so the patient's habits should be evaluated. Finally, because alcohol and drug use, or their withdrawal, adversely impact cardiac function, they should also be considered.

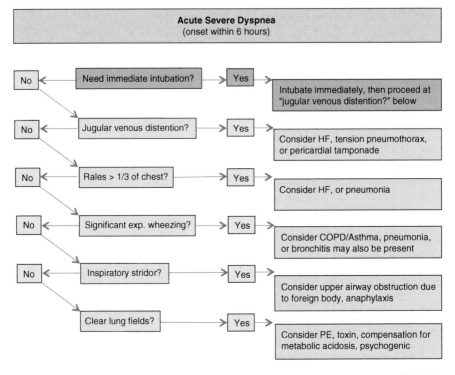

Fig. 16.1 Approach to the rapid evaluation of a patient presenting with acute dyspnea. The decision to intubate a patient with severe dyspnea is not determined by the results of any objective testing. Rather it is a clinical decision based solely on the physicians' impression that the patient is either currently, or imminently will, suffer acute respiratory failure. In cooperative but distressed patients, a limited trial of BiPap or CPAP may allow enough time for immediate therapeutic interventions to take effect, thus avoiding the need for more invasive measures. However, non-invasive ventilatory measures are not definitive airway management and should be considered as short term temporary adjuncts. If improvement in clinical status is not seen relatively quickly after their implementation, endotracheal intubation should be considered

Table 16.2 Sensitivity and specificity of various aspects of the history and physical

Variable	Sensitivity	Specificity	Accuracy
Hx of HF	62	94	80
Dyspnea	56	53	54
Orthopnea	47	88	72
Rales	56	80	70
S3 (auscultation)	20	99	66
JVD	39	94	72
Edema	67	68	68

Table 16.3 Framingham criteria for the diagnosis of heart failure

Major criteria	Minor criteria
Paroxysmal nocturnal dyspnea	Extremity edema
Neck vein distention	Night cough
Rales	Dyspnea on exertion
Cardiomegaly	Hepatomegaly
Acute pulmonary edema	Pleural effusion
S_3 gallop	Vital capacity reduce by 1/3 of normal
Increased venous pressure (>16 cm H_2O)	Tachycardia ($\geq$120)
Positive HJR	

Table 16.4 Boston criteria for diagnosing congestive heart failure

History	
Dyspnea at rest	4
Orthopnea	4
Paroxysmal nocturnal dyspnea	3
Dyspnea while walking	2
Dyspnea while climbing stairs	1
Chest X-ray	
Alveolar pulmonary edema	4
Interstitial pulmonary edema	3
Bilateral pleural effusions	3
Cardiothoracic ratio >0.5	3
Kerley A lines	2
Physical exam	
HR 91–110 bpm	1
HR >110 bpm	2
JVD >6 cm H_2O	2
JVD & edema or hepatomegaly	3
Basilar rales	1
Rales >basilar	2
Wheezing	3
S_3 gallop	3

Physical Examination Limitations

The initial part of the exam focuses on the vital signs and airway stability. Lung sounds, peripheral edema, JVD, abdominal jugular reflux (AJR), and the presence of extra heart sounds can help identify volume overload. Skin mottling, indicative of poor peripheral perfusion, is ominous, with a 17.5 odds ratio for hospital mortality [5]. Locating the point of maximal impulse (PMI) helps estimate the chronicity of HF. In chronic HF the PMI is shifted laterally due to ventricular remodeling. It is important to recognize that the exam has critical limits and variable performance metrics. In one study JVD and AJR had a predictive accuracy of only 81 % for pulmonary artery obstructive pressure > 18 mmHg, while rales had a positive predictive value of 100 %, versus a negative predictive value of only 35 % [6]. In another study, AJR had a sensitivity of 24 %, but a specificity of 94 % [4].

> *On physical, although she has audible wheezes to the extent that the cardiac exam is limited, Mrs. Macaroni's breathing pattern does not exemplify an difficulties in expiration (which if present, would have suggested an exacerbation of her prior COPD). Further, she has rales about half-way up her lung fields, greater on the right than the left, and although her obesity makes the interpretation of JVD difficult, she does have 1+ lower extremity edema. At this point the physician has enough information to initiate treatment.*

> *Clearly, antihypertensive therapy would be appropriate as it may optimize hemodynamics if ultimately a diagnosis of HF is made. Since HF is a likely cause of her presentation, sublingual, transdermal, or intravenous nitroglycerin could all be considered. Furthermore, aerosol bronchodilators may be utilized. While they provide minimal benefit in the setting of HF, their use may provide some improvement in the likely possibility that the patient's history of COPD is contributing to her dyspnea. At this point, an ECG and portable x-ray should be obtained, and lab testing initiated.*

Chest Radiography

Although negative films do not exclude abnormal LV function, a chest x-ray (CXR) is necessary as it can eliminate other diagnoses (e.g., pneumonia) from the differential. The x-ray findings of HF are, in descending frequency: dilated upper lobe vessels, cardiomegaly, interstitial edema, enlarged pulmonary artery, pleural effusion, alveolar edema, prominent superior vena cava, Kerley lines [7]. Since abnormalities lag the clinical appearance by hours, therapy is not withheld pending a film.

In chronic HF, CXR signs of congestion have unreliable sensitivity, specificity, and predictive value in identifying those with high pulmonary artery occlusive pressure (PAOP) [8]. Radiographic pulmonary congestion was absent in 53 % of mild to moderately elevated PAOP's (16–29 mmHg) and in 39 % of those with markedly elevated PAOP (>30 mmHg).

Cardiomegaly is useful in diagnosing HF. A cardiothoracic ratio > 60 % correlates with higher 5-year mortality [9]. However, CXRs have poor sensitivity for cardiomegaly [10]. In echocardiographically proven cardiomegaly, 22 % had cardiothoracic ratios <50 % [10]. Poor CXR detection of cardiomegaly is explained by intrathoracic cardiac rotation.

Pleural effusions are missed by CXR, especially if intubated and performed supine. In patients with pleural effusions, sensitivity, specificity, and accuracy of the supine CXR was 67 %, 70 %, and 67 %, respectively [11].

The sensitivity for HF findings with a portable CXR is poor. In mild HF, only dilated upper lobe vessels were found in greater than 60 % of patients. The frequency that CXR HF parameters are found increases with the severity of HF. With severe HF, x-ray findings occurred in at least 2/3's, except for Kerley lines in 11 % and a prominent vena cava in 44 % [12].

Echocardiography

Bedside ultrasound, when performed by the emergency physician, provides a rapid, non-invasive, inexpensive measure to assist in determining the etiology of dyspnea. It can evaluate for the presence of pneumothorax, provide information on myocardial contractility, and determine the presence of a pericardial effusion. And by looking at the lungs, ultrasound can aid in differentiating between the HF and the COPD by the identification of B-lines. It may also give information on pulmonary volume overload by direct lung imaging or by the evaluation of vena cava diameter changes that occur as a result of the respiratory cycle. Finally, ejection fraction can be measured, and while it helps defines the etiology and type of HF, there is no correlation between EF and symptoms.

Lab Testing

A number of lab tests may be performed, but with the exception of cardiac markers (natriuretic peptides and troponin), the causes of shortness of breath are not commonly identified by the lab. Unsuspected anemia, renal failure, severe electrolyte abnormalities, or perturbations of acid base status may contribute to shortness of breath, but rarely do severe symptoms arise from these factors alone.

Of note, while ABG's may be determine acid–base status and be of use when managing an intubated patient, their results are rarely of any diagnostic assistance in the acute setting. They should not be used to evaluate the airway or the need for intubation at the acute presentation. While they may be of use later in the management, at the time of presentation the time wasted obtaining ABG's is better spent performing a clinical assessment and initial interventions.

Natriuretic Peptides

Since they became commercially available late in the twentieth century, natriuretic peptides have been an important part of the emergency physician's armamentarium to help discriminate a potential heart failure presentation from that of the large number of its mimics. Natriuretic peptides represent a rapid and accurate test to assist in the evaluation of patients presenting with acute dyspnea. In the Breathing Not Properly trial [13] of >1500 patients presenting to an emergency department with undifferentiated dyspnea, the physician's diagnostic accuracy by clinical judgment was only 74%, but improved to 81.6% when the results of BNP testing were considered.

In Mrs. Macaroni's case, her BNP level returned from the point of care lab 23 minutes after her arrival in the ED. A result of 400 pg/mL requires some interpretation considerations, as this is considerably lower than might have been otherwise expected.

It is well described that BNP is found at levels lower than clinically expected in several situations relevant to the ED. First is in the setting of flash pulmonary edema, where an otherwise compensated patient experiences an acute episode of severe and nearly immediate onset dyspnea. In this setting it is not uncommon for the initial NP measurement to be lower than expected. This has been hypothesized to simply be the result of insufficient time for the protein to be synthesized and released into the circulation by the stressed myocardium and may explain the relatively low natriuretic peptide level of Mrs. Macaroni.

A second cause of unexpectedly low NP levels is reported to occur with obesity [14, 15]. It is unclear why this occurs, but it is well described with all NP and is an important consideration as most of the developed world struggles with an overwhelming obesity epidemic. Some have recommended doubling the BNP level while using the standard cutpoints in patients with a BMI above 35. In the case of Mrs. Macaroni, this would result in a corrected BNP level of 800, and clearly in the HF range.

Other factors can confound the interpretation of NP. This includes the fact that NP levels are critically affected by renal function, as circulating levels of both peptides markedly increase with declining kidney function [16]. In subjects with normal kidney function, 1/6th of secreted BNP is cleaved by the kidney with the remainder either bound by its receptors or inactivated by neutral endopeptidase. Additionally, as deterioration in kidney function has a greater impact on NT-proBNP than BNP levels, kidney function should be taken into account when interpreting data on BNP or NT-proBNP.

Of greatest importance when interpreting NP levels is the consideration of an alternative non-HF diagnosis. Because NP's are released in the setting of ventricular overload, it is commonly a heart failure test. However, a consideration of the differential diagnosis list of causes of shortness of breath finds that many are associated with ventricular wall stretch (e.g., myocardial infarction, pulmonary embolus, etc.). In these settings, while NP's may be elevated, it is not the result of a HF diagnosis, but rather caused by other etiologies (e.g., AMI, PE, etc.). Therefore, it is important to consider alternative explanations for the clinical picture rather than assuming an elevation of NP is always due to AHF.

Secondly, while the presence of an elevated NP can be suggestive of ventricular stress in the setting of heart failure, it is important to consider the possibility that multiple conditions may be present. For example, if a patient presents with pneumonia and has HF, they will have an elevated NP. It is critical that both underlying pathologies are diagnosed and treated. This is an important consideration as occurs most commonly in an older population that frequently suffers multiple co-morbidities. To assume that an elevated NP represents the solitary cause of dyspnea is done so at the patient's risk. It is thus the responsibility of the physician to consider that the possibility of multiple sources of dyspnea may exist, and implement appropriate therapy for their treatment.

Lastly, when interpreting the clinical meaning of the NP test result in a patient presenting to the emergency department with an elevated level, it is extremely valuable to have some knowledge of their baseline. It is common that patients with chronic HF will have a persistently elevated NP level and that it will exceed the rule out HF cutpoint. When a previously unknown patient presents to the emergency department, whether an elevated NP represents a new elevation, or is simply their chronic dry weight baseline requires knowledge of their usual status.

Further, when HF patients with a known chronically elevated NP level present to the emergency department, the significant relative change value (RCV) must be considered. The RCV is the amount of change in a lab test that is associated with an increased probability of a clinically relevant change in the patient's underlying status, as opposed to a normal variation of the lab result. It is generally supported that a NP elevation exceeding twice the patient's baseline is suggestive of a clinically relevant HF exacerbation. Increases less than a doubling of their baseline dry weight NP should prompt an investigation of other potential causes of patient's presentation. For decreasing NP levels, the clinically relevant change is generally felt to be a 50% decrease, with decreasing levels of less than 50% not representing clinically significant improvements of baseline status [17].

The Need for Diagnostic Speed

The emergency department represents a clinical environment where gravely ill patients may present mixed among large numbers of moderately sick individuals. Thus a sorting process is required to identify, as rapidly as possible, those who need immediate intervention, hospitalization, or therapy from those in who discharge for outpatient therapy would be appropriate. The need for rapid diagnosis and treatment is supported by one analysis [18] of 14,900 hospitalized acute decompensated heart failure patients who were stratified by BNP and the time it took to receive treatment with loop diuretics. Data from this study demonstrate that the greatest acute mortality was seen in the group of patients with the highest BNP levels and who suffered the longest delay in treatment (Fig. 16.2). In fact, treatment delays of as little as 4 h resulted in a subsequent 250% relative mortality increase in the group with BNP levels exceeding 1865 pg/mL.

Unique to emergency medicine practice is the concept that all patients must go somewhere within as little as 4 h after their arrival. This further complicates the sorting process that is an integral part of emergency medicine. Natriuretic peptides have unique utility in helping to decide on where patients will be optimally served. This is because presentation NP levels are directly associated with short term

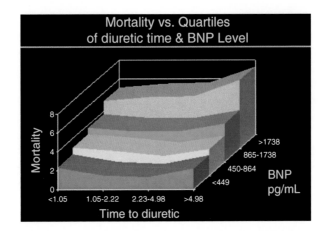

Fig. 16.2 Mortality vs. time to diuretic in quartiles of presentation BNP Level (From Maisel et al. [18], with permission)

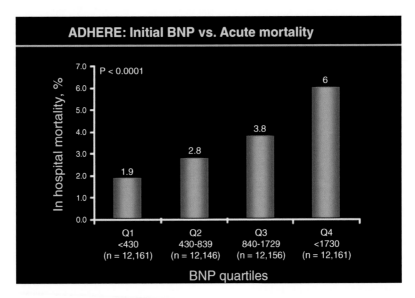

Fig. 16.3 Outcomes vs presentation natriuretic peptide level (From Fonarow et al. [19], with permission)

mortality and can help identifying a subset of patients who may potentially benefit from ICU admission. In an analysis of over 45,000 patients [19], higher BNP levels were reported to be reflective of greater acute mortality risk (Fig. 16.3). In this analysis, the lowest inpatient mortality (subsequently 1.9 %) was seen when the initial BNP was below 430 pg/mL, but increased to 6 % in the cohort with a BNP exceeding 1730 pg/mL (p < 0.0001). As a mortality rate of 6 % exceeds the contemporary mortality rate of myocardial infarction, early knowledge of the NP level may help emergency physician's to decide if a patient is an ICU candidate or could be appropriately served in regular medical floor unit.

In our case of Mrs. Macaroni, since she is a new presentation, consideration of her baseline status is unknowable. However, it is common in the emergency department for patients to present with a clear history of a prior HF diagnosis, and no knowledge of their baseline NP levels. When this occurs, the physician must consider the acuity of the patient's presentation, and the severity of their symptoms, when making diagnostic and disposition decisions

References

1. Wuerz RC, Meador SA. Effects of prehospital medications on mortality and length of stay in congestive heart failure. Ann Emerg Med. 2002;21(6):669–74. Maisel AS et al. N Engl J Med. 2002;347(3):161-7.
2. McKee PA, Castelli WP, McNamara PM, et al. The natural history of congestive heart failure: the Framingham study. N Engl J Med. 1971;285:1441–6.
3. Ho KKL, Anderson KM, Kannel WB, Grossman W, Levy D. Congestive heart failure/myocardial responses/valvular heart disease: survival after the onset of congestive heart failure in Framingham heart study subjects. Circulation. 1993;88(1):107–15.
4. Marantz PR, Kaplan MC, Alderman MH. Clinical diagnosis of congestive heart failure in patients with acute dyspnea. Chest. 1990;97(4):776–81.
5. Le Conte P, Coutant V, N'Guyen JM, Baron D, Touze MD, Potel G. Prognostic factors in acute cardiogenic pulmonary edema. Am J Emerg Med. 1999;17:329–32.
6. Butman SM, Ewy GA, Standen JR, Kern KB, Hahn E. Bedside cardiovascular examination in patients with severe chronic heart failure: importance of reset or inducible jugular venous distention. JACC. 1993;22(4):968–74.
7. Cohn JN, Johnson G, Ziesche S, Cobb F, Francis G, Tristani F, et al. A comparison of enlapril with hydralazine-isosorbide dinitrate in the treatment of chronic congestive heart failure. NEJM. 1991;325:303–10.
8. Chakko S, Woska D, Marinez H, et al. Clinical, radiographic, and hemodynamic correlation's in chronic congestive heart failure: conflicting results may lead to inappropriate care. Am J Med. 1991;90:353–9.
9. Koga Y, Wada T, Toshima H, Akazawa K, Nose Y. Prognostic significance of electrocardiographic findings in patients with dilated cardiomyopathy. Heart Ves. 1993;8:37–41.
10. Kono T, Suwa M, Hanada H, Hirota Y, Kawamura K. Clinical significance of normal cardiac silhouette in dilated cardiomyopathy–evaluation based upon echocardiography and magnetic resonance imaging. Jpn Circ J. 1992;56(4):359–65.
11. Ruskin JA, Gurney JW, Thorsen MK, Goodman LR. Detection of pleural effusions on supine chest radiographs. AJR. 1987;148:681–3.
12. Chait A, Cohen HE, Meltzer LE, VanDurme JP. The bedside chest radiograph in the evaluation of incipient heart failure. Radiology. 1972;105:563–6.
13. Maisel AS, Krishnaswamy P, Nowak RM, McCord J, Hollander JE, Duc P, Omland T, Storrow AB, Abraham WT, Wu AH, Clopton P, Steg PG, Westheim A, Knudsen CW, Perez A, Kazanegra R, Hermann HC, McCullough PA, Breathing Not Properly Multinational Study Investigators, et al. Rapid measurement of B-type natriuretic peptide in the emergency diagnosis of heart failure. N Engl J Med. 2002;347(3):161–7.

14. Das SR, Drazner MH, Dries DL, Vega GL, Stanek HG, Abdullah SM, et al. Impact of body mass and body composition on circulating levels of natriuretic peptides results from the Dallas Heart Study. Circulation. 2005;112:2163–8.
15. McCord JM, Mundy BJ, Hudson MP, Maisel AS, Hollander JE, Abraham WT, et al. Relationship between obesity and B-type natriuretic peptide levels. Arch Intern Med. 2004;164:2247–52.
16. Maisel A, Mueller C, Adams Jr K, Anker SD, Aspromonte N, Cleland JG, Cohen-Solal A, Dahlstrom U, DeMaria A, Di Somma S, Filippatos GS, Fonarow GC, Jourdain P, Komajda M, Liu PP, McDonagh T, McDonald K, Mebazaa A, Nieminen MS, Peacock WF, Tubaro M, Valle R, Vanderhyden M, Yancy CW, Zannad F, Braunwald E. State of the art: using natriuretic peptide levels in clinical practice. Eur J Heart Fail. 2008;10(9):824–39. doi:10.1016/j. ejheart.2008.07.014. Epub 2008 Aug 29.
17. Di Somma S, Magrini L, Ferri E. In-hospital brain natriuretic peptide and N-terminal prohormone brain natriuretic peptide variations are predictors of short-term and long-term outcome in acute decompensated heart failure. Crit Care. 2011;15(1):116.
18. Maisel AS, Peacock WF, McMullin N, Jessie R, Fonarow GC, Wynne J, Mills RM. Timing of immunoreactive B-type natriuretic peptide levels and treatment delay in acute decompensated heart failure: an ADHERE (Acute Decompensated Heart Failure National Registry) analysis. JACC. 2008;52(7):534–40.
19. Fonarow GC, Peacock WF, Phillips CO, Givertz MM, Lopatin M, ADHERE Scientific Advisory Committee and Investigators. Admission B-type natriuretic peptide levels and in-hospital mortality in acute decompensated heart failure. J Am Coll Cardiol. 2007;49(19):1943–50.

Chapter 17
Heart Failure: Natriuretic Peptide Use in the Hospital

Kevin Shah and James Iwaz

Abstract Acute decompensated heart failure (ADHF) is a leading cause of hospitalization amongst elderly in the U.S. The role of natriuretic peptides (NPs) is clear in the evaluation of acute dyspnea to help diagnose ADHF. NPs are quantitative markers of wall stress and reflect severity of heart failure. In the inpatient management of ADHF, serial sampling and recognition of down-trending NPs is a powerful indicator of patients who are at lower risk for future adverse events. Serial monitoring at least once during hospitalization (or if clinical uncertainty exists) and a pre-discharge NP should be checked to ensure patients are appropriate for discharge. If persistent elevation occurs, alternate etiologies for this should be considered and medications should be further up-titrated and optimized prior to discharge.

Keywords Natriuretic peptide • Heart failure • Prognosis in heart failure • Monitoring in heart failure • Mortality in heart failure • Cardiac Biomarkers • Acute decompensated heart failure

Background and Physiology

The natriuretic peptides (NPs), B-type natriuretic peptide (BNP) and N-terminal proBNP (NT-proBNP), have an established role in the approach to undifferentiated dyspnea. As discussed in earlier chapters, BNP and NT-proBNP are secreted from cardiac myocytes in response to increased wall tension, usually from volume overload and expansion. While NPs have a powerful relationship with cardiac pressure,

K. Shah, MD (✉)
Department of Internal Medicine, University of California San Diego, San Diego, CA, USA
e-mail: kevinshah@gmail.com

J. Iwaz, MD
Department of Internal Medicine, UCSD Medical Center, San Diego, CA, USA

© Springer International Publishing Switzerland 2016
A.S. Maisel, A.S. Jaffe (eds.), *Cardiac Biomarkers*,
DOI 10.1007/978-3-319-42982-3_17

Fig. 17.1 Rational for inpatient NP-guided therapy

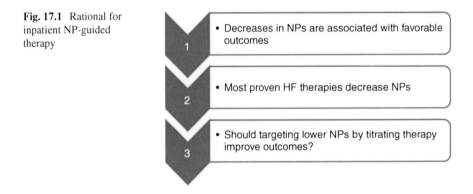

1. • Decreases in NPs are associated with favorable outcomes

2. • Most proven HF therapies decrease NPs

3. • Should targeting lower NPs by titrating therapy improve outcomes?

they have a relationship with valvular heart disease, pulmonary artery pressure, heart rhythm abnormalities and coronary ischemia. BNP is the biologically active hormone with a half-life of about 21 min, while NT-proBNP is not biologically active and has an estimated half-life of 70 min.

Signs and symptoms in the diagnosis of heart failure can be non-specific and the NPs have a role in the diagnosis of acute decompensated HF (ADHF). Patients with heart failure who suffer acute decompensations are admitted and decongested to a point where they appear near euvolemia with medication optimization and then discharged with outpatient follow up. Although these patients may feel symptomatically improved, they have high rates of readmission for heart failure, possibly due to inadequate decongestion and subclinical hypervolemia [1]. Risk stratification for future events in patients with ADHF is difficult since prognosis is often determined by factors such as New York Heart Association (NYHA) and functional class.

Readmissions for HF contribute greatly to the cost of medical care in the United States. Thus, if one could find ways to optimize medical therapy for those with ADHF, one could lower the rates of readmissions and decrease associated healthcare costs. The inpatient management of heart failure and incorporation of NPs is evolving. The rationale behind the routine use of NPs for inpatient HF monitoring is simple. Most proven HF therapies have been shown to decrease NP concentrations [2–5] and decreases in NP concentration over time have also demonstrated favorable outcomes. Therefore, strategies involving titration of therapy towards specific NP targets may improve outcomes (Fig. 17.1).

Value of NPS in ADHF

One of the difficulties in our ability to optimize patients admitted with ADHF is our limitations in clinical assessment of volume status. Accurate assessment of volume status is difficult. We rely on exam findings including jugular venous pressure, crackles on pulmonary exam, S3 gallop on cardiovascular exam, and lower extremity edema. Additionally, weights are often checked as an indicator of total body volume depletion with diuresis and decongestion. Therefore, accurate volume status can be considered to some extent an art with low inter-rater reliability. In contrast, NPs are quantitative, reproducible, and can serve as a potential surrogate for hypervolemia. In studies with invasive hemodynamic monitoring, NPs have had a positive relationship with pulmonary capillary wedge pressure (PCWP) [6]. However, placement of a pulmonary artery catheter has complications and as such is mainly reserved for patients with severe decompensations usually requiring ino-trope therapy and/or those in undifferentiated shocks. Appropriate management can be difficult with over-diuresis running the risk of significant electrolyte abnormali-ties, acute kidney injury, orthostatic hypotension, syncope, and acute renal failure. Under-diuresis may lead to non-optimization of volume status prior to discharge with subsequent re-hospitalizations and increased cost, hypoxia, or cardiorenal syn-drome. Thus, a more objective guide to management of fluid status would be benefi-cial. NPs may represent subclinical congestion that is difficult to assess on exam and persistently elevated concentrations may indicate mild hypervolemia.

In addition to volume status estimation, NPs also indicate persistent elevation of the renin-angiotensin aldosterone system (RAAS). The NPs are in fact the counter-regulatory measure to the deleterious overactivation of RAAS in ADHF [7]. Treatment of ADHF decreases NPs, endothelin, and circulating norepinephrine [8]. Therefore, the persistent elevation of the deleterious systems including RAAS and catecholamines are also indicated by elevations of NPs during treatment of ADHF. Therapies which lower NPs would indirectly indicate down-regulation of RAAS.

When assessing elevated concentrations of NPs, it is important to note that there is no cutoff that is 100 % diagnostic of HF. Alternate etiologies for elevation of NPs should always be considered. It should be noticed that heart failure with reduced ejection fraction (HFrEF) is known to have greater NP concentrations than in pre-served ejection fraction (HFpEF). Alternate causes of NP elevation include dys-rhythmias, cor pulmonale, pulmonary embolism, pulmonary hypertension and valvular heart diseases. Furthermore, renal dysfunction may cause higher concen-trations of NPs and obesity may cause falsely lower concentrations. It is important to keep these caveats in mind when interpreting initial NP concentrations and dur-ing hospitalization when assessing response to therapy.

Prognostic Value of NPS

Knowledge of which patients admitted with ADHF are at highest risk for future adverse events is important in a disease with such morbidity and mortality. The NPs have a significant role in prognostication; many believe BNP values have two com-ponents. One represents the "dry" or euvolemic component, and the other repre-sents the "wet" or hypervolemic component due to acute congestion.

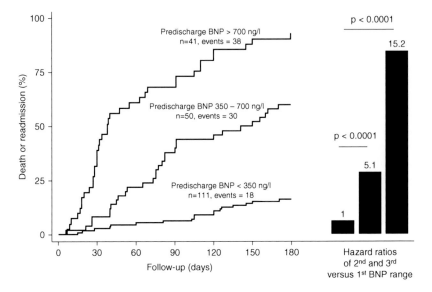

Fig. 17.2 BNP levels less than 350 pg/mL on discharge have the improved long-term outcomes (From Logeart et al. [14], with permission)

BNP measured on admission in ADHF is an independent predictor of in-hospital and future mortality and cardiovascular events in patients who presented with acute heart failure [9–12]. Given its association with reduced left ventricular ejection fraction (LVEF) and worsened NYHA functional status, this is not an unexpected finding but important for identifying high risk patients and establish closer follow up. Interestingly, NPs measured on discharge from HF hospitalization have been increasingly more useful. Multiple studies have demonstrated persistently elevated NPs on discharge (absolute and as compared to admission) portend poor outcomes [13–15]. Those with pre-discharge BNP less than 350 pg/mL have the lowest incidence of 6 month events [14] (Fig. 17.2). Incorporation of a pre-discharge NT-proBNP has also demonstrated similar prognostic ability as BNP [15]. Whether admission, discharge, or change in NP during hospitalization, is the most significant prognostic indicator has also been analyzed. The most important indicator in an analysis of 7,039 elderly patients with ADHF demonstrated discharge BNP was the most important characteristic for predicting 1-year mortality or re-hospitalization [16]. In addition to assessment of decrease prior to discharge, individuals have also studied whether an absolute versus percent change of NP has greater prognostic value. One study demonstrated that a percent change of NT-proBNP is more important for prediction of HF hospitalization-free survival than absolute value [15] while others demonstrated that a lower absolute BNP on discharge is more predictive than a percent decrease [16]. These data provide us the framework for creating an algorithm for how to utilize inpatient NP monitoring for those with ADHF (Fig. 17.3). Timely prognostic information by serial NP measurements allows clinicians to intensify treatment during hospitalization and improve prognosis.

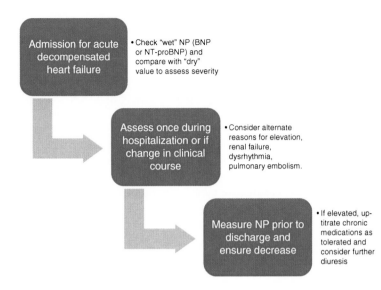

Fig. 17.3 Algorithm for inpatient NP use in ADHF

Case 1

A 63-year-old male with a history of ischemic cardiomyopathy (LVEF 48%, dry BNP 180 pg/mL), chronic kidney disease (baseline serum creatinine 1.5 mg/dL), persistent atrial fibrillation (on novel anticoagulant rivaroxaban), presents with shortness of breath at rest, 8 lb of weight gain, and leg swelling. His exam is significant for elevated jugular venous pressure (14 cm H2O), bibasilar rales, S3 gallop and peripheral edema. His labs are unchanged from baseline except for BNP of 930 pg/mL.

The patient was admitted to general cardiology service and started on afterload reduction with his home dose of ACE inhibitor, beta blocker, and was diuresed with IV bumetanide with appropriate response. Patient's symptoms and exam findings improved on hospital day 2, with a decrease in weight by 3 lb. His BNP on hospital day 2 was 860 pg/mL.

Patient's current regimen was continued with mild improvement of signs and symptoms of congestion on hospital day 3. Patient was ambulating without symptoms and his BNP was 870 pg/mL.

Alternate etiologies for persistence of NP elevation were considered which included renal failure, pulmonary embolism, and dysrhythmia. There was no suggestion of any of these alternate causes, therefore it was concluded that the patient was far from optimization even though his symptoms and exam findings have improved. Patient's medications were reviewed and his beta blocker dose was increased and addition of low-dose mineralocorticoid antagonist was initiated given this persistence of BNP elevation. His diuresis was continued and on discharge his BNP had decreased to 380 pg/mL with resolution of his initial symptoms and exam findings.

Conclusion

The natriuretic peptides have a solidified role in the diagnosis of ADHF in those with undifferentiated dyspnea. Their measurement at baseline in those with ADHF correlates with degree of HF severity and reflect long-term prognosis. While active treatment of HF ensues, NPs have been shown to downtrend reflecting improvement of hemodynamics and the RAAS system as well. During hospitalization, re-check of NP concentration during hospitalization should be considered if a patient's clinical status is in question. More importantly, NPs should be checked prior to discharge and if a decrease is not observed these patients should be considered highest risk for adverse event and aggressive medical up-titration should be considered.

References

1. Maisel AS. Use of BNP levels in monitoring hospitalized heart failure patients with heart failure. Heart Fail Rev. 2003;8:339–44.
2. Troughton RW, Richards AM. Outpatient monitoring and treatment of chronic heart failure guided by amino-terminal Pro-B-type natriuretic peptide measurement. Am J Cardiol. 2008;101(Suppl):72A–5.
3. Tsutamoto T, Wada A, Maeda K, et al. Effect of spirinolactone on plasma brain natriuretic peptide and left ventricular remodeling in patients with congestive heart failure. J Am Coll Cardiol. 2001;37:1228–33.
4. Rousseau MF, Gurne O, Duprez D, et al. Beneficial neurohormonal profile of spirinolactone in severe congestive heart failure: results from the rales neurohormonal substudy. J Am Coll Cardiol. 2002;40:1596–601.
5. Kohno M, Minami M, Kano H, et al. Effect of angiotensin-converting enzyme inhibitor on left ventricular parameters and circulating brain natriuretic peptide in elderly hypertensives with left ventricular hypertrophy. Metabolism. 2000;49:1356–60.
6. Kazanegra R, Cheng V, Garcia A, et al. A rapid test for B-type natriuretic peptide correlates with falling wedge pressures in patients treated for decompensated heart failure: a pilot study. J Card Fail. 2001;7:21–9.
7. Munagala VK, Burnett Jr JC, Redfield MM. The natriuretic peptides in cardiovascular medicine. Curr Probl Cardiol. 2004;29:707–69.
8. Johnson W, Omland T, Hall C, Lucas C, Myking OL, Collins C, Pfeffer M, Rouleau JL, Stevenson LW. Neurohormonal activation rapidly decreases after intravenous therapy with diuretics and vasodilators for class IV heart failure. J Am Coll Cardiol. 2002;39(10):1623–9.
9. Fonarow GC, Peacock WF, Phillips CO, Givertz MM, Lopatin M. Admission B-type natriuretic peptide levels and in-hospital mortality in acute decompensated heart failure. J Am Coll Cardiol. 2007;49:1943–50.
10. Yu CM, Sanderson JE. Plasma brain natriuretic peptide—an independent predictor of cardiovascular mortality in acute heart failure. Eur J Heart Fail. 1999;1:59–65.
11. Tamura K, Takahashi N, Nakatani Y, Onishi S, Iwasaka T. Prognostic impact of plasma brain natriuretic peptide for cardiac events in elderly patients with congestive heart failure. Gerontology. 2001;47:46–51.
12. Harrison A, Morrison LK, Krishnaswamy P, Kazanegra R, Clopton P, Dao Q, et al. B-type natriuretic peptide predicts future cardiac events in patients presenting to the emergency department with dyspnea. Ann Emerg Med. 2002;39:131–8.

13. O'Brien RJ, Squire IB, Demme B, Davies JE, Ng LL. Pre-discharge, but not admission, levels of NT-proBNP predict adverse prognosis following acute LVF. Eur J Heart Fail. 2003;5(4):499–506.
14. Logeart D, Thabut G, Jourdain P, Chavelas C, Beyne P, Beauvais F, Bouvier E, Solal AC. Predischarge B-type natriuretic peptide assay for identifying patients at high risk of re-admission after decompensated heart failure. J Am Coll Cardiol. 2004;43(4):635–41.
15. Bettencourt P, Azevedo A, Pimenta J, Frioes F, Ferreira S, Ferreira A. N-terminal-pro-brain natriuretic peptide predicts outcome after hospital discharge in heart failure patients. Circulation. 2004;110:2168–74.
16. Kociol RD, Horton JR, Fonarow GC, Reyes EM, Shaw LK, O'Connor CM, Felker GM, Hernandez AF. Admission, discharge, or change in B-type natriuretic peptide and long-term outcomes: data from Organized Program to Initiate Lifesaving Treatment in Hospitalized Patients with Heart Failure (OPTIMIZE-HF) linked to Medicare claims. Circ Heart Fail. 2011;4(5):628–36.

Chapter 18
Natriuretic Peptide Guided Therapy in Outpatient Heart Failure Management

Matthew N. Peters and Christopher R. deFilippi

Abstract An increased focus on precision outpatient heart failure management has the potential to decrease the significant morbidity, mortality and cost associated with heart failure hospitalization. Natriuretic peptides represent an objective and reproducible surrogate measurement of cardiac function and volume status which is widely available in the ambulatory setting. Initial trials using natriuretic peptides to guide therapy in ambulatory heart failure patients have shown promise in decreasing associated morbidity and mortality, however, have been limited by significant inter-study variability in inclusion criteria, threshold natriuretic peptide levels and implementation of therapeutic intervention.

Keywords Heart failure • Ambulatory • Outpatient • Natriuretic peptides • BNP • NT-proBNP • Hospitalization for heart failure • All-cause mortality • Heart failure therapy • HFrEF • HFpEF

Considerable morbidity, mortality and cost are associated with hospitalization for heart failure (HF) that extends well beyond the duration of the admission. Accordingly a concentrated focus on intervention in the ambulatory setting has potentially tremendous therapeutic implications. Evidence based therapies such as beta blockers (BB) and renin-angiotensin system inhibitors (RAS) have been repeatedly shown to improve HF outcomes. However, it is widely felt that many patients are not sufficiently treated. A likely explanation for the under treatment of HF in the outpatient setting is the fact that HF symptoms are often subtle, subjective and under-recognized. The natriuretic peptides (NP) B-type natriuretic peptide (BNP)

M.N. Peters, MD (✉)
Department of Cardiovascular Medicine, University of Maryland Medical Center, Baltimore, MD, USA
e-mail: mattpeters25@gmail.com

C.R. deFilippi, MD
Department of Medicine, University of Maryland School of Medicine, Maryland Heart Center University of Maryland Medical Center, Baltimore, MD, USA

© Springer International Publishing Switzerland 2016
A.S. Maisel, A.S. Jaffe (eds.), *Cardiac Biomarkers*,
DOI 10.1007/978-3-319-42982-3_18

and N-terminal pro-B-type natriuretic peptide (NT-proBNP) represent a sensitive and non-invasive surrogate measurement of cardiac function and volume which is objective, reproducible and widely available in the outpatient setting.

Potential for Intervention

The therapeutic benefit of NP monitoring in the outpatient setting is two-fold. First, an interval increase in a serial NP level can be an indication of worsening HF status and can identify patients who need increased attention and potentially, intervention. Second, NP levels can actually be used to track response to therapy and allow for more aggressive up-titration of medications than might be attempted based on symptom status despite sub guideline doses of medications.

Medication Titration

Monitoring of NP levels in HF outpatients affords the ability to individualize therapy or what to now is often referred to as precision medicine. Patients who are at high risk for HF complications are targeted to receive higher doses of guideline-directed medical therapies (GDMT), many of which are routinely administered at lower doses than those studied in clinical trials. Fortunately, many HF therapies have been associated with predictable NP responses including a decrease in levels with adequate titration of angiotensin converting enzyme inhibitors (ACE-I), angiotensin receptor blockers (ARB), mineralocorticoid receptor antagonists (MRA), beta blockers (BB) (following an initial transient increase), diuretics (loop and thiazide), exercise, effective rate control of atrial arrhythmias and even chronic resynchronization therapy (CRT) [1]. Consequently, elevated NP levels, in addition to demonstrating progressively worsening congestion, may represent inadequacy of treatment and fluctuating patterns may identify patients who are not medically optimized and require enhanced levels of observation. Conversely, patients with low or normal NP levels may be potentially weaned down in order to decrease potential adverse medication side effects.

Clinical Trials: What We Know

The first randomized controlled trial to evaluate NP-guided treatment for HF was published in 2000 and showed a dramatic benefit [2]. Unfortunately subsequent randomized control studies have not consistently duplicated this initial study and have had widely variable results. The primary reason for the wide variation in outcomes has been attributed to the difference in study designs and patient populations. Published randomized clinical trials can be divided into two main categories: general HF outpatients and immediate post-discharge HF outpatients. A summary of the randomized clinical trials with primary clinical outcomes which have been included in previous meta-analysis is presented in Table 18.1.

META Analysis

Between 2009 and 2014 a total of 4 meta-analyses have been published in an attempt to provide NP utilization guidance. The first meta-analysis, in 2009, reported on 6 studies covering 1627 patients and demonstrated a 0.69 hazard ratio for all-cause mortality [12]. Limitations of this initial meta-analysis included the inclusion of 3 unpublished studies and the lack of any analysis of all-cause or HR-related hospitalizations [12]. A subsequent meta-analysis, published in 2010, covered 8 studies and 1726 patients and demonstrated a relative risk of 0.79 for all-cause mortality [13]. The same study found no difference in all-cause hospitalization and interestingly found the reduction in all-cause mortality was only apparent in patients under age 75 [13]. A major reported limitation was that the decrease in all-cause mortality was apparently driven by the Trial of Intensified versus Standard Medical Therapy in Elderly Patients with Congestive Heart Failure Trial (TIME-CHF) [4] without which all statistical significance was erased [13].

In 2013 Savarese published a meta-analysis of 2686 patients in 12 randomized clinical trials [14]. Important findings included significant reductions in all-cause mortality (which unlike the findings in the previous Porpakkham, et al. meta-analysis, were not solely attributed to one sub-study), HF-related hospitalization but not in all-cause hospitalization [14]. Similar to the previous meta-analysis, this study also only showed mortality benefit in patients younger than 75 years of age [14]. An additional important finding in the Savarese study was that the reduction in all-cause mortality and HF-related hospitalizations were only found with NT-proBNP and not BNP [14]. Finally, in 2014, an 11 study, 2000 patient meta-analysis was performed, which unlike previous meta-analyses used actual patient level (as opposed to aggregate) data allowing for more rigorous testing, incorporation of standard outcome definitions and detailed analysis of individual patient characteristics (Fig. 18.1) [15]. This study demonstrated the most convincing evidence for benefit of NP surveillance -guided therapy to date with a nearly 40 % reduction in all-cause mortality and a nearly 20 % reduction in both HHF and hospitalization for any cardiovascular disease [15]. Once again a significant decrease in all-cause mortality was only seen in patients younger than 75 [15]. Importantly, this 2014 meta-analysis demonstrated that ACE-I/ARB were the only medication classes to differ between NP-guided and standard of care arms and an increase in medications in both arms were similarly associated with improved outcomes [15].

Table 18.1 Summary of the randomized clinical trials with primary clinical outcomes which have been included in previous four meta-analyses incorporating NP-guided outpatient HF management

Trial	Years	n	Inclusion	HFpEF	F/U	NP Target	Primary end	Results
Outpatient								
Christchurch Pilot [2]	1997–1999	69	LVEF <40 % NYHA II-IV	No	9.5 months	NT-pro-BNP<1700	Death+CV hospitalization+outpatient HF	Positive
STARS-BNP [3]	2001–2005	220	LVEF ≤45 % NYHA II-III	No	15 months	BNP<100	HF mortality+HF hospitalization	Positive
TIME-CHF [4]	2001–2006	499	LVEF<40% HF prev 12 months NTproBNP >400/800 in <75 and >75 years	No	18 months	NT-proBNP>400 in age 60-74 >800 pg/mL in patients>75	Hospitalization free survival	Neutral
SIGNAL-HF [5]	2006–2009	252	LVEF<50% NT-proBNP>800 (M) and >1000 (F)	No	9 months	-NT-pro-BNP<50 % baseline	Composite of days alive, days out of hospital and symptom score	Neutral
UPSTEP [6]	2006–2009	279	LVEF<40%, NYHA II-IV BNP>150 (<75) and >300 (≥75) No HF prev 30 day	No	≥12 months	BNP<150 in younger and <300 in elderly:	Composite of all-cause mortality, hospitalization or HF worsening	Neutral
PROTECT [7]	2006–2010	151	NYHA III-IV EF <40% HHF in prev 6 months	No	≥6 months	NT pro-BNP <1000	Total Cardiovascular events	Positive

Trial	Years	n	Inclusion	HFpEF	F/U	NP Target	Primary end	Results
GUIDE-IT [1]	2014-pres		EF<40% HF event in past 12 months NTproBNP>2000 or BNP>400 during 30 days prior to randomization	No	12–24 months		CV death or HF hospitalization	TBD
Post-Discharge								
BATTLESCARRED [8]	2001–2006	364	Symptomatic HF, NT-proBNP>400	Yes	24 months	NT-pro-BNP<1270	All- cause mortality	Neutral
Berger et al. [9]	2003–2004		EF<40% NYHA III-IV	No	>12 months	NT-pro-BNP <2200	Days alive outside of hospital	Positive
STARBRITE [10]	2003–2005	122	LVEF<35%	No	>3 months	Individual BNP at discharge		Neutral
PRIMA [11]	2004–2007	345	Decompensated H and NT-proBNP>1700 at admission	Yes	≥12 months	Individual lowest NT-proBNP at discharge or at 2-week follow-up	Days alive outside of hospital	Neutral

BATTLESCARRED NT-pro BNP-assisted treatment to lessen serial cardiac readmissions and death, *CV* cardiovascular, *HABIT* Heart Failure Assessment With BNP in the Home, *HF* heart failure, *LVEF* left ventricular ejection fraction, *PRIMA* Can PRo-brain-natriuretic peptide guided therapy of chronic heart failure IMprove heart fAilure morbidity and mortality study, *PROTECT* Use of NT-proBNP Testing to Guide Heart Failure Therapy in the Outpatient Setting, *SIGNAL-HF* Swedish Intervention study: guidelines and NT-proBNP AnaLysis in Heart Failure, *STARBRITE* Strategies for Tailoring Advanced Heart Failure Regimens in the Outpatient Setting, *STAR-BNP* Plasma Brain Natriuretic Peptide-Guided Therapy to Improve Outcome in Heart Failure, *TIME-CHF* Trial of Intensified versus Standard Medical Therapy in Elderly Patients with Congestive Heart Failure, *UPSTEP* Use of PeptideS in Tailoring hEart failure Project

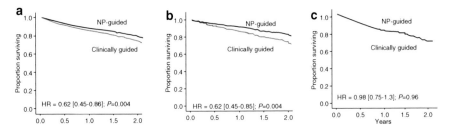

Fig. 18.1 Kaplan-Meier survival curves for the primary endpoint, overall mortality: (**a**) total group; (**b**) (below age 75 (n = 982) and (**c**) 75 years and above (n = 1018) as represented in the 2014 Troughton, et al. meta-analysis, the most recently published meta-analysis on NP-guided outpatient HF management (From Troughton et al. [15], with permission)

Limitations and Pitfalls with Previous Clinical Trials

Variation in Clinical Trial Design

The large extent of heterogeneity in previous clinical trial results can be mostly attributed to a combination of variability in clinical trial design (including differences in treatment strategies), alternating use of BNP and NT-pro-BNP, inconsistent NP cut-off values and differences in inclusion criteria leading to variability in patient populations.

Two types of interventional strategies have been employed using NP-guided therapy: the previously discussed pharmacologic intervention; as well as referral intervention such as in the North-Star Adherence Study where patients were referred to either specialty clinics or returned to their general practitioner based on NP results [16]. NP-guided pharmacologic therapy trials have enrolled patients beginning in 1997 [2]. Over the subsequent 20 years there have been concurrent alterations in recommended GDMT based on evolving guidelines for HF therapy including continued prevalence of ACE-I/ARB and BB, large increases in MRA and CRT therapy and substantial decreases in the use of digoxin. Further discrepancies in treatment strategies has been seen in TIME-CHF and Use of PeptideS in Tailoring hEart failure Project (UPSTEP) which contained no specific algorithm for adjusting GDMT which was rather arbitrarily decided by the investigators [4, 6].

Table 18.1 depicts the dramatic variability in NP threshold and cut-off values which have been employed to initiate therapy. Not only do the absolute value cut-offs differ but some studies use individual percentage change (as opposed to a universal cut-off value) as threshold for treatment as in the Swedish Intervention study guidelines and NT-proBNP AnaLysis in Heart Failure Trial (SIGNAL-HF) where intervention was focused on achieving NT-proBNP<50% of baseline [5]. It is theorized that many trials utilized conservative NP goals that were too high which translated to less aggressive intervention in patients who were able to meet their respective NP goals while still carrying residual risk associated with insufficient HF treatment. Evidence behind this theory is supported by the fact that the cohorts of patients in two of the neutral/non-positive result studies (SIGNAL-HF) and Can PRo-brain-natriuretic peptide guided therapy of chronic heart failure IMprove heart fAilure morbidity and mortality study (PRIMA) who significantly decreased their NP values (regardless of pre-specified study target value) had substantially better outcomes [5, 11].

Not only were varying NP levels utilized to make clinical decisions in various studies but both BNP and NT-pro-BNP have been utilized, which based on the evidence presented in several studies, are not interchangeable. In Savarese et al's 2013 meta-analysis only NT-proBNP (and not BNP guided therapy) was found to be significantly associated with improved survival and reduced hospitlizaiton [14]. It has been hypothesized that NT-proBNP may serve as a better intervention-guided biomarker due to its higher circulating levels and enhanced chemical stability [14].

Variability in Patient Population

Inter-study variability is also created by differences in inclusion criteria and the resulting differences in patient population have a considerable confounding effect. In the Porapakkham et al. 2010 meta-analysis it was found that patients <75 years of age were much more responsive to NP-directed therapy in comparison to those older than 75 [13]. This finding has been hypothesized to be due to less aggressive up-titration of ACE/ARB and BB in the elderly population. Support for this hypothesis was provided by Troughton et al's 2014 meta-analysis (which also demonstrated dramatically decreased utility of NP guided therapy in the patients over 75) whereby ACE/ARB and BB increases were much more prominent in the under 75 population.

An additional confounding factor is the concurrent presence of multiple significant comorbidities. While confounding comorbidities have varied, the majority of studies have completely excluded many common comorbid conditions in HF including acute coronary syndrome previous coronary revascularization, hemodynamic instability, significant valvular disease, pulmonary hypertension, candidacy for cardiac transplant, chronic renal failure, severe hepatic or pulmonary disease and life expectancy less than 6 months [4].

In addition to age and comorbidities, the specific types of HF patients included may also have a confounding role. Numerous studies have enrolled varying proportions of heart failure with reduced ejection fraction (HFrEF) and heart failure with preserved ejection fraction (HFpEF). While HFrEF has been more frequently studied in comparison to HFpEF, one 2010 study actually showed trends towards worse outcomes in HFpEF patients allocated to NT-pro-BNP guided management compared to standard of care [8]. Hypotheses for the worsened outcome in HFpEF compared HFrEF include the notion that there are no known effective therapies for HFrEF and thus increasing medication dosage may be ineffective or even harmful. Furthermore, it has been speculated that elevations of NP in HFpEF may be alternatively due to cardiorenal dysfunction as opposed to myocardial stretch as in HFrEF.

Optimization of NP-Guided Therapy and Potential Impact on Readmission

Important components to optimization of NP-guided therapy include identification of patient cohorts at elevated risk for readmission and establishment of appropriate time intervals in which to evaluate NP levels.

It has been previously demonstrated that NT-pro-NBP variations offer the greatest diagnostic yield at 2 weeks after a change in therapy [17]. Unfortunately it has been shown that that by post discharge day 7, 32 % of all 30 day readmissions have already occurred [18]. Consequently, waiting a full 2 weeks to evaluate changes in NP level may be too late to prevent a large proportion HF readmissions. While more frequent screening intervals may not be necessary in the entire HF patient cohort, more frequent screening may be warranted in patients with elevated NP levels before or shortly after discharge (which have been shown to predict higher rates of early readmission).

Feasibility and Tolerability

In order for NP guided therapy to be truly cost effective costs, of readmission and associated decreased morbidity must outweigh elevating costs of medical visits and laboratory studies as well any treatment of side-effects related to aggressive up-titration of HF medications. Encouragingly, a post-hoc analysis of TIME-CHF demonstrated no differences in withdrawal rate or adverse events between NP-guided and clinically guided groups, which importantly included similar incidences of worsening renal function and hyperkalemia [19]. Of similar importance was a subsequent TIME-CHF extended follow-up study extended to 5 years where effects of NT-proBNP guided therapy were maintained long after cessation of the intervention suggesting that even short-term NT-pro-BNP guided therapy may have long term effects [20]. Additional cost-saving effect may be obtainable if the results found in the recent pilot study, Heart Failure Assessment with BNP in the Home (HABIT) (which demonstrated enhanced clinical outcomes with NP home monitoring) can be duplicated [21].

Future Study

Primarily due to the heterogeneity in previously conducted NP-guided studies there are currently no NP-guided therapy recommendations endorsed in national and international guidelines. The most recent American College of Cardiology/American Heart Association guidelines for heart failure management give NP guided outpatient therapy a level IIb recommendation [22]. Similarly, the most recent European Society of Cardiology recommendations state that NP assisted management of HF patients is still uncertain [23]. However, both guidelines from both organizations endorse a potentially expanded role following publication of additional data.

Thankfully the ongoing National Heart, Lung and Blood Institute sponsored Guiding Evidence Based Therapy Using Biomarker Evidence Based Therapy Using Biomarker Intensified Treatment in Heart Failure Trial (GUIDE-IT) has been enrolling patients since 2014 and will hopefully fill much of the current knowledge gaps [1]. GUIDE-IT is a prospective randomized, multicenter trial which will seek to enroll 1100 high risk HFrEF patients with NT-proBNP level of <1000 pg/mL. Not only will the study be the largest for HF biomarker-guided therapy performed to date, but it will eliminate potentially confounding HFpEF patients and address the efficacy of an NP guided strategy in adults >75 years. It is hoped that the study will provide an aggressive target NT-proBNP level and substantially reduce the risk for under treatment.

Conclusions

Due to variations in inclusion criteria, treatment strategy and NP cut points no current guidelines recommend for the use of serial measurement of NP levels to guide titration of therapy. Moving forward, more precise and clinically attainable NP targets must be defined. It is important for serial NP monitoring to be appropriately evaluated and utilized in across specific age groups, specified systolic function and across a wide range of medical comorbidities. While NP-guided therapy has the potential to provide significant therapeutic benefit, it is currently unknown whether hypothesized mortally benefits from aggressive NP lowering can outweigh potential costs of monitoring and associated side effects.

References

1. Felker GM, Ahmad T, Anstrom KJ, et al. Rationale and design of the GUIDE-IT study: guiding evidence based therapy using biomarker intensified treatment in heart failure. JACC Heart Fail. 2014;2(5):457–65. doi:10.1016/j.jchf.2014.05.007.
2. Troughton RW, Frampton CM, Yandle TG, Espiner EA, Nicholls MG, Richards AM. Treatment of heart failure guided by plasma aminoterminal brain natriuretic peptide (N-BNP) concentrations. *Lancet (London, England)*. 2000;355(9210):1126–1130. http://www.ncbi.nlm.nih.gov/pubmed/10791374. Accessed December 27, 2015.
3. Jourdain P, Jondeau G, Funck F, et al. Plasma brain natriuretic peptide-guided therapy to improve outcome in heart failure: the STARS-BNP Multicenter Study. J Am Coll Cardiol. 2007;49(16):1733–9. doi:10.1016/j.jacc.2006.10.081.
4. Pfisterer M, Buser P, Rickli H, et al. BNP-guided vs symptom-guided heart failure therapy: the Trial of Intensified vs Standard Medical Therapy in Elderly Patients With Congestive Heart Failure (TIME-CHF) randomized trial. JAMA. 2009;301(4):383–92. doi:10.1001/jama.2009.2.

5. Persson H, Erntell H, Eriksson B, Johansson G, Swedberg K, Dahlström U. Improved pharmacological therapy of chronic heart failure in primary care: a randomized Study of NT-proBNP Guided Management of Heart Failure–SIGNAL-HF (Swedish Intervention study–Guidelines and NT-proBNP AnaLysis in Heart Failure). Eur J Heart Fail. 2010;12(12):1300–8. doi:10.1093/eurjhf/hfq169.
6. Karlström P, Alehagen U, Boman K, Dahlström U. Brain natriuretic peptide-guided treatment does not improve morbidity and mortality in extensively treated patients with chronic heart failure: responders to treatment have a significantly better outcome. Eur J Heart Fail. 2011;13(10):1096–103. doi:10.1093/eurjhf/hfr078.
7. Januzzi JL, Rehman SU, Mohammed AA, et al. Use of amino-terminal pro-B-type natriuretic peptide to guide outpatient therapy of patients with chronic left ventricular systolic dysfunction. J Am Coll Cardiol. 2011;58(18):1881–9. doi:10.1016/j.jacc.2011.03.072.
8. Lainchbury JG, Troughton RW, Strangman KM, et al. N-terminal pro-B-type natriuretic peptide-guided treatment for chronic heart failure: results from the BATTLESCARRED (NT-proBNP-Assisted Treatment To Lessen Serial Cardiac Readmissions and Death) trial. J Am Coll Cardiol. 2009;55(1):53–60. doi:10.1016/j.jacc.2009.02.095.
9. Berger R, Moertl D, Peter S, et al. N-terminal pro-B-type natriuretic peptide-guided, intensive patient management in addition to multidisciplinary care in chronic heart failure a 3-arm, prospective, randomized pilot study. J Am Coll Cardiol. 2010;55(7):645–53. doi:10.1016/j.jacc.2009.08.078.
10. Shah MR, Califf RM, Nohria A, et al. The STARBRITE trial: a randomized, pilot study of B-type natriuretic peptide-guided therapy in patients with advanced heart failure. J Card Fail. 2011;17(8):613–21. doi:10.1016/j.cardfail.2011.04.012.
11. Eurlings LWM, van Pol PEJ, Kok WE, et al. Management of chronic heart failure guided by individual N-terminal pro-B-type natriuretic peptide targets: results of the PRIMA (Can PRo-brain-natriuretic peptide guided therapy of chronic heart failure IMprove heart fAilure morbidity and mortality?) study. J Am Coll Cardiol. 2010;56(25):2090–100. doi:10.1016/j.jacc.2010.07.030.
12. Felker GM, Hasselblad V, Hernandez AF, O'Connor CM. Biomarker-guided therapy in chronic heart failure: a meta-analysis of randomized controlled trials. Am Heart J. 2009;158(3):422–30. doi:10.1016/j.ahj.2009.06.018.
13. Porapakkham P, Porapakkham P, Zimmet H, Billah B, Krum H. B-type natriuretic peptide-guided heart failure therapy: a meta-analysis. Arch Intern Med. 2010;170(6):507–14. doi:10.1001/archinternmed.2010.35.
14. Savarese G, Trimarco B, Dellegrottaglie S, et al. Natriuretic peptide-guided therapy in chronic heart failure: a meta-analysis of 2,686 patients in 12 randomized trials. PLoS One. 2013;8(3), e58287. doi:10.1371/journal.pone.0058287.
15. Troughton RW, Frampton CM, Brunner-La Rocca H-P, et al. Effect of B-type natriuretic peptide-guided treatment of chronic heart failure on total mortality and hospitalization: an individual patient meta-analysis. Eur Heart J. 2014;35(23):1559–67. doi:10.1093/eurheartj/ehu090.
16. Schou M, Gislason G, Videbaek L, et al. Effect of extended follow-up in a specialized heart failure clinic on adherence to guideline recommended therapy: NorthStar Adherence Study. Eur J Heart Fail. 2014;16(11):1249–55. doi:10.1002/ejhf.176.
17. Pascual-Figal DA, Domingo M, Casas T, et al. Usefulness of clinical and NT-proBNP monitoring for prognostic guidance in destabilized heart failure outpatients. Eur Heart J. 2008;29(8):1011–8. doi:10.1093/eurheartj/ehn023.
18. Dharmarajan K, Hsieh AF, Lin Z, et al. Diagnoses and timing of 30-day readmissions after hospitalization for heart failure, acute myocardial infarction, or pneumonia. JAMA. 2013;309(4):355–63. doi:10.1001/jama.2012.216476.
19. Sanders-van Wijk S, van Asselt ADI, Rickli H, et al. Cost-effectiveness of N-terminal pro-B-type natriuretic-guided therapy in elderly heart failure patients: results from TIME-CHF (Trial

of Intensified versus Standard Medical Therapy in Elderly Patients with Congestive Heart Failure). JACC Heart Fail. 2013;1(1):64–71. doi:10.1016/j.jchf.2012.08.002.

20. Sanders-van Wijk S, Maeder MT, Nietlispach F, et al. Long-term results of intensified, N-terminal-pro-B-type natriuretic peptide-guided versus symptom-guided treatment in elderly patients with heart failure: five-year follow-up from TIME-CHF. Circ Heart Fail. 2014;7(1):131–9. doi:10.1161/CIRCHEARTFAILURE.113.000527.

21. Maisel A, Barnard D, Jaski B, et al. Primary results of the HABIT Trial (heart failure assessment with BNP in the home). J Am Coll Cardiol. 2013;61(16):1726–35. doi:10.1016/j.jacc.2013.01.052.

22. Jessup M, Abraham WT, Casey DE, et al. 2009 focused update: ACCF/AHA Guidelines for the Diagnosis and Management of Heart Failure in Adults: a report of the American College of Cardiology Foundation/American Heart Association Task Force on Practice Guidelines: developed in collaboration with t. Circulation. 2009;119(14):1977–2016. doi:10.1161/CIRCULATIONAHA.109.192064.

23. McMurray JJV, Adamopoulos S, Anker SD, et al. ESC guidelines for the diagnosis and treatment of acute and chronic heart failure 2012: the task force for the diagnosis and treatment of acute and chronic heart failure 2012 of the European Society of Cardiology. Developed in collaboration with the Heart. Eur Heart J. 2012;33(14):1787–847. doi:10.1093/eurheartj/ehs104.

Chapter 19
Caveats Using Natriuretic Peptide Levels

Trenton M. Gluck, Kevin Shah, and Alan S. Maisel

Abstract Acute heart failure is difficult to diagnosis by history and physical exam alone. B-type natriuretic peptide and N-terminal pro-B-type natriuretic peptide are useful in both the diagnosis and prognosis of heart failure. However, there are various clinical situations that can cause elevations and depressions in the concentrations of natriuretic peptides. This can make clinical diagnoses very difficult, especially in patients with mildly elevated, or "gray zone" levels. Understanding the caveats of using natriuretic peptides is essential for predicting, diagnosing, and treating heart failure. This chapter discusses the causes of "gray zone" natriuretic peptide levels, establishes adjusted cutoffs to be used in patients with specific comorbidities, and applies the information to the interpretation of a case study.

Keywords Natriuretic Peptides • Caveats • B-type Natriuretic Peptide • N-terminal pro-B-type Natriuretic Peptide • Heart Failure • HFpEF • Obesity and acute heart failure • Diagnosis of Acute heart failure • Prognosis of Acute heart failure • Biomarkers • Cutoffs in natriuretic peptide levels

T.M. Gluck, BS
Department of Medicine, Division of Cardiovascular Medicine, Veterans Affairs San Diego Healthcare System, San Diego, CA, USA

K. Shah, MD
Department of Internal Medicine, University of California San Diego, San Diego, CA, USA

A.S. Maisel, MD, FACC (✉)
Department of Medicine, Division of Cardiovascular Medicine, University of California San Diego, San Diego, CA, USA

Department of Medicine, Coronary Care Unit and Heart Failure Program, Veterans Affairs San Diego Healthcare System, San Diego, CA, USA
e-mail: amaisel@ucsd.edu

© Springer International Publishing Switzerland 2016
A.S. Maisel, A.S. Jaffe (eds.), *Cardiac Biomarkers*,
DOI 10.1007/978-3-319-42982-3_19

An accurate heart failure ("HF") diagnosis relies on a number of factors, most importantly the clinical assessment done by the evaluating physician. The diagnosis of HF is difficult, however, due to the non-specific clinical presentations and various comorbidities commonly associated with HF. B-type natriuretic peptide (BNP) and N-terminal pro-B-type natriuretic peptide (NT-proBNP) are important tools for diagnosing and prognosticating patients with HF.

In order to interpret natriuretic peptide ("NP") levels, thresholds or "cutoffs" are used to help establish or exclude HF in acutely dyspneic patients. Patients being investigated for possible acute HF, however, often have comorbidities that reduce the diagnostic accuracy of NP cutoffs. These include but are not limited to mild HF, ischemia, dysrhythmias, cor pulmonale, obesity, renal dysfunction, age, and gender. In this chapter, we discuss the caveats to using NPs in the setting of acute HF, and use the available clinical data to establish appropriately adjusted cutoffs.

Case Study

A 45 year old male with a history of diastolic dysfunction presents to the ED with dyspnea on exertion for the past 2 weeks and dyspnea at rest for 1 day. The patient is obese with a BMI of 32, and has gained 10 lb since his last primary care checkup 3 months ago. On evaluation rales and an S3 gallop are heard, but because the patient is obese, a JVP cannot be properly estimated. No clear evidence of peripheral edema is noted. A chest radiography shows mild interstitial edema. The patient has a BNP of 60 pg/ml and an NT-proBNP of 270 pg/ml. His BNP was 20 pg/ml at his primary care provider visit 3 months ago. No previous NT-proBNP results are available. Given these findings, what would be the best way to interpret and understand these seemingly normal NP levels? The rest of the chapter will explain the caveats to using NPs and how to interpret their values within the context of various clinical scenarios.

Causes of NP Elevation

Age and Gender

Both BNP and NT-proBNP increase with age. Many factors have been proposed as a cause for these elevations including decreased renal function, increased cardiac size, hormonal modulation, and age-related subclinical heart diseases, specifically those that alter ventricular structure and reduce function. Most young and healthy individuals have BNP and NT-proBNP levels below 25 and 70 pg/ml, respectively [1]. Therefore the use of single, age-independent cutoffs, while having good diagnostic value in younger patients with relatively low values, is not recommended.

Table 19.1 NT-proBNP age dependent cutoffs for establishing heart failure in acutely dyspneic patients

Age	Below 50	50–75	Above 75
NT-proBNP (pg/ml)	450	900	1800

Data from Januzzi et al. [3, 4]

While BNP levels indeed increase with age, using a 100 pg/ml cutoff results in minimal loss of specificity in older patients [2]. However, NT-proBNP age-dependent cutoffs are recommended for establishing HF (Table 19.1). These cutoffs maintain 90 % sensitivities and 84 % specificities in HF diagnosis [3, 4]. Additionally, an age-independent NT-proBNP value of 300 pg/ml is used for exclusion of HF in acutely dyspneic patients [3–5].

With respect to gender and its effect on NP measurements, BNP and NT-proBNP concentrations are higher on average in women than in men, at all ages [6]. This may be caused by a combination of increased estrogen or decreased testosterone [7]. However, the existing NT-proBNP and BNP cut offs are still accurate for HF diagnosis in both men and women presenting with acute symptoms.

Renal Dysfunction

Renal disease is typically seen in about 40 % of patients with HF [8]. Both BNP and NT-proBNP concentrations are elevated in patients with renal dysfunction. Patients with chronic kidney disease ("CKD") generally have higher intravascular volumes, reduced renal clearance, and an overactive renin-angiotensin endocrine response. All of these factors are thought to contribute to the increase in NPs, but BNP elevation is most strongly correlated with myocardial structural abnormalities, and indicators of left ventricular ("LV") overload, independent of the severity of renal dysfunction [9]. Therefore, it is likely that the increased ventricular pressures and resulting ventricular stress cause NP elevations seen in these patients.

CKD patients are more likely to have intermediately elevated NPs, which can be difficult to interpret. Often times, CKD patients with mild BNP elevation do not have acute HF. However, moderately elevated BNP levels in these patients are strong predictors of eventual HF onset [10]. An increased BNP cut point of 200 pg/ml should be used to rule out HF in CKD patients, especially for those with severe renal dysfunction (GFR < 44 mL/min/1.7 m^2).

NT-proBNP elevation is strongly correlated to reduced GFR. However, the accuracy of NT-proBNP cut offs is not significantly reduced in patients with moderate renal dysfunction, and NT-proBNP, like BNP, maintains its prognostic value independent of renal dysfunction [11]. Patients with severe renal dysfunction may benefit from the use of adjusted NT-pro-BNP cutoffs, however none have been established.

Acute Coronary Syndrome ("ACS")

BNP is elevated in patients with acute myocardial infarction independent of concurrent HF [12]. The degree of left ventricular dysfunction may be correlated to BNP elevation, as seen in patients with various degrees of renal failure. NT-proBNP may also be elevated in acute myocardial infarction and has been shown to correlate with cardiac troponin I levels [13]. Although NPs have no role in the diagnosis of ACS, they can help diagnose concomitant HF and are excellent prognosticators of 30 day mortality in ACS patients, even in those without HF [13].

Pulmonary Disease

NPs may be elevated in the setting of pulmonary disease. It may be clinically challenging to distinguish between HF and a pulmonary etiology in dyspneic patients. NP elevation in pulmonary disease is thought to reflect the level of right ventricular strain, as in the cases of pulmonary hypertension and an acute pulmonary embolism [14]. Other primary pulmonary causes of dyspnea (e.g., chronic obstructive pulmonary disease, bronchitis, pneumonia) have lower levels of NPs than in pulmonary embolism and pulmonary hypertension. Studies in animal models have shown that in response to hypoxia, decreased expression of the NPR-C BNP clearance receptor can lead to elevated levels [15].

Patients suffering from pulmonary disease without HF, however, will only have intermediately elevated NPs [16]. NP rule in cut points are still useful for the diagnosis of HF in patients with concomitant pulmonary disease because NPs are typically higher in these patients than in those with pulmonary disease alone.

Increased Cardiac Output Conditions

Sepsis, hyperthyroidism, cirrhosis, and other etiologies of elevated cardiac output can cause NP elevation. The reason for this elevation is not fully understood, but evidence has suggested that underlying myocardial dysfunction and possible inflammatory mechanisms are responsible [5, 17]. NPs are only moderately elevated in patients with cirrhosis or hyperthyroidism, but patients with severe sepsis and shock often have NP levels that are indistinguishable from patients with acute HF. Clinical judgement, therefore, is the best tool for differentiating between these patients and those with HF.

Atrial Fibrillation

NPs are elevated in patients with atrial fibrillation ("AF"). BNP, NT-proBNP, and mid regional pro atrial natriuretic peptide (MR-proANP) have reduced diagnostic accuracies in the setting of acute HF [18]. An increased BNP cutoff of 200 pg/ml may increase the specificity of HF diagnosis in AF patients suspected of concomitant HF. While NT-proBNP is elevated in setting of AF, patients with AF and acute HF have indistinguishable NT-proBNP levels as compared to HF patients without AF. AF patients with HF have significantly higher NT-proBNP levels than in patients with AF alone [19].

Causes of NP Depression

Obesity

In patients who are overweight, and especially those who are obese, it is often very difficult to perform a physical exam that elucidates the clear clinical manifestations of HF. Therefore, it important to understand how to evaluate NPs in the obese patient.

BNP and NT-proBNP levels are lower in obese patients (body mass index, or BMI > 30) in comparison to overweight (BMI 25–29.9) and lean patients (BMI < 25). This inverse relationship between elevated BMI and depressed NPs is seen in patients both with and without HF [20]. The cause of lowered NP levels is still unknown. Increased expression of the NPR-C receptor in adipocytes may cause rapid breakdown and clearance of BNP in obese patients [21]. However, NT-proBNP, which is not believed to bind to the NPR-C receptor, is also depressed in patients with elevated BMI [22]. According to the Dallas Heart Study, BNP and NT-proBNP were lower in people with increased BMI, but BNP depression was inversely correlated with increased lean body mass, not fat body mass, suggesting another possible etiology for NP depression [22]. A number of factors including decreased synthesis, hormonal modulation, and increased clearance likely play a role in such depression.

Adjusted cutoffs should be used when interpreting NPs in dyspneic patients with obesity. BNP levels of 170 pg/ml in lean patients, 110 pg/ml in overweight patients, and 54 pg/ml in obese patients maintain 90 % sensitivity in ruling out HF [20]. Regardless of BMI, BNP is correlated with the severity of HF symptoms, and it is still an excellent predictor of mortality. Despite the slight correlation of decreased NT-proBNP levels in patients with increased BMI, adjusted cutoffs have not been implemented to compensate for the possible reduction in sensitivity of HF diagnosis.

Diastolic Heart Failure

Diastolic heart failure, also called heart failure with preserved ejection fraction ("HFpEF") is a common subtype of HF. Up to 50 % of HF patients may have HFpEF, and a higher incidence of associated risk factors such as diabetes, obesity, and hypertension may be causing this percentage to increase [23]. Currently, the gold standard for diagnosing HFpEF is an echocardiogram that shows the characteristic diastolic dysfunction along with signs and symptoms of HF. HFpEF and systolic HF, or heart failure with reduced ejection fraction ("HFrEF"), are usually clinically indistinguishable. While NPs cannot be used to differentiate between the two HF phenotypes, both BNP and NT-proBNP can be elevated to a lesser extent in patients with HFpEF compared to those with HFrEF. However, BNP and NT-pro BNP are significantly elevated in patients with HFpEF compared to those without HF [24]. Therefore, a BNP cutoff of 100 pg/ml is still accurate at differentiating between symptomatic patients with HFpEF and those without HF [25].

Even though less NT-proBNP elevation may be seen in HFpEF patients compared to those with HFrEF, existing rule in cutoffs retain fairly high sensitivity in differentiating between HFpEF and non HF patients. A lower NT-proBNP cutoff of 120 pg/ml, however, is suggested for excluding HFpEF. NT-proBNP has an added prognostic value in HFpEF patients, as the level of NT-proBNP elevation correlates to the severity of associated symptoms [24, 25].

Other Causes of NP Depression

There are a number of comorbidities and conditions that can cause lower NPs in patients with acute heart failure. When HF onset occurs rather rapidly as in flash pulmonary edema, NPs do not have enough time to be upregulated and detected in the blood [5, 26]. Causes of flash pulmonary edema include acute valvular insufficiency, coronary ischemia, arrhythmia, and diastolic dysfunction.

When the cause of HF occurs upstream of the left ventricle, as in acute mitral regurgitation or mitral stenosis, the absence of significant ventricular stress causes NPs to remain only moderately elevated [27]. Patients with cardiac tamponade or constrictive pericarditis may have HF symptoms, but normal or only slightly elevated NP levels. The Increased pericardial pressure in these patients prevents the myocardium from stretching, which decreases the amount of NPs released [5, 28].

The "Gray Zone"

Patients presenting with symptoms of acute HF with BNP levels 100–400 pg/ml, and NT-proBNP levels in between the previously mentioned rule out cut off (300 pg/ ml) and the age-specific rule in values (450, 900, or 1800 pg/ml) are considered to be in the "gray zone" (Table 19.2). Interpreting gray zone NP levels poses the

Table 19.2 Common causes of NP elevation and depression

NP elevation	NP depression
Low body weight	Obesity
Acute coronary syndrome	Flash pulmonary edema
Renal dysfunction	Acute mitral regurgitation
Dysrhythmias	Mitral stenosis
LV dysfunction	Cardiac tamponade
Obstructive sleep apnea	Constrictive pericarditis
Acute pulmonary embolism	Young age
Pulmonary hypertension	HFpEF
RV dysfunction	
Sepsis	
Cirrhosis	
Cor pulmonale	
Hyperthyroidism	
Old age	

greatest challenge to correctly diagnosing acute HF. The common comorbidities previously discussed can cause NP elevation in patients without HF and NP depression in those with HF.

It is important to note that even though gray zone NP levels have reduced diagnostic accuracy in the acute setting, patients with elevated gray zone levels have poorer outcomes (e.g., reduced mortality, increased hazard) than dyspneic patients without elevated NPs [29]. Patients with gray zone values may have subclinical or intermediate HF, cardiac ischemia, severe pulmonary disease, or other diseases that cause intermediate NP elevation [30]. Gray zone NPs, therefore, should not be discarded as a negative result because of their associated prognostic usefulness.

Patients with previous histories of HF also can have intermediately elevated NPs. After an acute HF exacerbation, hospitalization and treatment do not always return NP levels back to normal. Therefore, physicians should interpret NPs in comparison to a patient's individual dry baseline levels, measured when that patient is asymptomatic and euvolemic. BNP or NT-proBNP levels above a patient's dry baseline could be indicative of an acute HF exacerbation [5].

Case Study NP Interpretation

Understanding the caveats to using NPs may resolve the case of the 45 year old patient with seemingly normal NPs. NP levels are negative according to the standard cutoffs, BNP < 100 pg/ml and NT-proBNP < 450 pg/ml (for patients less than 50 years old), which could be misleading (Fig. 19.1). Because this patient has a BMI > 30, his BNP is actually elevated using the recommended 54 pg/ml obesity cutoff. One must also consider that if this patient has HFpEF (which an echocardiogram would help determine), his NPs may not be as elevated as they would be in the setting of systolic HF. His NT-proBNP is not normal and actually is elevated using the recommended HFpEF rule out threshold of 120 pg/ml. Due to the patient's

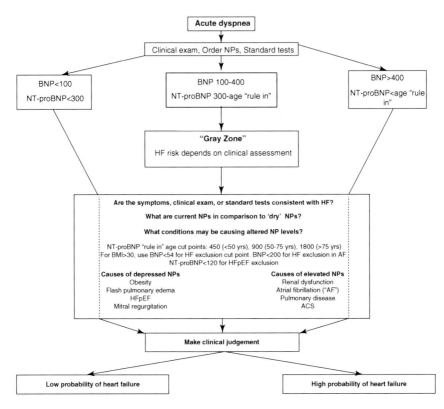

Fig. 19.1 An algorithm for evaluating patients with acute dyspnea using BNP and NT-pro BNP. Accurate interpretation of NPs depends on knowledge of the common comorbidities and clinical situations that cause NP elevation and depression. BNP and NT-proBNP values are measured in pg/ml

history of HF, it is necessary to compare his current "wet" BNP to the dry BNP taken 3 months ago, which is now elevated by 200%. Accordingly, it would appear that his NP levels are indicative of acute HF.

Conclusion

Heart failure is often difficult to diagnose clinically, and natriuretic peptides add diagnostic and prognostic value to the assessing physician. Knowledge of the various caveats to BNP and NT-proBNP interpretation is crucial to ensuring their clinical efficacy. As seen in the previously described case study, a proper and thorough understanding of using natriuretic peptide levels may resolve what appears to be discordant and misleading data. Factors such as age, gender, obesity, renal disease, ischemia, previous HF, preserved ejection fraction, dysrhythmia, and pulmonary disease should determine how to interpret NP cutoffs to avoid false-positives and the more harmful false-negatives, especially in patients with "gray zone" levels. Natriuretic peptides when used properly in conjunction with appropriate clinical judgement will aid in the accurate diagnosis and effective management of heart failure.

References

1. Daniels LB, Allison MA, Clopton P, et al. Use of natriuretic peptides in pre-participation screening of college athletes. Int J Cardiol. 2008;124(3):411–4.
2. Maisel AS, Clopton P, Krishnaswamy P, et al. Impact of age, race, and sex on the ability of B-type natriuretic peptide to aid in the emergency diagnosis of heart failure: results from the Breathing Not Properly (BNP) multinational study. Am Heart J. 2004;147(6):1078–84.
3. Januzzi JL, van Kimmenade R, Lainchbury J, et al. NT-proBNP testing for diagnosis and short-term prognosis in acute destabilized heart failure: an international pooled analysis of 1256 patients: the International Collaborative of NT-proBNP Study. Eur Heart J. 2006;27(3):330–7.
4. Januzzi JL, Camargo CA, Anwaruddin S, et al. The N-terminal Pro-BNP investigation of dyspnea in the emergency department (PRIDE) study. Am J Cardiol. 2005;95(8):948–54.
5. Daniels LB, Maisel AS. Natriuretic peptides. J Am Coll Cardiol. 2007;50(25):2357–68.
6. Redfield M, Rodeheffer RJ, Jacobsen SJ, et al. Plasma brain natriuretic peptide concentration: impact of age and gender. J Am Coll Cardiol. 2002;40(5):976–82.
7. Maffei S, Del Ry S, Prontera C, Clerico A. Increase in circulating levels of cardiac natriuretic peptides after hormone replacement therapy in postmenopausal women. Clin Sci (Lond). 2001;101:447–53.
8. Hillege HL, Girbes AR, de Kam PJ, et al. Renal function, neurohormonal activation, and survival in patients with chronic heart failure. Circulation. 2000;102(2):203–10.
9. Cataliotti A, Malatino LS, Jougasaki M, et al. Circulating natriuretic peptide concentrations in patients with end-stage renal disease: role of brain natriuretic peptide as a biomarker for ventricular remodeling. Mayo Clin Proc. 2001;76(11):1111–9.
10. McCullough PA, Duc P, Omland T, et al. B-type natriuretic peptide and renal function in the diagnosis of heart failure: an analysis from the Breathing Not Properly Multinational Study. Am J Kidney Dis. 2003;41(3):571–9.
11. Anwaruddin S, Lloyd Jones DM, Baggish A, et al. Renal function, congestive heart failure, and amino-terminal pro-brain natriuretic peptide measurement: results from the ProBNP Investigation of Dyspnea in the Emergency Department (PRIDE) Study. J Am Coll Cardiol. 2006;47(1):91–7.
12. Morita E, Yasue H, Yoshimura M, et al. Increased plasma levels of brain natriuretic peptide in patients with acute myocardial infarction. Circulation. 1993;88(1):82–91.
13. Zdravkovic V, Mladenovic V, Colic M, et al. NT-proBNP for prognostic and diagnostic evaluation in patients with acute coronary syndromes. Kardiol Pol. 2013;71(5):472–9.
14. Nagaya N, Nishikimi T, Okano Y, et al. Plasma brain natriuretic peptide levels increase in proportion to the extent of right ventricular dysfunction in pulmonary hypertension. J Am Coll Cardiol. 1998;31(1):202–8.
15. Klinger JR, Arnal F, Warburton RR, et al. Downregulation of pulmonary atrial natriuretic peptide receptors in rats exposed to chronic hypoxia. J Appl Physiol. 1994;77(3):1309–16.
16. Morrison LK, Harrison A, Krishnaswamy P, et al. Utility of a rapid B-natriuretic peptide assay in differentiating congestive heart failure from lung disease in patients presenting with dyspnea. J Am Coll Cardiol. 2002;39(2):202–9.

17. Rudiger A, Gasser S, Fischler M, et al. Comparable increase of B-type natriuretic peptide and amino-terminal pro-B-type natriuretic peptide levels in patients with severe sepsis, septic shock, and acute heart failure. Crit Care Med. 2006;34(8):2140–4.
18. Richards M, Di Somma S, Mueller C, et al. Atrial fibrillation impairs the diagnostic performance of cardiac natriuretic peptides in dyspneic patients: results from the BACH Study (Biomarkers in ACute Heart Failure). JACC Heart Fail. 2013;1(3):192–9.
19. Morello A, Lloyd Jones DM, Chae CU, et al. Association of atrial fibrillation and amino-terminal pro-brain natriuretic peptide concentrations in dyspneic subjects with and without acute heart failure: results from the ProBNP Investigation of Dyspnea in the Emergency Department (PRIDE) study. Am Heart J. 2007;153(1):90–7.
20. Daniels LB, Clopton P, Bhalla V, et al. How obesity affects the cut-points for B-type natriuretic peptide in the diagnosis of acute heart failure. Results from the Breathing Not Properly Multinational Study. Am Heart J. 2006;151(5):999–1005.
21. Sarzani R, Dessì Fulgheri P, Paci VM, et al. Expression of natriuretic peptide receptors in human adipose and other tissues. J Endocrinol Invest. 1996;19(9):581–5.
22. Das SR, Drazner MH, Dries DL, et al. Impact of body mass and body composition on circulating levels of natriuretic peptides: results from the Dallas Heart Study. Circulation. 2005;112(14):2163–8.
23. Owan TE, Hodge DO, Herges RM, et al. Trends in prevalence and outcome of heart failure with preserved ejection fraction. N Engl J Med. 2006;355(3):251–9.
24. O'Donoghue M, Chen A, Baggish AL, et al. The effects of ejection fraction on N-terminal ProBNP and BNP levels in patients with acute CHF: analysis from the ProBNP Investigation of Dyspnea in the Emergency Department (PRIDE) study. J Card Fail. 2005;11(5 Suppl):S9–14.
25. Maisel AS, McCord J, Nowak RM, et al. Bedside B-Type natriuretic peptide in the emergency diagnosis of heart failure with reduced or preserved ejection fraction. Results from the Breathing Not Properly Multinational Study. J Am Coll Cardiol. 2003;41(11):2010–7.
26. Rimoldi SF, Yuzefpolskaya M, Allemann Y, et al. Flash pulmonary edema. Prog Cardiovasc Dis. 2009;52(3):249–59.
27. Kerr AJ, Raffel OC, Whalley GA, et al. Elevated B-type natriuretic peptide despite normal left ventricular function on rest and exercise stress echocardiography in mitral regurgitation. Eur Heart J. 2008;29(3):363–70.
28. Minai K, Komukai K, Arase S, et al. Cardiac tamponade as an independent condition affecting the relationship between the plasma B-type natriuretic peptide levels and cardiac function. Heart Vessels. 2013;28(4):510–3.
29. van Kimmenade RR, Pinto YM, Januzzi JL. Importance and interpretation of intermediate (gray zone) amino-terminal pro-B-type natriuretic peptide concentrations. Am J Cardiol. 2008;101(3A):39–42.
30. Brenden CK, Hollander JE, Guss D, et al. Gray zone BNP levels in heart failure patients in the emergency department: results from the Rapid Emergency Department Heart Failure Outpatient Trial (REDHOT) multicenter study. Am Heart J. 2006;151(5):1006–11.

Chapter 20
Gaps in Our Biomarker Armamentarium: What Novel Biomarkers Might Be Synergistic in Patients with Acute Disease

Bertil Lindahl

Abstract We have seen dramatic improvements of the acute cardiac care in the last 20 years, which have led to a substantial reduction in short and long term mortality after acute myocardial infarction (AMI) as well as after heart failure (HF) [1, 2]. These impressive successes have been achieved mainly by improved treatments but also through improved diagnostic methods. During this time period we have got access to some very strong new biomarkers, cardiac troponins (cardiac troponin I and cardiac troponin I) and natriuretic peptides (BNP and NT-proBNP). Their success and widespread use are based upon their excellent diagnostic properties rather than their similarly excellent prognostic properties. The introduction and development of more and more sensitive cTn assays have revolutionized the diagnosis of AMI.

Keywords Biomarkers in cardiology • Novel biomarkers in cardiology • Acute myocardial infarction and biomarkers • Cardiac troponins • Heart failure and biomarkers

We have seen dramatic improvements of the acute cardiac care in the last 20 years, which have led to a substantial reduction in short and long term mortality after acute myocardial infarction (AMI) as well as after heart failure (HF) [1, 2]. These impressive successes have been achieved mainly by improved treatments but also through improved diagnostic methods. During this time period we have got access to some very strong new biomarkers, cardiac troponins (cardiac troponin I and cardiac troponin I) and natriuretic peptides (BNP and NT-proBNP). Their success and widespread use are based upon their excellent diagnostic properties rather than their similarly excellent prognostic properties. The introduction and development of more and more sensitive cTn assays have revolutionized the diagnosis of AMI. AMI can now be ruled-in or ruled-out within a few hours, rather than within a day in the

B. Lindahl, MD, PhD
Uppsala Clinical Research Center and Department of Medical Sciences, Uppsala University Hospital, Uppsala, Sweden
e-mail: bertil.lindahl@ucr.uu.se

© Springer International Publishing Switzerland 2016
A.S. Maisel, A.S. Jaffe (eds.), *Cardiac Biomarkers*,
DOI 10.1007/978-3-319-42982-3_20

pre-troponin era. Furthermore, in a large proportion of patients previously classified as having unstable angina, elevated levels of cardiac troponin can be detected, and hence, these patients are now classified as having AMI. Similarly, the natriuretic peptides, BNP and NT-proBNP, markers increasing in response to pressure and/or volume overload of the heart, have been established as a first line diagnostic test both in acute and chronic HF.

However, despite these impressive advances, there are many remaining gaps in our diagnostic arsenal for acute cardiac patients. Numerous new biomarkers have been suggested during the last decades to close these gaps. However, very few of those, if any, are in routine clinical use, why is that? The key question for every biomarker is: will knowledge of the level of the marker in an individual patient lead to a change in the treatment or management of the patient?

A biomarker does not exist in isolation; the clinical usefulness of the marker is heavily dependent on available therapeutic options. That a marker provides independent prognostic (independent of already available risk markers) information is important; it tells that the level of the marker reflects some pathophysiological process of importance. However, that is seldom enough for a marker to be clinically useful. It must be possible to implement measures, based on the biomarker information, that improve the outcome for the patient. Unfortunately, that is seldom the case. That is why so many proposed markers in cardiology have failed to reach widespread use. It stands in contrast to in oncology where a number of biomarkers (mostly genetic markers) are decisive for the selection of adequate treatment because they classify the tumors into therapeutically meaningful subgroups [3].

Another important aspect of biomarkers is that there is a world of difference between being able to show statistical differences between disease and non-disease at group level, and being able to reliably identify or exclude the disease in an individual patient. There is an important difference in thinking between markers for diagnostic use and prognostic use. For diagnosis we tend to think in a dichotomous way – you either have, or not have the disease; or belong, or not belong to a diagnostic subgroup (e.g., ischemic or non-ischemic heart failure). In contrast, for prognosis we think in probabilities, e.g., the risk of dying within 1 year increases from 5 to 20%. Many of the "new" biomarkers have been evaluated regarding their prognostic capacity and shown to be prognostic. However, more seldom are the studies appropriately designed to be able to show added value above established clinical risk markers and biomarkers, nor are proper diagnostic studies or prospective treatment studies stratified on the biomarker results performed.

Gaps in Our Biomarker Armamentarium: Patients with Suspicion of an Acute Coronary Syndrome

With the introduction of more sensitive cTn assays it has become painfully evident for clinicians that myocardial injury, and thereby cTn elevation, is present also in many acute and chronic conditions other than classical AMI [4]. Only a small minority of patients seeking acute care for symptoms indicative of an acute coronary syndrome will eventually be diagnosed with classical (type 1) AMI. Typically, less than 10% of chest pain patients seen in the emergency department (ED) will have AMI [5] and in this population the positive predictive value for AMI of an elevation of cTn above the 99th percentile of healthy individuals is less than 50%. Including also patients with other more vague symptoms causing enough suspicion to lead to cardiac troponin testing, an even lower proportion will be diagnosed with AMI. Therefore, it is important to be able to separate cTn elevation due to acute myocardial injury from cTn elevation due to chronic myocardial injury; and cTn elevation due to myocardial ischemia from cTn elevation due to non-ischemic causes. Furthermore, it is important to distinguish between ischemic myocardial injury caused by a athero-thrombo-embolic coronary event (type 1 AMI) from an ischemic myocardial injury secondary to oxygen supply–demand imbalance of other reasons (type 2 AMI) [4].

Gap 1: Separation of Acute and Chronic Myocardial Injury (Case 1)

Chronic elevations of cTn, as well as ST-T changes in the ECG, are common among patients with stable angina, stable congestive heart failure or atrial fibrillation. These patients often visit the emergency department and have cTn measured and therefore represent a diagnostic challenge. In one study of stable CAD patients without any acute symptoms, as much as 7% would have been labeled AMI following the Universal Definition of AMI when diagnostic classification had been based on a single cTn result and ECG changes [6]. The obvious solution is to repeat cTn measurements and look for an increase or decrease in cTn levels. However, also patients with elevated cTn due to an acute AMI sometimes lack significant changes over a 3–6 h period, e.g., late presenters [7]. Therefore, a biomarker that could tell whether the cTn elevation represents an acute injury or a chronic condition would be very helpful. Simultaneous elevation of Copeptin and cTn indicates that the damage is acute and has started within the last few hours [8]. However, the opposite is not true, a non-elevated Copeptin level in conjunction with an elevated cTn do not exclude an acute injury, especially in cases with small acute AMIs or when the injury occurred for more than a few hours ago. Copeptin is therefore of limited value for this purpose. In the future, measuring different posttranslational modified subforms of cTn may be a way to determine the age of the myocardial injury [9]. Another future possibility may be measurement of single microRNAs or clusters of microRNAs (see below).

Gap 2: Separation of Acute Myocardial Infarction (=Acute Ischemic Injury) from Acute Non-ischemic Myocardial Injury

To differentiate myocardial damage and cTn elevation of ischemic from non-ischemic origin is a common problem facing clinicians, especially in the emergency department or in the intensive care unit (ICU). cTn is very often elevated in critically ill patients, e.g., studies of patients in the ICU show that the majority of the patients will have elevated cTn, although ischemia or a classical AMI (type 1) will only be possible to prove in a minority of these cases [10]. However, this problem is also frequent outside the ICU, e.g., myocarditis with an atypical presentation, especially when lacking a history of recent viral infection, can be very difficult to separate in the acute phase from a non-ST elevation myocardial infarction. Cardiac magnetic resonance imaging at a later stage is often required to separate the two entities.

A reliable marker of myocardial ischemia would also be valuable for identifying the remaining, but rare, cases of true unstable angina, i.e., patients with new onset of myocardial ischemia at rest or at minimal exertion and without concomitant elevation of cTn.

Therefore, a biomarker able to detect myocardial ischemia would be of great value to complement measurement of cTn. However, the proposed markers of ischemia, have so far been a disappointment. There was great hope around ischemia modified albumin (IMA) some 10 years ago, but studies failed to prove IMA as a reliable marker of ischemia and IMA is no longer on the market. Since microRNAs seem to be involved in the myocardium's response to ischemia certain microRNA may emerge as a useful marker of myocardial ischemia in the future.

Gap 3: Separation of Type 1 AMI from Type 2 AMI (Case 2)

In type 1 AMI the ischemia and necrosis are caused by an insufficient blood supply due to a primary athero-thrombo-embolic event in the coronary artery completely or partially blocking the blood flow. In contrast, in type 2 AMI the myocardial ischemia and necrosis arise secondary to a non-coronary, triggering factor that provokes an imbalance in the supply and demand of oxygen to the myocardium [4]. In the former case the immediate therapeutic measures are focused on restoring and maintaining sufficient blood supply and in the latter case the immediate therapeutic measures are focused on removing the triggering factor causing the imbalance in the supply and demand of oxygen. Type 2 AMI is not uncommon, especially in more unselected populations. Depending on the type of population, the proportion of AMI patients with type-2 AMI varies tremendously in the literature, from 2 to over 30 % [11]. However, it may be very difficult to separate a type 1 and type 2 AMI from each other just from the clinical presentation and history. Therefore, it would be of great value to have a biomarker able to separate type 1 and 2 AMI already on admission. Possible candidates would be markers able to detect the underlying plaque rupture or plaque erosion, which will be a formidable challenge given the minimal size of the ruptured plaque. Alternative, and possibly more likely, candidates would be markers of the thrombotic process in the coronary artery. However, at present the markers of activation of the coagulation system have severe preanalytical limitations, are too insensitive or have very large inter individual variability, making them not useful for use on individual patients in clinical routine.

Gaps in Our Biomarker Armamentarium–Patients with Suspected or Verified Heart Failure

HF is a heterogeneous syndrome, with many different underlying causes and manifests itself in everything from mild unspecific symptoms and signs to very severe and typical symptoms and signs. Consequently, no single diagnostic test provides 100 % accuracy, e.g., natriuretic peptides provide a very high negative predictive value, but an only modest positive predictive value for the diagnosis. Once diagnosed, etiological considerations include ischemic (post myocardial infarction and chronic coronary artery disease) and nonischemic causes (e.g., hypertensive, valvular, genetic cardiomyopathies, metabolic, infiltrative, toxins, infectious, arrhythmic, and pericardial). Furthermore, comorbidities such as chronic kidney disease or chronic obstructive pulmonary disease are common. Obviously, knowing the underlying cause and any significant comorbidity has large prognostic and therapeutic consequences. It is therefore important to develop new diagnostic methods, and not least new biomarkers, that improve the diagnosis of HF, identify underlying causes, enhance risk assessment and guide therapy.

The natriuretic peptides (discussed in depth in Chaps. 13, 14, 15. 16, 17, 18, 19) have gained widespread use the last 15–20 years, and are undoubtedly valuable for diagnosis, prognosis and to some extent for guiding therapy. However, there are several areas in which additional biomarkers would be valuable. Several biomarkers, reflecting other pathophysiological mechanisms than the natriuretic peptides, have been suggested and evaluated, such as Soluble ST2 (sST2) (Chap. 21), Growth differentiation factor (GDF)-15, Mid-regional pro adrenomedullin (MR-proADM), Galectin-3 and cardiac troponins (Chaps. 7, 8, 9). All these markers have been shown to provide prognostic information in heart failure patients, in some studies independent of the natriuretic peptides and thus, providing additional prognostic information. However, the main limitations of these markers are that no one has shown any clinically meaningful added value for diagnosis of heart failure or selection of heart failure treatment. Hence, it is doubtful that these markers will gain widespread clinical use in heart failure patients, except cardiac troponins. Cardiac troponins are routinely used in patients with suspected acute heart failure to verify or exclude concomitant myocardial infarction or injury.

Gap 1: Heart Failure in Patients with Comorbidities

Patients with heart failure often have coexisting diseases that complicate the diagnostic process, e.g., the interpretation of the level of BNP or NT-proBNP is difficult in patients with depressed renal function. Other examples of diagnostic difficulties are patients with known chronic heart failure and chronic obstructive pulmonary disease, or with known chronic heart failure and signs of a respiratory infection that comes to the ED with worsening symptoms of dyspnea. In these situation multimarker approaches probably is the way forward; intelligent combinations of new and existing markers.

Gap 2: Heart Failure with Reduced Ejection Fraction Versus Preserved Ejection Fraction (Case 3)

Approximately, half of the heart failure population has heart failure with reduced ejection fraction (HFrEF), and the other half has heart failure with preserved ejection fraction (HFpEF). However, there is a gender difference; HFpEF is more common than HFrEF in women and vice versa in men. Both patients with HFpEF and HFrEF still have a poor prognosis, although patients with HFpEF have a slightly lower long term mortality compared to HFrEF, hazard ratio (95 % confidence interval) 0.86 (0.77-0.97) [12]. There is a strong evidence based foundation for the treatment recommendations in HFrEF. In contrast, there is no specific evidence based treatment for HFpEF. Hence, it is clinically important to separate these two entities. Furthermore, it may be challenging to diagnose heart failure in patients with HFpEF, especially in patients with an abnormal relaxation filling pattern in whom the levels of natriuretic peptides may be normal. Consequently, a limited utility of natriuretic peptides for the detection of mild systolic and diastolic dysfunction was found in a large unselected population [13].

Gap 3: Heart Failure of Ischemic Origin Versus Non-ischemic Origin (Case 3)

Identification of the underlying cause of the heart failure has important therapeutical consequences. In case of underlying coronary artery disease it is critical to determine whether there are signs of hibernating myocardium and thus a potentially reversible cause of the depressed ventricular function. Heart failure of nonischemic origin includes a wide variety of causes such as hypertension, genetic cardiomyopathies, valvular, congenital, metabolic, infiltrative, infectious, arrhythmic diseases, all with different treatment and different prognosis. It can sometimes be difficult and cumbersome to identify the cause. However, to make it even more complex, the causes of heart failure are not mutually exclusive; not seldom two or more causes exist in parallel and it can be very difficult to determine their relative importance. Therefore, biomarkers capable of identifying specific underlying causes would potentially be clinically useful.

What Novel Biomarkers Might Be Synergistic in Patients with Acute Disease

The Road to a Clinically Useful and Widely Adopted Biomarker

As discussed previously, to be clinically useful a novel biomarker must provide information that ultimately improves the management and treatment of the individual patient.

- The new biomarker improves the diagnostic accuracy compared to an already established marker or any other diagnostic test, provides the diagnosis faster (if time is critical in the decision making process) or provides similar accuracy but to lower costs.
- The new biomarker makes it possible to diagnose an entity where there currently is no useful biomarker or test, or makes it possible to subclassify the disease in a clinically meaningful way.
- The new biomarker makes it possible to select treatment or monitor treatment based on the biomarker levels.
- The new biomarker gives prognostic information of such magnitude that it directly affects the management of the patient, e.g., identifies a subgroup of such low risk that specific treatment can be avoided.

In the following a number of biomarkers will be discussed, biomarkers which may have the potential to meet any of the above claims. However, it is important to stress that all these markers still have a long way to go to prove their clinical usefulness. Appropriately sized prospective studies in appropriate populations and with robust endpoints and best available gold standards and comparators will be needed.

Micro RNA

MicroRNAs (miRNAs) are small, non-coding, RNA molecules consisting of approximately 22 nucleotides. Currently more than 2,500 miRNAs have been described in humans. miRNAs act as post-transcriptional regulators of gene expression and are key regulators of complex biological processes. Since some of the miRNAs are possible to measure in the circulation, they have been investigated as novel biomarkers for cardiovascular diseases, especially acute myocardial infarction and heart failure. The levels of miRNAs in patients are either elevated or decreased as compared to in healthy individuals. Measuring clusters of miRNAs, instead of single miRNA, identifying characteristic signatures of miRNA might increase the diagnostic and prognostic potential.

For quantification of miRNA, high throughput sequencing, real time PCR (qPCR) or microarrays is used, all time consuming methods not particularly suitable for measurements in daily practice. Furthermore, there is a lack of standardized protocols and automatized work flows.

For comprehensive reviews of miRNA in cardiovascular disease see reference [14, 15].

Acute Myocardial Infarction and Coronary Artery Disease

A number of circulating miRNAs have shown promising results for diagnosis of AMI in small studies (e.g., miR-1, miR-133a, miR-133b, miR-208a, miR-499, miR-499-5p); some studies have suggested that measurement of miRNA may allow earlier diagnosis of AMI compared to measurement of cardiac troponins. However, in one of the few larger clinical studies [16], none of the six evaluated miRNAs was able to out-perform, or add to, cardiac troponin. Other small studies have suggested that signatures of circulating miRNAs might be useful for separating patients with unstable angina from patients with stable angina pectoris. Maybe of potentially more importance is that a number of miRNAs has been linked to a diagnosis of coronary artery disease, a condition where we currently lack useful biomarkers. However, these initial results need to be verified in larger studies.

Heart Failure

An increasing number of miRNAs have been shown to exhibit altered circulating levels in the peripheral blood of patients with heart failure (e.g., miR-122, miR-210, miR-423-5p, miR-499 and miR-622). Particularly interesting is the possibility to subclassify heart failure patients according to underlying etiology. The expression of miRNA is a highly dynamic process; with different expression of miRNAs in different stages of the conditions leading to HF. Furthermore, different expression of miRNAs have been related to HF-associated pathologies, such as hypertrophy, hypertrophic cardiomyopathy, dilated cardiomyopathy and ischemic cardiomyopathy. Consequently, some small studies have verified different expression of miRNAs in patients suffering from heart failure of ischemic and nonischemic origin. In addition several miRNAs have shown potential as prognostic indicators.

However, the evaluation of miRNAs as clinically useful biomarkers in acute coronary syndromes/coronary artery disease as well in heart failure is still in its infancy; larger and appropriately designed trials are required to establish whether current candidates provide additional benefit, over and above those of existing biomarkers. Furthermore, to be clinically useful substantial technological development are required to enable rapid, reliable and reproducible results for the absolute quantification of circulating miRNAs.

Metabolomics

Metabolomics is a term used to describe the measurement of multiple small-molecule metabolites in biological specimens. The Human Metabolome Database contains to date over 41,000 metabolites (http://www.hmdb.ca/). Metabolites represent the end-products of multiple reactions and interactions in biological processes. Therefore, determination of metabolites may allow an integrated and dynamic measurement of phenotype and medical condition.

Although there is an increasing interest in metabolomics profiling for identification of novel biomarkers or signatures of biomarkers in cardiovascular diseases, metabolomics profiling may have its largest potential for identification of novel disease mechanisms.

Metabolomic profiling is most often performed with either nuclear magnetic resonance or mass spectrometry in combination with liquid chromatography or gas chromatography. Nuclear magnetic resonance is a simpler technique not requiring chemical manipulation of samples when working with biological fluids, while mass spectrometry offers a much better sensitivity. For comprehensive reviews of metabolomics in cardiovascular disease see references [17–19].

Acute Myocardial Ischemia and Coronary Artery Disease

Since it is well known that acute restrictions of coronary flow induce dramatic and immediate shifts in cardiac metabolism there are hopes that it will be possible to diagnose cardiac ischemia by metabolomics profiling. In a small study, 32 metabolites measured in serum showed dynamic changes after ischemia, of which four (Creatine, Glucose + taurine, Lactate and Triglycerides) displayed statistical significant differences 2 h after the induction of myocardial ischemia [20]. When testing this biosignature based on the 32 metabolites, on patients with acute chest pain, it was possible to reliably discriminate patients with myocardial ischemia from those with non-coronary ischemic chest pain. However, these results need to be confirmed in much larger studies. Other studies have shown a strong association of arginine and its downstream metabolites ornithine and citrulline with coronary artery disease and with future adverse cardiovascular events.

Heart Failure

Heart failure is associated with metabolic dysfunction. Therefore, metabolomics has been applied to studies of heart failure to discover valuable biomarkers. The studies so far are small and relatively few; and have reported a diverse array of molecular profiles, perhaps reflecting the heterogeneous nature of the heart failure syndrome, but also differences in selection of patients, study design, assays used, and statistical methodology. A recent study identified a cluster of 4 metabolites (histidine, phenylalanine, spermidine, and phosphatidylcholine C34:4) that separated stage C HF patients from healthy control subjects. The discriminatory ability of this combination was similar to that of B-type natriuretic peptide alone. A different combination of 4 metabolite parameters (dimethylarginine/arginine ratio, spermidine, butyrylcarnitine, and total essential amino acids) was associated with outcome after 1.3 years, and classified patients according to risk better than B-type natriuretic peptide [21].

Protein Markers

Several new protein markers of interest for diagnosis or prognosis in acute myocardial infarction or heart failure are described elsewhere in this book, e.g., Copeptin, ST2, and Galactin 3.

Growth Differentiation Factor 15 (GDF-15) is an additional marker of potential interest that has been evaluated extensively in recent years [22, 23]. GDF-15 is a member of the transforming growth factor β superfamily; it is also known as macrophage inhibitory cytokine-1, placental transforming growth factor-beta, gene placental bone morphogenic protein, prostate-derived factor, NSAID-activated gene 1, and placental transforming growth factor Beta. GDF-15 is expressed in virtually all tissues. The exact biological functions of GDF-15 are still poorly understood, however, its expression is up-regulated with many different pathological conditions including inflammation, cancer, cardiovascular diseases, pulmonary disease and renal disease.

Owing to the lack of tissue specificity, GDF-15 has a limited potential as a diagnostic marker. However, GDF-15 has been shown to be a strong and independent predictor of mortality and disease progression in patients with established disease such as acute coronary syndromes, angina pectoris, heart failure, stroke, chronic kidney disease, and different types of cancer. Also in community-dwellers, higher concentrations of GDF-15 have been associated with increased cardiovascular as well as non-cardiovascular mortality, and development and progression of a broad range of diseases including coronary artery disease and heart failure. Especially for prediction of mortality, GDF-15 has emerged as one of the strongest biomarker ("death marker"). There is however, no strong support so far that GDF-15 is useful for selection of specific treatment or for monitoring of treatment effects in cardiovascular diseases.

Concluding Remarks

The biomarker research is a rapidly evolving field and it is hard to predict exactly where the next break through will occur in cardiovascular diseases. However, undoubtedly we will get new useful biomarkers in our diagnostic and prognostic arsenal within the next few years. The more biomarkers we get, the more important it becomes for the diagnosing physician to use them properly and interpret the results wisely. Therefore, it will be very important that adequate training in using and interpreting of new biomarkers are conducted in parallel with the introduction of the markers.

Case 1

A woman, 84 years of age, with paroxysmal atrial fibrillation, congestive heart failure, renal dysfunction and chronic back pain, was admitted due to a new episode of atrial fibrillation and chest discomfort, but no typical ischemic chest pain. She has previously been hospitalized with an AMI 5 years ago and an episode of atrial fibrillation and worsening of heart failure 3 years ago.

On admission she had an oxygen saturation of 95 % on O_2 2 L/min, had no peripheral oedema, a blood pressure of 165/105 mmHg and a heart rate of 110 beats/min. The ECG showed atrial fibrillation, minor unspecific lateral ST-depression and was otherwise unchanged compared to previous recordings. Laboratory values on admission: cTnI 0.15 µg/L (Upper reference limit 0.022 µg/L); Hb 118 g/L, Creatinine 277 µmol/L.

Clinically relevant questions for the emergency physican: Is the elevation of troponin I caused by an acute ischemic event, e.g., a type 1 or type 2 AMI? Or is the elevation of troponin I expression of a chronic condition that causes a constant rise of troponin, like CHF and atrial fibrillation, or just high age? Does the elevation of troponin prompt any specific treatment?

The patient was given extra medication temporarily to control the heart rate. Sinus rhythm was restored spontaneously within a few hours and the chest discomfort disappeared. cTnI after 3 and 9 h were 0.19 and 0.14 µg/L, respectively. The patient's medical records revealed that the corresponding cTnI values during the previous hospitalization for atrial fibrillation and heart failures were 0.24, 0.22 and 0.19 µg/L.

The cTnI levels were interpreted as chronic elevation of cTnI in an elderly patient with atrial fibrillation, CHF and renal dysfunction and not as expression of an AMI. Therefore, no coronary angiogram was performed. She was discharged in her habitual state and with unchanged medication after a couple of days to her home.

A biomarker able to detect already on admission, ongoing ischemia or to separate acutely released cardiac troponin from cardiac troponin chronically released would be helpful in this situation for the immediate management of the patient.

Case 2

A man, 75 years of age, with known hypertension and diabetes mellitus, was admitted due to 1 h of chest pain, dyspnea and palpitations. On admission he had no peripheral oedema, a blood pressure of 140/60 mmHg and a heart rate of 150 beats/min. The ECG showed atrial fibrillation and ST segment depression in inferior and lateral leads. On admission cTnI was 0.02 (upper reference limit 0.022 µg/L), Creatinine 85 µmol/L and Hb 139 g/L.

Clinically relevant questions for the emergency physician: Has the patient ongoing ischemia? In case of ischemia, is it a type 1 or a type 2 AMI? Is there an indication of acute or subacute coronary angiography?

Cardiac TnI values after 6 and 24 h were 1.9 and 7.8 µg/L, respectively. After restoring sinus rhythm the patient was without symptoms. A coronary angiogram performed day three showed minor atherosclerotic changes in proximal and mid LAD and RCA, and a stenosis of around 50 % in LCX. No PCI was attempted. Warfarin was added to the previous medication for hypertension and diabetes mellitus and the patient was discharged home. Interpretation: Type 2 AMI in a man with moderate coronary artery disease but no culprit lesion, in which the acute ischemia was triggered by an episode of rapid atrial fibrillation.

In this patient biomarkers capable of detecting ischemia and to early differentiate between type 1 and type 2 AMI, respectively, would have been valuable for the further management, e.g., for determining the need and timing of coronary angiography.

Case 3

A woman, 60 years of age, with chronic treatment with warfarin due to repeated episodes of deep venous thrombosis, was examined at the outpatient clinic because of episodes of chest pain and palpitations, and dyspnea. The chest pain and dyspnea occur at moderate exertion. The examination showed no dyspnea at rest; no oedema; heart rate 80, ordinary first and second heart sound, a systolic murmur grade 2 with maximum in I3 sinister; blood pressure 110/60; no pulmonary crepitations. ECG showed sinus rhythm, supra ventricular ectopic beats, no Q wave or ischemic ST-T changes. Laboratory values: NT-proBNP 3790 ng/L, cardiac troponin I, potassium, sodium and creatinine within normal limits. Chest X-ray showed minor to moderate amount of pleural effusion and minor signs of interstitial pulmonary oedema.

The condition was interpreted as heart failure, possibly on the basis of ischemic heart disease. The patient was referred for echocardiography and myocardial scintigraphy.

The myocardial scintigraphy showed moderately reduced working capacity and chest pain during exercise that slowly vanished at rest. No significantly reduced myocardial uptake of the isotope, neither at rest nor during exercise. The left ventricular had normal size and a calculated ejection fraction of 62 %. Echocardiography showed also normal ejection fraction but clear signs of diastolic dysfunction and moderate pulmonary hypertension. No evidence of significant valvular engagement.

The condition was interpreted as heart failure with preserved ejection fraction (HFpEF), ischemic heart disease or hypertension unlikely causes. Despite medication the patient showed progression of the symptoms and with continuously highly elevated NT-proBNP values. The patient was referred for further investigation with right sided catheterization including myocardial biopsy.

The right sided catheterization showed a picture consistent with restrictive cardiomyopathy and secondary pulmonary hypertension. The biopsy verified cardiac amyloidosis. The patient was treated with autologous stem cell transplantation.

References

1. Jernberg T, Johanson P, Held C, Svennblad B, Lindbäck J, Wallentin L. Association between adoption of evidence-based treatment and survival for patients with st-elevation myocardial infarction. JAMA. 2011;305(16):1677–84.
2. Gabet A, Juillière Y, Lamarche-Vadel A, Vernay M, Olié V. National trends in rate of patients hospitalized for heart failure and heart failure mortality in France, 2000–2012. Eur J Heart Fail. 2015;17(6):583–90.
3. Rodríguez-Antona C, Taron M. Pharmacogenomic biomarkers for personalized cancer treatment. J Intern Med. 2015;277(2):201–17.
4. Thygesen K, Alpert JS, Jaffe AS, Simoons ML, Chaitman BR, White HD, et al. Third universal definition of myocardial infarction. Eur Heart J. 2012;33(20):2551–67.
5. Backus BE, Six AJ, Kelder JC, et al. A Prospective validation of the HEART score for chest pain in the emergency department: a multinational validation study. Int J Cardiol. 2013;168(3): 2153–8.
6. Eggers KM, Lind L, Venge P, Lindahl B. Will the universal definition of myocardial infarction criteria result in an overdiagnosis of myocardial infarction? Am J Cardiol. 2009;103(5):588–91.
7. Bjurman C, Larsson M, Johanson P, Petzold M, Lindahl B, Fu MLX, et al. Small changes in troponin T levels Are common in patients with non–ST-segment elevation myocardial infarction and are linked to higher mortality. J Am Coll Cardiol. 2013;62(14):1231–8.
8. Möckel M, Searle J. Copeptin—marker of acute myocardial infarction. Curr Atheroscler Rep. 2014;16(7):1–8. English.
9. Streng AS, de Boer D, van der Velden J, van Dieijen-Visser MP, Wodzig WKWH. Posttranslational modifications of cardiac troponin T: an overview. J Mol Cell Cardiol. 2013;63:47–56.
10. Ostermann M, Lo J, Toolan M, Tuddenham E, Sanderson B, Lei K, et al. A prospective study of the impact of serial troponin measurements on the diagnosis of myocardial infarction and hospital and six-month mortality in patients admitted to ICU with non-cardiac diagnoses. Crit Care. 2014;18(2):R62. PubMed PMID: doi:10.1186/cc13818.
11. Collinson PO, Lindahl B. Type 2 myocardial infarction – the chimaera of cardiology? Heart. 2015;101(21):1697–703. In Press.
12. Gerber Y, Weston SA, Redfield MM, et al. A contemporary appraisal of the heart failure epidemic in Olmsted County, Minnesota, 2000 to 2010. JAMA Intern Med. 2015;175(6): 996–1004.
13. Redfield MM, Rodeheffer RJ, Jacobsen SJ, Mahoney DW, Bailey KR, Burnett JC. Plasma brain natriuretic peptide to detect preclinical ventricular systolic or diastolic dysfunction: a community-based study. Circulation. 2004;109(25):3176–81.

14. Romaine SPR, Tomaszewski M, Condorelli G, Samani NJ. MicroRNAs in cardiovascular disease: an introduction for clinicians. Heart. 2015;101(12):921–8.
15. Schulte C, Zeller T. microRNA-based diagnostics and therapy in cardiovascular disease—Summing up the facts. Cardiovasc Diagn Ther. 2015;5(1):17–36.
16. Devaux Y, Mueller M, Haaf P, Goretti E, Twerenbold R, Zangrando J, et al. Diagnostic and prognostic value of circulating microRNAs in patients with acute chest pain. J Intern Med. 2015;277(2):260–71.
17. Shah SH, Kraus WE, Newgard CB. Metabolomic profiling for the identification of novel biomarkers and mechanisms related to common cardiovascular diseases: form and function. Circulation. 2012;126(9):1110–20.
18. Senn T, Hazen SL, Tang WHW. Translating metabolomics to cardiovascular biomarkers. Prog Cardiovasc Dis. 2012;55(1):70–6.
19. Bodi V, Marrachelli V, Husser O, Chorro F, Viña J, Monleon D. Metabolomics in the diagnosis of acute myocardial ischemia. J Cardiovasc Transl Res. 2013;6(5):808–15. English.
20. Bodi V, Sanchis J, Morales JM, Marrachelli VG, Nunez J, Forteza MJ, et al. Metabolomic profile of human myocardial ischemia by nuclear magnetic resonance spectroscopy of peripheral blood serum: a translational study based on transient coronary occlusion models. J Am Coll Cardiol. 2012;59(18):1629–41.
21. Cheng ML, Wang C-H, Shiao M-S, Liu M-H, Huang Y-Y, Huang C-Y, et al. Metabolic disturbances identified in plasma Are associated with outcomes in patients with heart failure: diagnostic and prognostic value of metabolomics. J Am Coll Cardiol. 2015;65(15):1509–20.
22. Xu X, Li Z, Gao W. Growth differentiation factor 15 in cardiovascular diseases: from bench to bedside. Biomarkers. 2011;16(6):466–75.
23. Lindahl B. The story of growth differentiation factor 15: another piece of the puzzle. Clin Chem. 2013;59(11):1550–2.

Chapter 21
Biomarkers in Heart Failure: ST2

Antoni Bayes-Genis and Josep Lupón

Abstract Biomarkers have emerged as indispensable tools for diagnosis and prognosis in a variety of cardiovascular diseases, and several are now considered standard of care. New markers are constantly being developed, but very few are able to significantly improve upon already-established markers. ST2 is a marker of cardiomyocyte stress and fibrosis which provides incremental value to natriuretic peptides for risk stratification in heart failure. Based upon the totality of data, measurement of ST2 is now recommended for additive risk stratification in patients with acute or ambulatory heart failure in the 2013 ACCF/AHA Guidelines. Looking forward, ST2 levels may be useful for tailoring medical therapy and to predict ventricular reverse remodeling. This chapter provides an up-to-date overview of ST2 as a marker of heart failure, and provides illustrative clinical cases into the application of ST2 now and in the future.

Keywords ST2 biomarker • Biomarker ST2 • Cardiomyocyte stress and fibrosis • Risk prediction in chronic heart failure • Biomarkers in heart failure • Heart failure biomarkers

Biomarkers have an established role in aiding with diagnosis and prognosis in a number of cardiovascular diseases. Natriuretic peptides in particular have evolved over the past 10 years to become part of the standard of care for evaluating heart failure (HF) patients in both acute and ambulatory settings. Despite the

A. Bayes-Genis, MD, PhD (✉)
Department of Cardiology, Heart Failure Unit, Heart Institute, Hospital Universitari, Germans Trias i Pujol, Badalona, Barcelona, Spain

Hospital Universitari Germans Trias i Pujol, Badalona, Spain
e-mail: abayesgenis@gmail.com

J. Lupón, MD, PhD
Department of Medicine, Universitat Autònoma de Barcelona, Barcelona, Spain

Heart Failure Unit, Heart Institute, Hospital Universitari Germans Trias i Pujol, Badalona, Spain

© Springer International Publishing Switzerland 2016
A.S. Maisel, A.S. Jaffe (eds.), *Cardiac Biomarkers*,
DOI 10.1007/978-3-319-42982-3_21

well-documented successes and strengths of natriuretic peptides, there is plenty of room for improvement in the way we evaluate and risk-stratify patients with or at risk for HF. Although a large number of candidate biomarkers have been evaluated to help fill this gap, few have survived the rigorous studies that are a prerequisite to translation into the clinical realm. ST2 is a biomarker that has successfully navigated this course and is recently emerging as a bona fide tool for patient care.

ST2 is a member of the interleukin-1 receptor-like family of proteins. Through alternative splicing ST2 is found in multiple isoforms, including a transmembrane form (ST2 ligand, or ST2L) and a soluble form (sST2) [1]. In response to mechanical stress, cardiomyocytes and fibroblasts express both ST2L and sST2. Both isoforms of ST2 bind to interleukin-33 (IL-33), which is also induced by cellular stretch and is thought to protect against myocardial fibrosis, left ventricular hypertrophy and adverse cardiovascular remodeling in pressure-overload states. Soluble ST2, which is the isoform measured by current assays, is thought to act as a decoy receptor for IL-33. The presence of high levels of sST2 blocks the favorable effects of IL-33 by limiting activation of the cascade triggered by the IL-33/ST2L interaction. Higher levels of sST2 (hereafter referred to simply as "ST2") are associated with increased myocardial fibrosis, adverse cardiac remodeling, and worse cardiovascular outcomes [1].

Measurement of ST2 is accomplished via an enzyme-linked immunosorbent assay (ELISA). Only the Presage assay (Critical Diagnostics®) is FDA cleared and CE marked. The Presage assay has good precision (coefficient of variation <5 %) even at very low analyte concentrations, as well as high *in vitro* stability [2]. With this assay, ST2 levels are now detectable in 100 % of the population. ST2 levels appear to be stable over the long-term in frozen samples. Levels of ST2 are not significantly associated with body mass index, and seem to have a weaker association with age and renal insufficiency compared to the natriuretic peptides [3]. The upper reference limit for the Presage ST2 assay is 35 ng/mL (the recommended cut-point for risk stratification in chronic HF), and 95 % of normal individuals have levels below this threshold. A recent study evaluating the biological variation of ST2 and other cardiovascular biomarkers found that the long-term intra-individual variation for ST2 was only 11 %, considerably lower than that of the natriuretic peptides (33–50 %) [4]. This low biological variation suggests that ST2 may be a useful marker to follow serially to guide therapy.

ST2 in Assessing Heart Failure Risk

The recent 2013 AHA/ACC Guidelines for the Management of Heart Failure give a class IIb recommendation for the measurement of ST2 in acute or ambulatory HF patients, noting that ST2 is not only predictive of hospitalization and death in patients with HF, but is also additive to the natriuretic peptides in its prognostic value [5].

Acute Heart Failure

In the setting of acute HF, ST2 levels rise and provide important prognostic information, though they are not recommended for use in diagnosing HF. One of the earliest studies to establish this was the PRIDE study, which evaluated 593 patients who presented to the Emergency Department (ED) with acute shortness of breath [6]. The authors found that patients diagnosed with acute HF had higher ST2 levels compared to those whose dyspnea was due to some other cause. In addition, ST2 levels were higher in those with more advanced HF symptoms based upon the New York Heart Association (NYHA) classification. For ST2 concentrations above the median there was a graded relationship between decile of ST2 and risk of 1-year mortality; patients in the highest decile of ST2 concentration were at particularly high risk, with a 1 year mortality rate exceeding 40 %. In multivariable analyses, ST2 levels were strongly associated with risk of death at 1 year, even after adjusting for natriuretic peptide levels. More recently, a 5-center cohort study of acutely dyspneic patients in the ED found that ST2 but not NT-proBNP was associated with 1 year mortality after multivariable analysis, and this was also true among the subset of 200 patients with normal systolic function [7]. This was consistent with another study, which found that ST2 levels appear to be equally predictive among HF patients with preserved and reduced systolic function.

Clinical Case 1

Male patient, 75 years old, with a long history of past smoking habit, until 2 years ago. History of hypertension, dyslipidemia, and diabetes mellitus. The patient has suffered an anterior acute myocardial infarction in December 2013. Coronary angiography showed 80 % stenosis in left main coronary artery and 50 % in right coronary artery. A drug-eluting stent was placed in left main coronary artery. The echocardiography showed a LVEF of 33 %. He was on treatment with ASA 100 mg, clopidogrel 75 mg, carvedilol 12.5 mg bid, enalapril 5 mg bid and atorvastatin 10 mg.

He was admitted 2 months later due to acute pulmonary edema. Admission BP 149/84 mmHg, HR 106 bpm, and O_2 saturation 91 %. EKG: transient atrial fibrillation; no ischemic changes (Fig 21.1a, b).

Echocardiography showed: LVEF 34 %, LVEDD 65 mm, LVESD 54 mm. Coronary angiography displayed stent without stenoses and absence of new coronary lesions.

With i.v. diuretics and vasodilators the patient had a good in-hospital clinical course.

Admission biomarker levels: ST2 157 ng/mL, NT-proBNP 28100 ng/L
Discharge biomarker levels: ST2 22 ng/mL, NT-proBNP 3170 ng/L

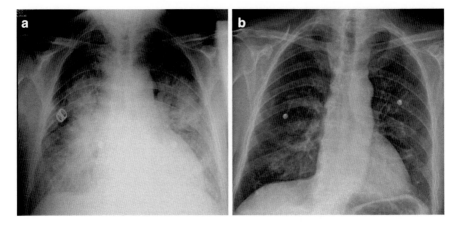

Fig. 21.1 Patient from case 1. (**a**) Admission X-ray. (**b**) Discharge X-ray

Discharge treatment: ASA 100 mg, warfarin, carvedilol 12.5 mg bid, enalapril 10 mg bid, eplerenone 25 mg, furosemide 40 and atorvastatin 40 mg.

Outcome

No HF readmissions or death during 1 year follow-up.

Comment

Patient with severe acute heart failure with very high levels of ST2 and NT-proBNP. Good early clinical course long with dramatic decrease of biomarker levels, both ST2 and NT-proBNP (Δ ST2 -86 % and Δ NT-proBNP -89 %). However, discharge levels of NT-proBNP were still significantly high. In contrast, ST2 levels fell below the recommended levels for stability (35 ng/mL). Despite the high NT-proBNP discharge levels, 1-year outcome was good.

Clinical Case 2

Male patient, 70 years old, non-smoker, obese (BMI 30 Kg/m^2). History of hypertension, dyslipemia, diabetes mellitus, COPD, and chronic anemia. Aortic valve replacement in the year 2000 because of aortic stenosis. Due to post-operative AV block, a pacemaker was implanted. In March 2013 he was admitted for acute decompensated HF. Echocardiography revealed LVEF 24 % with norm functioning aortic prosthesis. Upgrade to CRT was performed. The patient was on treatment with warfarin, furosemide 40 mg, carvedilol 25 mg bid, enalarpril 10 mg bid, bronchodilators, fluvastatin 80 mg.

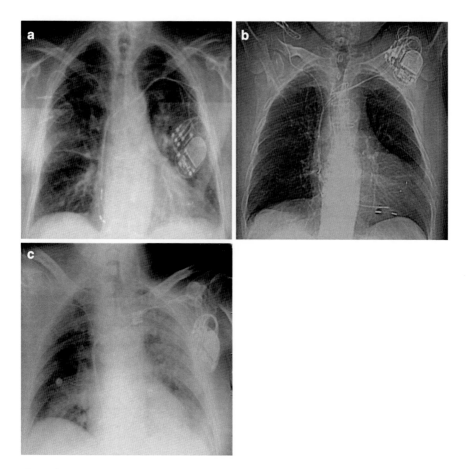

Fig. 21.2 Patient from case 2. (**a**) Admission X-ray. (**b**) Discharge X-ray. (**c**) Readmission x-ray

November 3rd 2013 he was admitted due to increased fatigue and right HF signs. Admission BP 131/78 mmHg, HR 70 bpm, and O_2 saturation 93 %.

Echocardiography showed LVEF 34 %, LVEDD 57 mm, LVESD 43 mm. Aortic prosthesis OK. PAP 35 mmHg. A coronary angiography was performed, that showed abnormal LAD origin from right coronary sinus, without significant stenosis (Fig. 21.2a, b). In-hospital course was favorable and discharged at day 6.

Admission biomarker levels: ST2 52 ng/mL, NT-proBNP 999 ng/L.

Discharge biomarker levels: ST2 60 ng/mL, NT-proBNP 515 ng/L

Discharge treatment: warfarin, furosemide 40 mg bid, carvedilol 25 mg bid, enalarpril 10 mg bid, eplerenone 25 mg, bronchodilators, fluvastatin 80 mg.

Outcome

The patient suffered a new HF readmission after 80 days and died during hospitalization (Fig. 21.2c).

Comment

Despite an initial favorable clinical course and also a favorable change in NT-proBNP levels (Δ –48 %) during the November 2013 admission, changes in ST2 levels during the last admission were not satisfactory (+15 %), remaining discharge ST2 levels above the recommended levels for stability (35 ng/mL). The persistence of high ST2 levels is a powerful predictor of increased risk of readmission and death.

Chronic Heart Failure

Consistent with the data in acute HF, studies in ambulatory HF patients have demonstrated the prognostic ability of ST2 across a wide range of cohorts. One large study of 891 outpatients demonstrated that ST2 provides incremental prognostic value to established HF mortality risk factors plus natriuretic peptides, with a significant improvement in reclassification and discrimination [8]. Other studies of ambulatory HF populations have found that ST2 levels are associated with functional capacity, and with both HF hospitalization and any cardiovascular hospitalization.

In a multicenter study of 1141 chronic heart failure patients, ST2 and NT-proBNP were compared with the Seattle Heart Failure Model (SHFM) for prediction of death or cardiac transplantation at 1 year. The combination of ST2 and NT-proBNP had similar risk discrimination as the SHFM. Although adding these biomarkers to the SHFM did not further improve risk discrimination, it did significantly improve risk classification [9]. There was a suggestion that ST2 levels were even more predictive of risk in patients with HF of non-ischemic etiology, compared to those with ischemic HF.

Clinical Case 3

Ambulatory female 75 years old. History of hypertension, diabetes mellitus, chronic kidney disease (creatinine 2.5 mg/dl) and iron deficiency-related anemia. Known atrial fibrillation since 2012 first diagnosis of dilated cardiomyopathy in December 2013: LVEF 35 %, moderate-severe mitral regurgitation and pulmonary artery pressure of 75 mmHg. Normal coronary angiography. The patient refused surgery. Treatment: warfarin, furosemide 40 mg bid, enalapril 5 mg bid, spironolactone 50 mg, oral iron supplements.

She was first attended at our HF Clinic in January 2015. Clinical examination showed mild hypotension (BP 95/60 mmHg), right HF signs, mild hepatomegaly and mild leg edema. EKG: Atrial fibrillation; no LBBB. Echocardiography showed LVEF 20 %, LVEDD 64 mm, LVESD 53 mm, severe mitral regurgitation, PAP

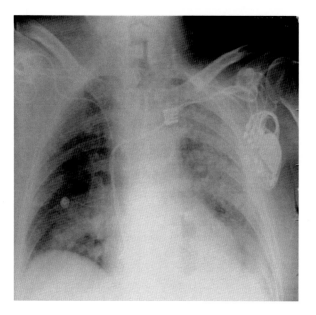

Fig. 21.3   Patient from case 3. First visit thorax X-ray

67 mmHg, e/e' 22, TAPSE 7 mm (Fig. 21.3). Now surgery was rejected by the heart team.

Biomarker levels: ST2 120 ng/mL, NT-proBNP 18,900 ng/L, eGFR 18 ml/min/1.73 m^2.

Digoxin 0.25 mg and spironolactone 12.5 mg od with careful supervision of renal function and K levels and low doses of carvedilol (3.125 mg bid) were added to the treatment, and flexible furosemide regimen was instituted. Intravenous Iron was administered.

Outcome

Despite close follow-up and treatment adjustments the patient died due to pump failure 6 months after her first visit to the HF Clinic.

Comment

This was an end-stage patient with poor prognosis. Biomarker levels were very highly elevated both NT-proBNP and ST2. However levels of NT-proBNP were disproportionally high due to severe renal dysfunction, hampering its interpretation. In contrast, ST2 levels are not significantly affected by renal function; 120 ng/mL is known to carry ominous prognosis in an ambulatory patient.

Multimarker Approach in Chronic HF

There has recently been an interest in multimarker strategies to examine panels of biomarkers that assess different pathophysiologic pathways. A report from the Pennsylvania Heart Failure Model (PHFM) tested the hypothesis that a group of seven biomarkers, each reflecting a different pathophysiologic pathway, could be combined into a multimarker score that would predict the risk of an adverse outcome, defined as death, cardiac transplantation or placement of a ventricular assist device [10]. Each of these seven biomarkers and their pathways were reported to be independently associated with the combined outcome. These biomarkers were: B-type natriuretic peptide (BNP; myocardial stretch), soluble fms-like tyrosine kinase receptor (vascular remodeling), high-sensitivity C-reactive protein (hsCRP; inflammation), ST2 (myocardial fibrosis-stretch), cardiac troponin I (cTnI; myocyte injury), uric acid (oxidative stress) and creatinine (renal function). The combined multimarker integer score provided an excellent assessment of risk with the hazard ratios of the intermediate- and high-risk tertiles (adjusted for clinical risk factors) significantly elevated to 3.5 and 6.8, respectively, compared with that of the lowest risk tertile. More recently, Lupón and colleagues investigated the value of combining NT-proBNP (myocardial stretch), highly sensitive cardiac troponin T (hsTnT; myocyte injury) and ST2 (myocardial fibrosis/strain) in a large, real-life cohort of 876 ambulatory patients with HF [11]. Overall, this study found that the three biomarkers were independently associated with all-cause mortality, although the combination of hsTnT plus ST2 performed better than the combination of all three added biomarkers (NT-proBNP + hs-cTnT + ST2). Additionally, the authors developed a web-based calculator, the Barcelona Bio-HF calculator that for the first time includes these three novel biomarkers, reflective of different pathophysiological pathways, on top of well-established clinical, echocardiographic and treatment variables for risk stratification [12]. In cross-validation studies, the average c-statistic of the new calculator was 0.79, which compared favorably to other models. The Barcelona Bio-HF calculator (www.BCN biohfcalculator.org) has the potential to provide risk assessment that is uniquely tailored to individual patients.

Clinical Case 4

Male, 68 years old, in NYHA functional III. LVEF 30 %. Routine blood test: hemoglobin 12 g/dl, sodium 130, eGFR 45 ml/min/1.73 m^2. Treatment: furosemide 60 mg, betablockers, ACEI and statins.

Using the Barcelona-Bio-HF risk calculator (www.bcnbiohfcalculator.org) the risk of death within the following 3 years for this patient based on clinical data + treatment is: 22 % at 1 year, 42 % at 2 years and 60 % at 3 years; and the life expectancy is 3 years.

Figure 21.4a shows the web-page of the biocalculator with clinical and treatment data. Risk of death at 1-2- and 3-years is depicted in the right panel (top). In the middle the prediction over time is shown in a graphical area (blue line). Life expectancy is depicted at the bottom.

If we incorporate data on 3 biomarkers such as NT-proBNP, high-sensitivity troponin T (hs-TnT) and ST2, the prognosis significantly varies whether a "benign" or an "adverse" biomarker profile is drawn.

Benign Biomarker Profile

NT-proBNP 1000 ng/L, hs-TnT 14 ng/L and ST2 34 ng/mL. The risk of death within the next 3 years falls significantly and life expectancy doubles (Fig. 21.4b). In the graphical area two survival curves are depicted in different colors: blue for the prediction with clinical + treatment alone and red for the model containing biomarkers.

Adverse Biomarker Profile

NT-proBNP 5000 ng/L, hs-TnT 80 ng/L, and ST2 120 ng/mL. The risk of death within the next 3 years increases very significantly and life expectancy decreases, (Fig 21.4c). Again differences in survival curves underline the prognostic importance of biomarkers:

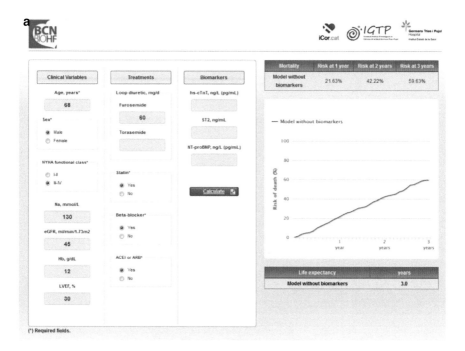

Fig. 21.4 (a–c) The web-page of the biocalculator with clinical and treatment data for the patient in case 4

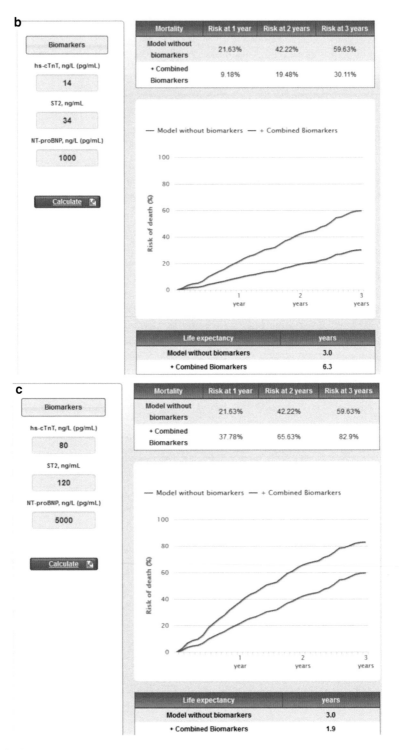

Fig. 21.4 (continued)

Comment

These two scenarios of circulating biomarkers (adding biomarker data on top of clinical evaluation) significantly modify risk estimation. It is important to underline two aspects: first, risk prediction accuracy is better with addition of biomarkers into the risk prediction model (discrimination, calibration and reclassification perform better); second, biomarker levels are dynamic and may vary with treatment; thus, patients' prognosis can be updated in every visit with newly obtained biomarker measurements

ST2 in Monitoring

Serial Monitoring

The low long-term intra-individual variation in levels gives ST2 a potential advantage for serial testing in HF patients. Boisot et al. first showed that among patients hospitalized with an acute HF decompensation, failure of the ST2 level to drop at least 15 % over the course of the hospitalization was associated with an increased risk of death at 90 days [13]. More recently, Llibre et al. [14] examined 185 patients admitted with acute HF and measured admission, discharge and ST2 dynamics. Admission and discharge ST2 levels and ST2 kinetics were useful for 1-year risk stratification. After adjustment for age, sex, ischemic etiology of HF, LVEF, creatinine, hemoglobin and concomitant NT-proBNP levels, discharge ST2 levels and ST2 kinetics provided the most valuable information.

Clinical Case 5

Ambulatory male 65 years old. History of smoking, hypertension and diabetes mellitus. Diagnosed of dilated cardiomyopathy on 2012, and on treatment with torasemide 10 mg, enalapril 10 mg bid, carvedilol 6.25 mg bid.

May 2015 he was admitted at the hospital due to decompensated HF (Fig. 21.5a).

EKG: Sinus rhythm, AQRS -60°, LBBB, QRS duration 150 ms (Fig. 21.5b).

Admission biomarker levels: ST2 135 ng/mL.

Echocardiogram: LVEF 27 %, LVEDD 64 mm, LVESD 48 mm, moderate mitral regurgitation, PAP 40 mmHg, abnormal interventricular septum movement. Normal coronary angiography.

With i.v. diuretics and vasodilator treatment the patient had a good clinical course. RCT was decided and implanted before discharge. Discharge treatment: carvedilol 6.25 mg bid, enalapril 10 mg bid, eplerenone 25, and furosemide 40.

Discharge ST2 levels: 70 ng/mL.

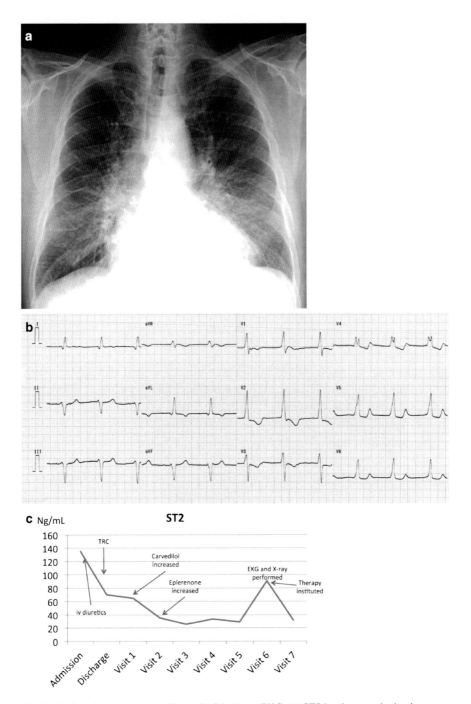

Fig. 21.5 Case 5. (**a**) Admission X-ray. (**b**) Discharge EKG. (**c**) ST2 levels were obtained at every visit after discharge, after 1 month and every 3 months thereafter. (**d, e**) At visit 6, an ST2 increase was detected. EKG and chest X-ray were performed

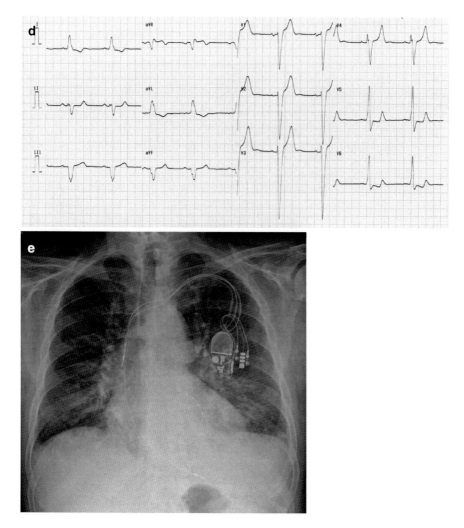

Fig. 21.5 (continued)

The patient was visited at the HF Clinic one week after discharge, after 1 month and every 3 months thereafter. ST2 levels were obtained at every visit (Fig. 21.5c), together with treatment changes:

At visit 6, an ST2 increase was detected. The patient only complained of some nocturnal cough. EKG and chest X-ray were performed (Fig. 21.5d, e):

EKG: spontaneous sinus rhythm and own AV conduction; no pacemaker spike visible on EKG; changes in the pattern of QRS relative to post-discharge EKG.
Chest X-ray: signs of left HF and atrial electrode displacement.
Diuretic dose was increased and the atrial electrode replaced. The patient had a favorable clinical course, and ST2 levels fell back to 32 ng/mL.

ST2 and Ventricular Remodeling

In a post-hoc analysis of the EPHESUS trial, in which acute MI patients (mostly STEMI) with left ventricular dysfunction were randomized to receive either the mineralocorticoid antagonist (MRA) eplerenone or placebo, individuals with high ST2 levels were found to have an increased risk of adverse ventricular remodeling at 24 weeks [15]. However, the risk of adverse remodeling was attenuated in the patients with high ST2 who were randomized to eplerenone. In contrast, patients with low ST2 levels had low levels of remodeling regardless of which arm they were randomized to. As this was not a prospective analysis the results are merely hypothesis-generating. Nonetheless, the results suggest a potentially important use for ST2: targeting MRA therapy to patients with elevated ST2 levels who are most likely to benefit could be a way to intelligently personalize post-MI care.

Very recently a remodeling score has been developed. Lupón et al. examined whether clinical variables plus serum concentrations of ST2, NT-proBNP, hs-cTnT, and galectin-3 predicted reverse remodeling (R2) [16]. Its is remarkable that among the studied biomarkers only ST2 emerged as a good surrogate of R2. The ST2R2 score developed contained 5 clinical variables: non-ischemic etiology, absence of LBBB, HF duration <12 months, LVEF <24%, and β-blocker treatment plus ST2<48 ng/mL. The score had an area under the curve of 0.79 in the derivation cohort and 0.73 in a separate validation cohort.

Clinical Case 6

Ambulatory male, 52 years old, ex-smoker. History of mild arterial hypertension, gout, knee osteoarthritis and glaucoma. In April 2013 begun with shortness of breath at moderate exercise, that progressively increased to mild effort.

In May 2013 he suffered of palpitations, rest dyspnea and a wide QRS tachycardia. He was admitted in the Cardiology ward: BP 145/80 mmHg. HR 60 bpm. No lung crackles. No 3rd heart sound. Mild mitral regurgitation murmur. No peripheral edema. No hepatomegaly. No jugular ingurgitation.

Echocardiography: LVEF 27%, LVEDD 59 mm, LVESD 45 mm, left atrium 44 mm, mild mitral regurgitation, PAP 45 mmHg. Normal coronary angiogram. Cardiac-MRI: LV dilatation (LVEDV 207 ml, LVESV 154 ml), LVEF 26%. No fibrosis. No signs of amyloid. EP Study: normal A-V conduction; No induction of VT/VF (Fig. 21.6).

Medication was uptitrated to: enalapril 10 mg bid, carvedilol 12.5 mg bid, furosemide 40 mg, and spironolactone 25 mg.

Follow-up at the HF Clinic: NYHA class II, ST2 20.6 ng/mL, NT-proBNP 430 ng/L.

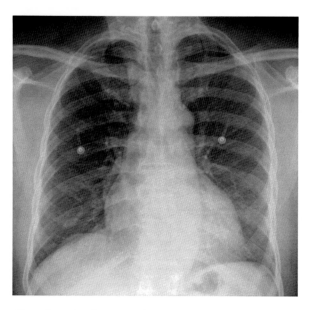

Fig. 21.6 Chest X-ray for patient from case 6

ST2-R2 Score		
Non-ischemic etiology:	5	(If yes: 5)
Absence of LBBB:	4	(If yes: 4)
ST2 < 48 ng/mL:	3	(If yes: 3)
HF duration < 12 months:	2	(If yes: 2)
Beta-blocker treatment:	2	(If yes: 2)
LVEF < 24 %:	0	(If yes: 1)
Total ST2-R2 Score	**16**	

Outcome

Twelve month follow-up Echocardiography: LVEF: 58 %, LVEDD: 55 mm, LVESD: 41 mm, left atrium: 35 mm, mild mitral regurgitation, PAP 35 mmHg.

Comment

A ST2-R2 score of 16 yields an 86 % of clinically relevant reverse ventricular remodeling (LVEF increase by ≥ 15 points). Indeed, this patient showed a very significant improvement after 1 year of treatment.

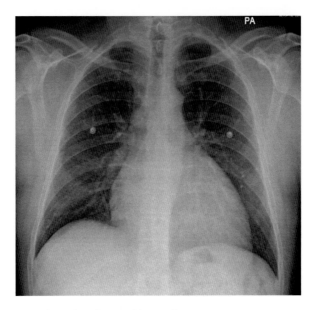

Fig. 21.7 Chest x-ray for patient discussed in case 7

Clinical Case 7

A 44 year old male, smoker of 30 cig/day until 2003. History of arterial hypertension, diabetes mellitus, dyslipidemia, gastric ulcer, and pneumonia. He suffered an anterior AMI in 2010. LVEF was 35%. Coronary angiography showed 99% proximal LAD stenosis, which was treated with a DES implant. In May 2012 was admitted due to progressive dyspnea and NYHA class IV. MRI showed LVEF 20%. Coronary angiography did not show restenosis nor new coronary lesions.

First visit at HF Clinic in March 2013: NYHA class III. orthopnea. BP 110/73 mmHg, HR 68 bpm. No signs of congestion (Fig. 21.7).

EKG: Sinus rhythm. QS V1-V4. QRS 100 ms, no LBBB.

Biomarker levels: ST2 80 ng/mL, NT-proBNP 1180 ng/L

Echocardiogram: LVEF 25%, anterior and apical akinesis, LVEDD 71 mm, LVESD 68 mm, left atrium 45 mm, mild mitral regurgitation, PAP 43 mmHg.

Medication: enalapril 10 mg bid, carvedilol 12.5 mg bid, furosemide 40 + 20 mg, AAS 100 mg, isosorbide mononitrate 40 mg tid, eplerenone 50 mg, digoxin 0.25 mg 3 d/w, atorvastatin 40 mg.

ST2-R2 Score		
Non-ischemic etiology:	0	(If yes: 5)
Absence of LBBB:	4	(If yes: 4)
ST2 < 48 ng/mL:	0	(If yes: 3)
HF duration < 12 months:	0	(If yes: 2)
Beta-blocker treatment:	2	(If yes: 2)
LVEF < 24%:	0	(If yes: 1)
Total ST2-R2 Score:	**6**	

Outcome

12 month follow-up echocardiogram: LVEF 29 %, LVEDD 66 mm, LVESD 62 mm, left atrium 45 mm, mild mitral regurgitation, PAP 38 mmHg.

Comment

With a ST2-R2 score of six, the probability of reverse remodeling (LVEF increase by $\geq$ 15 points) is 14 %. As expected, the patient did not show a clinically significant improvement after 1 year follow-up.

References

1. Kakkar R, Lee RT. The IL-33/ST2 pathway: therapeutic target and novel biomarker. Nat Rev Drug Discov. 2008;7:827–40.
2. Dieplinger B, Januzzi Jr JL, Steinmair M, et al. Analytical and clinical evaluation of a novel high-sensitivity assay for measurement of soluble ST2 in human plasma--the Presage ST2 assay. Clin Chim Acta. 2009;409:33–40.
3. Bayes-Genis A, Zamora E, de Antonio M, et al. Soluble ST2 serum concentration and renal function in heart failure. J Card Fail. 2013;19:768–7.
4. Wu AH, Wians F, Jaffe A. Biological variation of galectin-3 and soluble ST2 for chronic heart failure: implication on interpretation of test results. Am Heart J. 2013;165:995–9.
5. Yancy CW, Jessup M, Bozkurt B, et al. 2013 ACCF/AHA Guideline for the Management of Heart Failure: a report of the American College of Cardiology Foundation/American Heart Association Task Force on Practice Guidelines. J Am Coll Cardiol. 2013;62: e147–239.
6. Januzzi Jr JL, Peacock WF, Maisel AS, et al. Measurement of the interleukin family member ST2 in patients with acute dyspnea: results from the PRIDE (Pro-Brain Natriuretic Peptide Investigation of Dyspnea in the Emergency Department) study. J Am Coll Cardiol. 2007;50:607–13.
7. Shah KB, Kop WJ, Christenson RH, et al. Prognostic utility of ST2 in patients with acute dyspnea and preserved left ventricular ejection fraction. Clin Chem. 2011;57:874–82.
8. Bayes-Genis A, De Antonio M, Galan A, et al. Combined use of high-sensitivity ST2 and NT-proBNP to improve the prediction of death in heart failure. Eur J Heart Fail. 2012;14:32–8.
9. Ky B, French B, Mccloskey K, et al. High-sensitivity ST2 for prediction of adverse outcomes in chronic heart failure. Circ Heart Fail. 2011;4:180–7.
10. Ky B, French B, Levy WC, Sweitzer NK. Multiple biomarkers for risk prediction in chronic heart failure. Circ Heart Fail. 2012;5:183–90.
11. Lupón J, de Antonio M, Galán A, et al. Combined use of the novel biomarkers high-sensitivity troponin T and ST2 for heart failure risk stratification vs conventional assessment. Mayo Clin Proc. 2013;88:234–43.
12. Lupón J, de Antonio M, Vila J, et al. Development of a novel heart failure risk tool: the Barcelona bio-heart failure risk calculator (BCN bio-HF calculator). PLoS One. 2014;9:e85466.
13. Boisot S, Beede J, Isakson S, et al. Serial sampling of ST2 predicts 90-day mortality following destabilized heart failure. J Card Fail. 2008;14:732–8.
14. Llibre C, Zamora E, Caballero A, et al. The real-life value of ST2 monitoring during heart failure decompensation: impact on long-term readmission and mortality. Biomarkers. 2016;21(3):225–32.

15. Weir RA, Miller AM, Murphy GE, et al. Serum soluble ST2: a potential novel mediator in left ventricular and infarct remodeling after acute myocardial infarction. J Am Coll Cardiol. 2010;55:243–50.
16. Lupón J, Gaggin HK, de Antonio M, et al. Biomarker-assist score for reverse remodeling prediction in heart failure: the ST2-R2 score. Int J Cardiol. 2015;184:337–43.

Chapter 22
Biomarkers in Heart Failure: Procalcitonin

Martin Möckel and Julia Searle

Abstract Several studies have investigated procalcitonin (PCT) in the context of heart failure, both, as a prognostic marker but also as a marker to guide the decision on antibiotic treatment in acute heart failure. This chapter summarizes the current evidence on the value of PCT in the work-up of patients with acute heart failure and presents case reports, an algorithm and caveats to underline the potential use of PCT in this setting.

Keywords Procalcitonon (PCT) • Heart failure • Antibiotics • Diagnosis of heart failure • Risk stratification in heart failure • Biomarkers in heart failure

PCT Increase in Heart Failure and Underlying Hypotheses

In 1999, *The Lancet* published a prospective cohort study on endotoxin and immune activation in patients with chronic heart failure and recent onset of peripheral edema, analyzing a set of biomarkers connected with endotoxemia, inflammation and immune response and showing their elevated levels during the acute exacerbation. This was the first study where procalcitonin (PCT), a marker previously known in connection with bacterial infection and specifically sepsis, was connected to chronic heart failure and showed increased levels in patients as compared to healthy volunteers and even higher levels in patients with heart failure and peripheral edema, although patient numbers were small and findings on PCT non-significant [1]. As the study also showed raised endotoxin-levels in patients with heart failure, it added to the hypothesis that this might be caused by altered gut permeability due to edematous intestines, followed by bacterial translocation and endotoxin release into the blood stream [2–4].

Since then, several studies have investigated PCT as a marker in the context of heart failure, both, as a prognostic marker but also as a marker to guide the decision on antibiotic treatment in acute heart failure. This chapter will summarize the

M. Möckel, MD, PhD (✉) • J. Searle, MD, MPH
Division of Emergency Medicine and Department of Cardiology, Campus Virchow Klinikum and Campus Charité Mitte, Charité – Universitätsmedizin Berlin, Berlin, Germany
e-mail: martin.moeckel@charite.de

© Springer International Publishing Switzerland 2016
A.S. Maisel, A.S. Jaffe (eds.), *Cardiac Biomarkers*,
DOI 10.1007/978-3-319-42982-3_22

current evidence on the value of PCT and show case reports to underline the usefulness of PCT in heart failure.

Prognostic Value of PCT in Heart Failure

Inflammation plays an important role in chronic heart failure and seems to be connected to intestinal edema leading to an overexpression of pro-inflammatory cytokines with adverse effects on cardiac function and the general body metabolism [5]. Considering these hypotheses it is not surprising that PCT has been tested for its prognostic value in heart failure. Results of the BACH-study, a prospective, international trial with over 1,600 patients with dyspnea recruited in Emergency Departments [6], showed that PCT was significantly associated with 90-day mortality in patients diagnosed with acute heart failure (34.6% (n = 568) of all patients included in BACH). Patients in the fifth PCT quintile (>0.21 ng/ml) had a 90-day survival rate of only 80.5% as opposed to 92% for patients in the first PCT-quintile (<0.05 ng/ml) [7].

On the other hand, in a trial by Travaglino et al., conducted in 9 Italian EDs and analyzing data of 441 patients with acute dyspnea and an expected hospital stay of at least 72 h, PCT at admission was a significant, albeit modest predictor for 30- and 90-day mortality (AUC 0.70 and 0.73, respectively) in all patients, but sub-analysis showed that this was only true for patients without heart failure as their final diagnosis [8].

Recently, Villanueva et al. evaluated the association of PCT at admission and long-term outcome (median follow-up 2.0 years) in a cohort of 261 acute heart failure patients. Median PCT levels at admission to the Emergency Department were higher in the 41.4% of patients who died during the follow-up period (0.073 [0.047–0.111] vs. 0.051 [0.027–0.088] ng/ml). Mortality rate increased with PCT-quartiles, with a hazard ratio of 2.32 (1.18–4.55; p = 0.014) in Q4 as compared to Q1. The association was independent of white blood cell count, CRP, endotoxin and different interleukin levels [8]. In summary, evidence indicates a prognostic value of PCT in heart failure but is still sparse and inconclusive.

PCT as a Marker for Bacterial Infection in Heart Failure

Evidence for increased levels of PCT in patients with heart failure even in the absence of bacterial infection might question established diagnostic cut-off levels [9]. A large study from China with combined data sets of patients with heart failure or infection and re-adjudicated diagnoses (bacterial infection without heart failure, congestive heart failure without infection (heart failure only) and bacterial infection complicated by congestive heart failure) and healthy controls (n = 4,698 in total), showed significantly higher PCT levels in heart failure than in healthy controls. Likewise, patients with infections complicated by heart failure had higher PCT levels than patients with simple infections. As a consequence, the positive predictive value for bacterial infection, using a cut-off level of 0.1 ng/ml was highest in simple infection (95.1 %), lower in infection complicated by NYHA II and III heart failure (90.9 % and 87.6 % respectively) and lowest in infection complicated by NYHA IV heart failure (68.6 %).

PCT-Guided Antibiotic Treatment in the Emergency Department

Shortness of breath is a common chief complaint in the Emergency Department and is associated with a poor prognosis [10]. Studies show an equal distribution of cardiogenic and respiratory underlying diagnoses in emergency patients with dyspnea, with heart failure, pneumonia, chronic obstructive pulmonary disease and acute myocardial infarction in lead positions [6, 10, 11]. The similarity of symptoms and affected patients as well as the increasing rate of multi-morbidity with coexisting pulmonary and cardiac diseases pose a great challenge to the diagnostic work-up of patients with dyspnea, especially in the setting of an Emergency Department where fast decisions are indispensable. Additionally, early labelling of a patient into "cardiac" or "pulmonary" can set off the "wrong" algorithm for further patient work-up and thus lead to inadequate treatment.

Ray et al. were able to show that inappropriate treatment in elderly patients with acute respiratory failure in the Emergency Department significantly increased the risk of in-hospital death [11].

In 2004, Christ-Crain et al. published a trial evaluating PCT-guided antibiotic treatment in emergency patients with lower respiratory tract infections, and were able to show a significant reduction in antibiotics overuse. Bacterial infection was deemed excluded with PCT-levels below 0.1 ng/ml, unlikely with levels between 0.1 and 0.25 ng/ml, possible with levels between 0.25 and 0.5 ng/ml and likely above 0.5 ng/ml. Notably, of the 597 patients enrolled with dyspnea and/or cough and suspected lower respiratory tract infection, 68 had a final diagnosis of heart failure, but these were excluded from the analysis [12].

A sub-analysis of the BACH-data revealed that patients with a diagnosis of acute heart failure and an increased value of PCT above 0.21 ng/ml had a worse outcome if they did not receive antibiotic treatment. Likewise, patients with AHF and a PCT value below 0.05 ng/ml had a better prognosis if they were not given an antibiotic. In patients with PCT values between these two cut-points, antibiotic treatment did not affect survival. Interestingly the BACH-data showed that emergency physician estimation of the presence of pneumonia was unreliable and especially in patients, where the emergency physicians judged the probability of pneumonia as "low" or "medium", information on the patient's PCT value had the potential to guide re-adjustment of the underlying diagnosis [7].

Recently, Schuetz et al. analyzed data from the ProHOSP trial, a randomized, interventional study where patients with suspected lower respiratory tract infections were randomized to standard or PCT-guided antibiotic treatment decision. Antibiotic treatment was discouraged if PCT was below 0.25 ng/ml and strongly discouraged if PCT was below 0.1 ng/ml. Antibiotic treatment was recommended if PCT was above 0.25 ng/ml and strongly recommended if PCT was above 0.5 ng/ml. The authors now analyzed data of a subset of 233 patients with a history of chronic heart failure, who were evenly distributed in the two study groups. Primary endpoint of the analysis was an adverse outcome (mortality and ICU-admission) within 30 days of ED presentation. The combined endpoint was non-significantly lower in the PCT-group (16.4 % [19/116] versus 22.2 % [26/117], p = 0.26), but antibiotic exposure was significantly shorter in the PCT-guided group, as were antibiotic side effects. In patients with a low initial PCT-value, the PCT-guided group had a significantly lower adverse outcome rate and significantly shorter antibiotic exposure than controls, indicating that excluding respiratory infection and avoiding inadequate antibiotic treatment has a great potential to improve patient outcome [13].

In April 2014, a large, international randomized trial was initiated to prospectively compare standard with PCT-guided antibiotic treatment for acute heart failure patients in the ED (IMPACT-EU, NCT02392689.gov) https://clinicaltrials.gov/ct2/show/NCT02392689?term=NCT02392689&rank=1).

Patients with suspected heart failure and increased natriuretic peptides (midregional pro atrial natriuretic peptide (MR-proANP) >300 pmol/L, brain natriuretic peptide (BNP) >350 ng/ml or N-terminal of the pro-hormone brain natriuretic peptide (NT-proBNP) >1800 ng/l) will be randomly assigned to a standard management group or a PCT-guided group where a cutoff level of 0.2 ng/ml will be used to support decision on antibiotic therapy initiation. Patients will be followed up 30 and 90 days after randomization to evaluate the survival status, re-hospitalizations and antibiotic therapies.

Case Reports

The following five case vignettes highlight the potential benefit of the use of PCT in combination with a natriuretic peptide. **Case 1:** Patient with pulmonary edema due to AHF in combination with pneumonia. **Case 2:** Patient with hypertensive pulmonary edema and antibiotic treatment despite a low PCT-level. **Case 3:** Patient with pulmonary edema due to AHF in combination with an acute exacerbation of a newly diagnosed chronic obstructive pulmonary disease. **Case 4:** Delayed antibiotic therapy in a patient with pneumonia combined with pulmonary edema due to AHF. **Case 5:** Patient with pulmonary edema due to AHF combined with renal failure and urinary tract infection

Case Report 1: Biomarkers in Herat Failure – PCT

Patient with pulmonary edema due to AHF in combination with pneumonia

Age, Gender

61 year-old, male patient

Current Reason for Visiting the Emergency Department

Presentation to the Emergency Department via the general practitioner with acute heart failure and known CAD-3, increasing use of nitroglycerin, increasing productive cough (clear sputum), increasing peripheral edema, chest pain

Medical History and Risk Factors

CAD-3, CABG 20 years previously, AMI 5 years previously
IDDM
pAVK with amputation of the lower right leg
M. Parkinson
Arterial hypertension, hypercholesterolemia, ex-smoker

Important Diagnostic Findings

SO_2 87 %, respiratory rate 30/min
Bedside chest X-ray: pulmonary edema, pulmonary infiltration possible

Laboratory Findings at Admission (Routine)

TnI 5.7 ug/l (norm < 0.1)
CRP 15.27 mg/dl (norm <0.5 mg/dl)
Leukocytes 12.32/nl (norm 4.5–11.0/nl)

Laboratory Findings (Blind)

PCT: 0.47 ng/ml at admission
ANP: 491 pmol/l

Therapeutic Measures

Admission to Cardiology ward with pulmonary edema. Troponin elevation probably due to AHF.
Fast recompensation with furosemide.
Initiation of antibiotic therapy (Sultamicillin + Clarithromycin) due to pneumonia.

Length of Hospital Stay

9 days
Patient died 3.5 months later (Sepsis and end-stage heart failure)

Comment

Patients with acute heart failure often have concomitant infections, either as "pre-cipitant" or caused by congestion and hypoxemia. Early recognition of infection is crucial and PCT may support this.

Case Report 2: Biomarkers in Heart Failure – PCT

Patient with hypertensive pulmonary edema and antibiotic treatment despite a low PCT-level

Age, Gender

81 year-old, female patient

Current Reason for Visiting the Emergency Department

Presentation to the Emergency Department via ambulance with shortness of breath, SO_2 on the ambulance 92 %, arterial hypertension (205/100 mmHg)

Increasing dyspnea since the previous day (now NYHA III), BP 170/120 mmHg at admission. No productive coughing or clinical signs of infection reported.

Medical History and Risk Factors

Chronic obstructive pulmonary disease (COPD)
Tachyarrhythmia absoluta with Coumarin-medication
Arterial hypertension

Important Diagnostic Findings

ECG: AA, HR 72/min, ST-depression V4-V6, signs of left ventricular hypertrophy
Physical examination: Basal rales, temperature 34.9 °C ax.
Respiratory rate 33/min
Chest X-ray: Cardiomegaly, cardiac decompensation combined with an infiltration
    in lower right lobe
Follow up Echo 4 months later: Normal ejection fraction

Laboratory Findings at Admission (Routine)

TnT <0.01 ug/l (norm <0.03 ug/l)
CRP 1.61 mg/dl (norm <0.5 mg/dl)
Leukocytes 11.47/nl (norm 4.5–11.0/nl)

Laboratory Findings (Blind)

PCT: 0.1 ng/ml at admission
MR-proANP: 340 pmol/l

Therapeutic Measures

Fast re-compensation after normalization of blood pressure with Nitroglycerine and Urapidil, Furosemid 20 mg i.v.

Initiation of antibiotic therapy (Sultamicillin + Clarithromycin) due to clinical suspicion of pneumonia.

Discharge after normalization of BP and exclusion of AMI

Length of Hospital Stay

Ambulatory patient

After 3 months alive, no re-hospitalization.

Comment

Clinicians tend to prescribe antibiotics (ABx) very liberally; probably this was no pneumonia and the patient would have had the same outcome without ABx, which pose the threat of side effects and resistancies.

Case Report 3: Biomarkers in Heart Failure – PCT

Patient with pulmonary edema due to AHF in combination with an acute exacerbation of a newly diagnosed chronic obstructive pulmonary disease

Age, Gender

71 year-old, male patient

Current Reason for Visiting the Emergency Department

Presentation to the Emergency Department in the morning via ambulance with acute shortness of breath since 4 h

Increasing dyspnea at exertion since a few weeks, now NYHA IV, no clinical signs of infection.

BP 214/110 mmHg, SO_2 77 %

Medical History and Risk Factors

CAD-3, CABG 7 years previously, last coronary angiography 3 months ago.

Diabetes mellitus

Arterial hypertension, hypercholesterolemia, ex-smoker

Important Diagnostic Findings

ECG: SVT, HR 150/min, probably atrial flutter

Physical examination: Dyspnoea and tachypnea, bilateral rales and pulmonary obstruction

Chest X-ray: pulmonary edema

Laboratory Findings at Admission (Routine)

TnI 0.05 ug/l (norm <0.01 ug/l)
CRP 3.5 mg/dl (norm <0.5 mg/dl)
Leukocytes 18.81/nl (norm 4.5–11.0/nl)

Laboratory Findings (Blind)

PCT: 1.29 ng/ml at admission
ANP: 394 pmol/l

Therapeutic Measures

Admission to Cardiology ward with hypertensive pulmonary edema and TAA.

Fast re-compensation after normalization of blood pressure with furosemide and after cardioversion.

Initiation of antibiotic therapy (Sultamicillin + Clarithromycin) due to acute exacerbation of chronic obstructive pulmonary disease, which was diagnosed with spirometry 2 days later.

Length of Hospital Stay

14 days
After 3 months alive, no rehospitalisation.

Conclusion

Pulmonary infection in combination with pulmonary edema is difficult to diagnose, PCT at admission was very high, patient might have profited from earlier initiation of antibiotic therapy.

Case Report 4: Biomarkers in Heart Failure – PCT

Age, Gender

72 year-old, male patient

Current Reason for Visiting the Emergency Department

Presentation to the Emergency Department from a dialysis practice with chest pain and dyspnea. No improvement after nitrate

Medical History and Risk Factors

CAD-1, multiple stents
Chronic renal insufficiency, hemodialysis

Echocardiography 1 month previously: left ventricular hypertrophy, LVEF 60%

Important Diagnostic Findings

SO2 96%, respiratory rate 25/min, heart rate 86/min
Bedside chest X-ray: beginning pulmonary infiltration
ECG: tachycardia, AV block I°, slight ST elevation V3/V4
Coronary angiography: diffuse CAD, no culprit lesion

Laboratory Findings at Admission (Routine)

TNT 0.14 ug/l (<0.03 ug/l)
CRP 0.84 mg/dl (norm <0.5 mg/dl)
Leukocytes 7.39/nl (norm 4.5–11/nl)

Laboratory Findings (Blind)

PCT: 1.03 ng/ml
ANP: 767 pmol/l

Therapeutic Measures

Exclusion of AMI, due to pneumonic infiltration an antibiotic therapy was initiated
(Sultamicillin).

Length of Hospital Stay

1 day
Patient died 5 months later (probably sepsis)

Comment

Clinical differentiation of pulmonary infection from ACS and decompensation can
be difficult and lead to delayed antibiotic treatment.

Case Report 5: Biomarkers in Heart Failure – PCT

Age, Gender

71 year-old, male patient

Current Reason for Visiting the Emergency Department

Presentation to the Emergency Department with increasing dyspnea at rest for 3
days (NYHA IV). Peritoneal dialysis for 3 weeks. Increase in weight of 5 kg within
the last 5 weeks. No fever or cough.

Medical History and Risk Factors

CAD-3 with reduced LVEF, multiple Stents and CABG
Chronic renal insufficiency, peritoneal dialysis (start 2 weeks previously)
Arterial hypertension, Diabetes mellitus Type 2
MI II°, TI II-III°, PFO, chronic atrial fibrillation

Important Diagnostic Findings

SO2 96 %, respiratory rate 16/min, heart rate 113/min
Bedside chest X-ray: pulmonary infiltration
U-Stix: erythrocytes ++++, leucocytes +++++, protein +
ECG: tachycardia, atrial fibrillation, pacemaker
Physical examination: arrhythmia, systolic murmur, peripheral edema, rales

Laboratory Findings at Admission (Routine)

TnI 0.06 ug/l (norm <0.01 ug/l)
CRP 8.17 mg/dl (norm <0.5 mg/dl)
Leukocytes 7.87/nl (norm 4.5–11/nl)

Laboratory Findings (Blind)

PCT 0.45 ng/ml
MR-proANP 707 pmol/l

Therapeutic Measures

Diuresis with furosemide and increase of peritoneal dialysis improved the clinical
situation and lead to loss of weight. Due to urinary tract infection an antibiotic
therapy was initiated (first Ciprofloxacin, then Sultamicillin).

Length of Hospital Stay

26 days
Patient died 3.5 months later (heart failure)

Comment

Besides pneumonia, urinary tract infection is common in patients with heart and
renal failure and early diagnosis can be supported with PCT-testing at admission.

Conclusion and Potential Algorithm for PCT-Guided Antibiotic Treatment

Increased PCT levels in heart failure patients can be triggered by pathophysiological mechanisms independent of bacterial infection but can also indicate concomitant bacterial, and most likely pulmonary bacterial infection. Likewise, severity of disease as well as inadequate antibiotic treatment seem to provide PCT with a prognostic capacity. PCT-guided antibiotic treatment has got the potential to improve patient outcome, which is currently tested in a prospective randomized study (NCT02392689.gov). Definition of an appropriate cut-off level to diagnose infection in acute heart failure patients is an important prerequisite for its usefulness. The figure shows the algorithm for the potential use of PCT in acute patients with highly suspected acute heart failure, as it is currently tested in the IMPACT-EU trial.

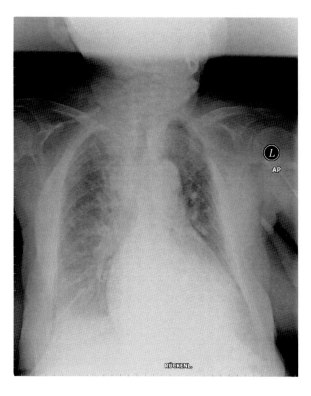

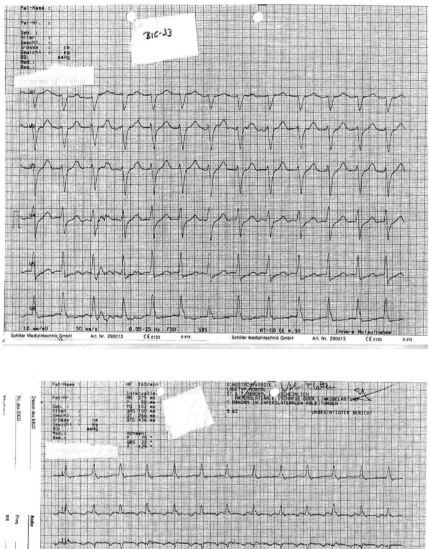

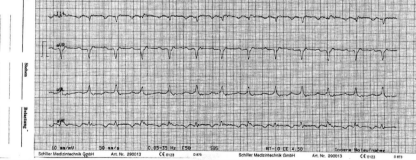

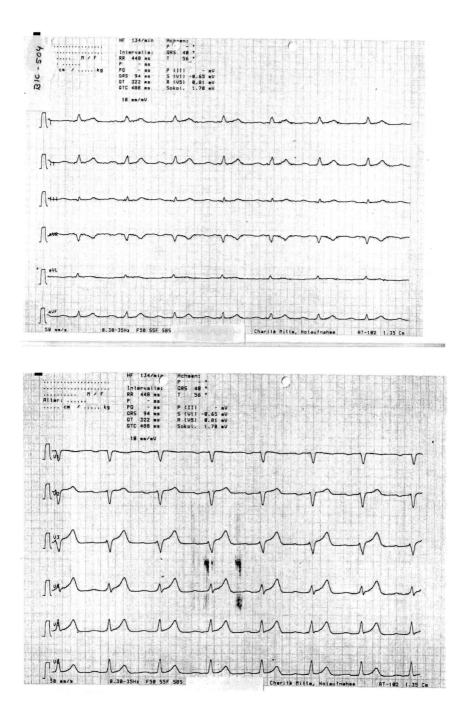

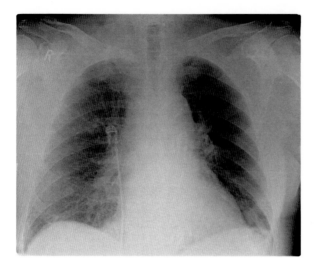

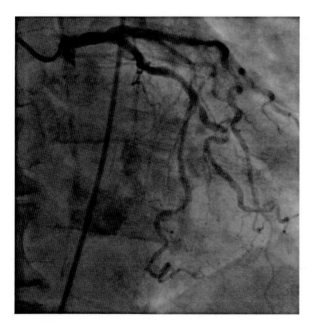

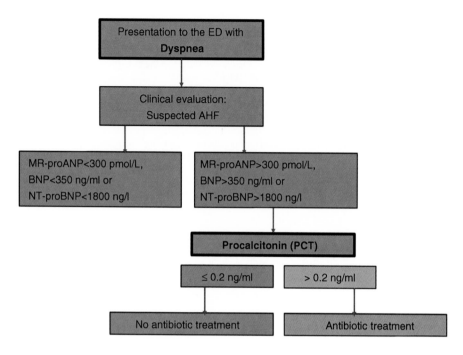

References

1. Niebauer J, Volk HD, Kemp M, et al. Endotoxin and immune activation in chronic heart fail-ure: a prospective cohort study. Lancet. 1999;353:1838–42.
2. Mann DL. Inflammatory mediators in heart failure: homogeneity through heterogeneity. Lancet. 1999;353:1812–3.
3. Anker SD, Egerer KR, Volk HD, Kox WJ, Poole-Wilson PA, Coats AJ. Elevated soluble CD14 receptors and altered cytokines in chronic heart failure. Am J Cardiol. 1997;79:1426–30.
4. Mollar A, Villanueva MP, Carratala A, Nunez E, Sanchis J, Nunez J. Determinants of procalci-tonin concentration in acute heart failure. Int J Cardiol. 2014;177:532–4.
5. Sandek A, Rauchhaus M, Anker SD, Von HS. The emerging role of the gut in chronic heart failure. Curr Opin Clin Nutr Metab Care. 2008;11:632–9.
6. Maisel A, Mueller C, Nowak R, et al. Mid-region pro-hormone markers for diagnosis and prognosis in acute dyspnea: results from the BACH (Biomarkers in Acute Heart Failure) trial. J Am Coll Cardiol. 2010;55:2062–76.
7. Maisel A, Neath SX, Landsberg J, et al. Use of procalcitonin for the diagnosis of pneumonia in patients presenting with a chief complaint of dyspnoea: results from the BACH (Biomarkers in Acute Heart Failure) trial. Eur J Heart Fail. 2012;14:278–86.
8. Travaglino F, Russo V, De BB, et al. Thirty and ninety days mortality predictive value of admission and in-hospital procalcitonin and mid-regional pro-adrenomedullin testing in patients with dyspnea. Results from the VERyfing DYspnea trial. Am J Emerg Med. 2014;32:334–41.
9. Sandek A, Springer J, Habedank D, Brunkhorst F, Anker SD. Procalcitonin-guided antibiotic treatment in heart failure. Lancet. 2004;363:1555–6.

10. Mockel M, Searle J, Muller R, et al. Chief complaints in medical emergencies: do they relate to underlying disease and outcome? The Charite Emergency Medicine Study (CHARITEM). Eur J Emerg Med. 2013;20:103–8.

11. Ray P, Birolleau S, Lefort Y, et al. Acute respiratory failure in the elderly: etiology, emergency diagnosis and prognosis. Crit Care. 2006;10:R82.

12. Christ-Crain M, Jaccard-Stolz D, Bingisser R, et al. Effect of procalcitonin-guided treatment on antibiotic use and outcome in lower respiratory tract infections: cluster-randomised, single-blinded intervention trial. Lancet. 2004;363:600–7.

13. Schuetz P, Kutz A, Grolimund E, et al. Excluding infection through procalcitonin testing improves outcomes of congestive heart failure patients presenting with acute respiratory symptoms: results from the randomized ProHOSP trial. Int J Cardiol. 2014;175:464–72.

Chapter 23
Novel Biomarkers in Heart Failure: Adrenomedullin and Proenkephalin

Daniel Chan and Leong Ng

Abstract Recently, two new neurohormonal systems have been implicated in cardiovascular disease, namely the adrenomedullin and enkephalin systems. New assay methodology has enabled measurement of the bioactive adrenomedullin peptide, and the more stable proenkephalin peptide (PENK) which is a surrogate for the enkephalin system. Both of these peptides are elevated in acute heart failure, and indicate poor prognosis. PENK in particular is related strongly to renal function. The future role of these novel biomarkers for heart failure management is discussed.

Keywords Adrenomedullin • Enkephalin • Opioids • Heart failure • Myocardial infarction • Acute kidney injury

Heart failure involves activation of a number of neurohormonal systems which could be used as biomarkers. Each of these biomarkers confers information about different aspects of the condition. Many of these peptides are unstable and have short half-lives, making study difficult. Recently, two novel biomarker systems have been described in heart failure, namely adrenomedullin and enkephalin, and development of sensitive and specific assays have enabled detection of the bioactive mature adrenomedullin [1] which is amidated at the C-terminal, and proenkephalin (PENK) [2], which is a surrogate for activation of the endogenous enkephalin system.

Adrenomedullin

Adrenomedullin (ADM) is a vasodilatory peptide which is elevated in many conditions including acute myocardial infarction, heart failure and sepsis. It is a 52 amino acid peptide originally isolated in human phaeochromocytoma cells and was found

D. Chan, BMedSci, BMBS • L. Ng, MD (✉)
Department of Cardiovascular Sciences, University of Leicester, Leicester, UK

NIHR Leicester Cardiovascular Biomedical Research Unit, Glenfield Hospital, Leicester, UK
e-mail: lln1@leicester.ac.uk

© Springer International Publishing Switzerland 2016
A.S. Maisel, A.S. Jaffe (eds.), *Cardiac Biomarkers*,
DOI 10.1007/978-3-319-42982-3_23

to elicit potent and long-lasting hypotensive effects. Beyond the cardiovascular system, ADM affects the respiratory, renal, endocrine and central nervous systems [3]. It functions as a paracrine/autocrine peptide, acting on tissue beds where it is synthesized.

To date, most of our understanding of the physiology of ADM's comes from work with vasculature. Intravenous infusion of ADM rapidly reduces total peripheral resistance and causes a dose-dependent reduction in blood pressure [4] in humans. This vasodilatory action is both caused by cyclic adenosine monophosphate(cAMP) generation through coupling of its receptor with adenylyl cyclase, and from nitric oxide production through phosphatidyl-inositol-3-kinase with subsequent nitric oxide synthase(NOS) activation. ADM administration to healthy adults and heart failure patients [5] increases cardiac output and decreases mean arterial pressure(MAP), increases heart rate and causes a natriuresis. ADM also reduces plasma aldosterone concentration, particularly in heart failure patients. Most studies agree that Adrenomedullin suppresses the renin-angiotensin-aldosterone(RAS) system, resulting in increased plasma renin but decreased aldosterone, vasopressin and endothelin production. Other cardioprotective actions of ADM is inhibition of cardiomyocyte apoptosis in the context of ischaemic/reperfusion injury.

Endogenous ADM increases under conditions of overhydration, hypertension, ischaemia, septic shock and endocrine and metabolic disorders [6]. Vascular endothelial cells, vascular smooth muscle cells and non-cardiac myocytes synthesize and secrete ADM in response to shear stress and stimulus from inflammatory cytokines [7], a response which can be modulated by glucocorticoids and thyroid hormone.

ADM acts through receptor complexes composed of the calcitonin receptor-like receptor and specific receptor-activity modifying proteins (RAMP). This generates cAMP which mediates ADM action. In addition, ADM also increases intracellular cGMP and its activity on NOS is enhanced by cAMP activated protein kinase A. In parallel ADM, also stimulates extracellular kinases via protein tyrosine kinase activation which may modulate the cell's mitogenic actions [3]. ADM is removed from circulation by neprilysin and other metalloproteases and aminopeptidases, with subsequent clearance from the lungs.

Measuring Adrenomedullin

ADM is synthesized from preproadrenomedullin, a 185-amino acid sequence which comprises a 21-amino acid signal peptide, a 20-amino acid proadrenomedullin-N-terminal 20 peptide (PAMP) (less biologically active than ADM), the mid-regional pro-adrenomedullin peptide, the ADM segment itself, and the C-Terminal pro-adrenomedullin. Preproadrenomedullin is enzymatically reduced by signal peptidase to form pro-adrenomedullin, which is then converted to mature ADM by prohormone convertase.

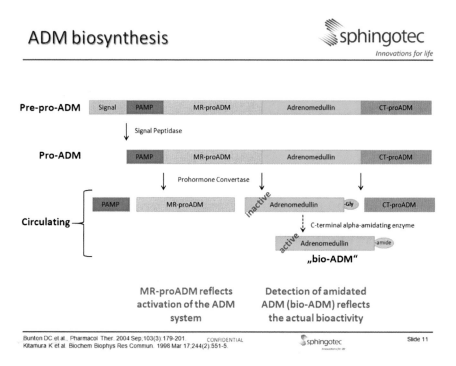

Fig. 23.1 Processing of preproadrenomedullin to bioactive mature adrenomedullin (Courtesy of Sphingotec, Hennigsdorf, Germany; Bunton DC, et al., *Pharmacol Ther.* 2004;103(3):179–201; Kitamura K, et al., *Biochem Biophys Res Commun.* 1998;244(2):551–5)

Measuring mature ADM in the plasma can be difficult. It has a short half-life (22 min). Circulating ADM can be bound to complement factor H, and has two forms - glycine-extended ADM (intermediate form which is the majority) and mature ADM (following enzymatic amidation). It is also produced where it is needed, and therefore is bound to target receptors near its production site, therefore hampering accurate peripheral sampling.

MRproADM is stoichiometrically generated with ADM. It has no physiological effect and is stable, and does not undergo any further transformation. It is generated in a 1:1 ratio with ADM and is therefore a good surrogate marker of the activation of the ADM system. Currently this peptide is measured by a novel commercial immunoluminetric assay [8]. However, its stability may be a disadvantage when levels are changing in a dynamic clinical situation.

Recently a novel double monoclonal sandwich immunoassay has been developed to measure bioactive human mature ADM which measures the active C-Terminal amidated form of ADM(mADM) instead of the inactive Glycine-extended variant of ADM (Fig. 23.1). In acute sepsis, compared to MRproADM, mADM is more predictive of 28-day mortality (mADM c-statistic 0.74 ($p < 0.00013$) vs MRproADM c-statistic 0.6 ($p < 0.22$) [1].

Adrenomedullin as a Biomarker of Risk in Heart Failure

ADM levels are elevated in the presence of traditional cardiovascular risk factors such as hypertension, diabetes, dyslipidaemia, myocardial infarction, stroke and active smoking. Cardiovascular disease, peripheral vascular disease, atrial fibrillation and reduced eGFR all increase MRproADM levels [9]. The presence of confounding disorders (such as diabetes) does not diminish the prognostic potential of MRproADM in the presence of heart failure [10], and importantly, even in apparently healthy individuals, elevated MRproADM alludes to elevated cardiovascular risk especially of incident heart failure [11].

ADM has emerged as an independent powerful marker of prognosis in heart failure, over and above traditional risk factors and natriuretic peptides. It is particularly helpful at predicting short term prognosis. Table 23.1 summarises the studies which have shown the prognostic value of ADM and its surrogates in heart failure [12–28]. Most of the studies demonstrate ADM's ability to predict heart failure individuals at the highest risk of mortality. This is true for both the patients with AHF (de novo or acute decompensation), and for the unselected patients presenting to emergency departments with breathlessness. Furthermore ADM seems to have the ability to predict reverse-remodelling in patients referred for cardiac resynchronisation therapy, although this finding will require further evaluation.

Proenkephalin

The enkephalin system is one member of the endogenous opioid family. The precursor proprotein proenkephalin is widely distributed in tissues, e.g., nervous and cardiovascular systems, adrenal medulla, immune system, kidneys [29]. The precursor protein is processed to met- and leu-enkephalins, as well as other products (Fig. 23.2), and these may have an autocrine/paracrine effect on tissues due to their efficient degradation. Enkephalins stimulate δ-opioid receptors, which are widely distributed in the nervous system, and also in the heart [30] and kidneys. Opioid receptors signal though modulation of cAMP, inositol phosphates and protein kinase C. They have been implicated in stress and immune responses, as well as antinociception. Enkephalins are co-released with catecholamines, being stored within nerve terminals. The effect on the cardiovascular system is mainly vasodepressor, with lowering of blood pressure and negative inotropy, as well as reduction of sympathetic activity and catecholamine release. Enkephalins also exhibit an inhibitory effect on cell proliferation [30] and may therefore affect tissue repair mechanisms.

Measuring PENK

As enkephalins are short-lived, measurement has been difficult. Enkephalins are degraded by peptidases, including neprilysin. Previous studies were unable to demonstrate changes in enkephalins post-myocardial infarction [31]. In animal models

Table 23.1 Studies relating to adrenomedullin as a biomarker

Author	N	Population	Endpoint and FU	Findings	Hazard ratio and AUC	Comments
Potocki (2009) [12]	287	ED pts with SOB (154 AHF)	Mortality at 30 days and 1 year	MRproADM predicts mortality	30 day OR 10.46 AUC 0.81 (0.73–0.9) 1 year AUC 0.75	MRproADM more powerful for short term prognosis
Maisel 2010–2011, Peacock (2011) [8, 13, 14]	1641	ED patients with SOB (568 AHF) BACH study	Mortality at 7,30 and 90 days	MRproADM predicts mortality	90 days – HR 2.4 (1.4–4.4) AUC 0.67 14 days AUC 0.742	If>1.98 nmol/L; Combining Copeptin and MRproADM increases 14 day AUC to 0.808
Shah (2012) [15]	560	ED patients with SOB (180 AHF) PRIDE study	Mortality at 1 year (4 years FU)	MRproADM predicts mortality	up to 1 year - HR 2.7 AUC 0.796	If>0.77 nmol/L
Cinar (2012) [16]	154	ED patients with SOB (65 AHF)	Mortality at 30 days	MRproADM predicts mortality	OR 8.5 AUC 0.81 (0.71–0.91)	If>1.5 nmol/L
Travaglino (2014) [17]	501	ED patients with SOB (162 AHF) VERDY study	Mortality at 90 days	MRproADM predicts mortality	baseline sample AUC 0.76; 72 hr sample AUC 0.7	Not statistically significant for prognosis at 30 days
Gegenhuber (2007) [18]	137	AHF	Mortality at 1 year	MRproADM predicts mortality	HR 2.11 (0.93–4.77) AUC 0.708	If>1.23 nmol/L
Lassus (2013) [19]	5306	AHF (MOCA study)	Mortality at 30 days and 1 year	MRproADM predicts mortality	30 day AUC 0.74; 1 year AUC 0.73	Net reclassification index (NRI) of 28.7% at 30 days and 9.1 % at 1 year
Neuhold (2010) [20]	181	Worsening HF	Mortality at 24 months	MRproADM predicts mortality	HR 2.79	MRproADM levels do not change with acute therapy
Pousset (2000) [21]	117	CHF	Death or Cardiac Transplant FU 237 day	Adrenomedullin predicts outcomes	HR 1.56 (1.05–2.32) p 0.03	

(continued)

Table 23.1 (continued)

Author	N	Population	Endpoint and FU	Findings	Hazard ratio and AUC	Comments
Richards (2001) [22]	297	CHF pts on Carvedilol or placebo	Death or Heart Failure events 18 months	Adrenomedullin predicts events	HR 2.4 (1.3–4.5)	If > 9.8 pmol/L: Carvedilol reduces events in patients with higher BNP or ADM
Gardner (2005) [23]	150	Severe CHF on transplant waiting list	Death or urgent transplant 666 days FU	Adrenomedullin predicts events	Not significant	ADM not prognostic in advanced heart failure
Adlbrecht (2009) [24]	786	CHF	Death at 4 months	MRproADM predicts death in NYHA I and II	HR 2.12	MRproADM not independently prognostic in severe heart failure
von Haehling (2010) [25]	501	CHF	Death at 1 year	Log_{10} MRproADM predicts mortality	HR 1.82 (1.24–2.66) AUC 0.72 (0.67–0.76)	
Bosselmann (2013) [26]	424	CHF	Death at 4.5 years	MRproADM predicts mortality	HR 2.37 (1.66–3.38)	If > 679 pmol/L; prognosis independent of renal function
Xue (2013) [27]	724	CHF	Death at 6 years	MRproADM predicts mortality dependant on HR stage	Stage A HR 3.78 (p 0.001); Stage B HR 1.579 (pNS); Stage C/D HR 2.74 (p 0.001)	
Morales (2010) [28]	50	CHF all assigned to CRT	Reverse remodelling at 22 months	MRproADM at baseline predicts reverse remodelling	27.2 vs 17.9 pmol/L (p 0.0003)	Independent of symptoms
Funke-Kaiser (2014) [11]	8444	General population FINRISK1997	Incident HF (14 years FU)	MRproADM predicts incident Heart Failure and death	HR 1.67 (1.49–1.87) for heart failure; HR 1.18 (1.08–1.28) for death	if > 0.59 nmol/L

ED Emergency department, *AHF* acute heart failure, *CHF* chronic heart failure, *AUC* area under the ROC curve, *CRT* cardiac resynchronisation therapy, *OR* odds ratio

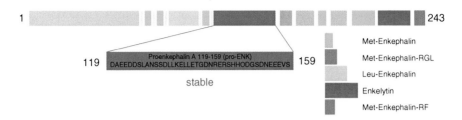

Fig. 23.2 Processing of proenkephalin to active short lived enkephalin peptides. The PENK peptide 119–159 is stable (Courtesy of Sphingotec, Hennigsdorf, Germany)

of heart failure, administration of a δ-opioid receptor antagonist led to increased blood pressure, cardiac output, and blood flow to kidney, heart, and other organs [32]. A role for endogenous opioids in humans with acute heart failure was also suggested following antagonism of opioid receptors using naloxone, which led to increased levels of the counter-regulatory hormones atrial natriuretic peptide(ANP) and catecholamines, with corresponding increases in heart rate and blood pressure [33]. However, these effects were not seen in patients with less severe heart failure, and naloxone may actually reduce levels of ANP in these patients [33]. Thus activation of the enkephalin system may be beneficial in moderate degrees of heart failure, where enkephalins could restrain excessive activation of the sympathetic nervous system, but detrimental in severe heart failure when overactivation of this system could lead to vascular collapse and renal impairment.

The recent development of an assay for a fragment of PENK comprising amino acids 119–159, suggested that this peptide is stable [2], has paved the way for more studies on the enkephalin system in cardiovascular disease. Initial studies of plasma PENK were performed in acute myocardial infarction [34]. PENK was strongly and negatively correlated to eGFR (r_s-0.583), and was an independent predictor of major adverse events, including death, heart failure and re-myocardial infarction. PENK-adjusted GRACE scores reclassified patients successfully, predominantly by upclassifying risk in those with endpoints.

Preliminary Studies with mADM and PENK in Acute Heart Failure

There are not many published studies using mADM and PENK as biomarkers in cardiovascular disease and none in acute heart failure. We recruited 515 (58.6% male, 43.9% with ischaemic heart disease, 59.2% with hypertension, 31.5% with diabetes) patients with acute decompensated heart failure, and obtained plasma samples on admission. Major adverse events were observed over the following year (140 deaths, 304 death/heart failure hospitalisation). Plasma mADM was elevated over two fold on admission (median [range] 50 [11.7–1772.8] pg/mL; normal subjects 20.7 pg/mL) as was plasma PENK (99.7 [14.8–641.3] pmol/L; normal subjects 44 pmol/L). Plasma mADM and PENK were correlated to eGFR (r_s −0.31 and −0.73 respectively). Plasma mADM at discharge was 44.2 [11.7–734.2] pg/mL, and PENK was 102.3 [18–736] pmol/L.

Table 23.2 Cox regression analysis for the endpoint of death/HF at 1 year, using ADHERE scores and mADM or PENK. Hazard ratios refer to Log_{10} biomarker levels normalised to one SD increment

Model with mADM	Univariable HR (95 % CI)	P	Multivariable HR (95 % CI)	P
Adhere 1	Reference	0.0005	Reference	0.0005
Adhere 2	1.47 (1.15–1.87)	0.002	1.43 (1.05–1.94)	0.023
Adhere 3	2.22 (1.70–2.91)	0.0005	1.99 (1.38–2.87)	0.0005
Adhere 4	2.80 (2.01–3.92)	0.002	2.65 (1.75–4.01)	0.0005
Adhere 5	3.85 (2.05–7.26)	0.0005	3.25 (1.33–7.94)	0.01
Log mADM (pg/ml)	1.51 (1.31–1.68)	0.0005	2.06 (1.68–2.52)	0.0005
Loop Diuretic	0.41 (0.34–0.51)	0.0005	0.66 (0.48–0.91)	0.01
Loop Diuretic* mADM	1.33 (1.18–1.50)	0.0005	0.60 (0.47–0.76)	0.0005
Model with PENK	**Univariable HR (95 % CI)**	**P**	**Multivariable HR (95 % CI)**	**P**
Adhere 1	Reference	0.0005	Reference	0.0005
Adhere 2	1.47 (1.15–1.87)	0.002	1.45 (1.06–1.97)	0.019
Adhere 3	2.22 (1.70–2.91)	0.0005	1.67 (1.14–2.44)	0.008
Adhere 4	2.80 (2.01–3.92)	0.002	2.32 (1.52–3.54)	0.0005
Adhere 5	3.85 (2.05–7.26)	0.0005	2.66 (1.05–6.74)	0.039
Log PENK (pmol/L)	1.51 (1.34–1.71)	0.0005	1.54 (1.24–1.91)	0.0005
Loop Diuretic	0.41 (0.34–0.51)	0.0005	0.59 (0.44–0.79)	0.001
Loop Diuretic* PENK	1.41 (1.24–1.61)	0.0005	0.85 (0.66–1.10)	NS

* signifies interaction in statistical analysis (i.e. interaction between biomarker and the treatment)

Using the ADHERE score [35] in combination with either of these biomarkers for prediction of death/HF at 1 year, both mADM and PENK remained significant independent predictors (Table 23.2). There was also significant interaction between mADM levels and diuretic therapy, although the interaction with PENK levels was not significant. This is illustrated in Kaplan-Meier survival curves (Fig. 23.3) which show a progressive increase in risk in those in higher PENK and mADM tertiles, and also suggest a significant reduction of events in those treated with diuretics in the highest tertile of mADM and PENK (p<0.0005 for both).

A practical scheme for risk stratification in acute heart failure using the ADHERE score, mADM and PENK is presented in the following classification and regression tree (CART) analysis (Fig. 23.4), allowing patients to be classified as low and high risk individuals and enabling clinicians to target more intensive therapy at those with the highest risk.

Conclusions

The emergence of these two novel biomarker systems (mADM and PENK) may enable more accurate risk stratification of patients with acute heart failure and enable precision medicine in the future. In patients who may be prescribed

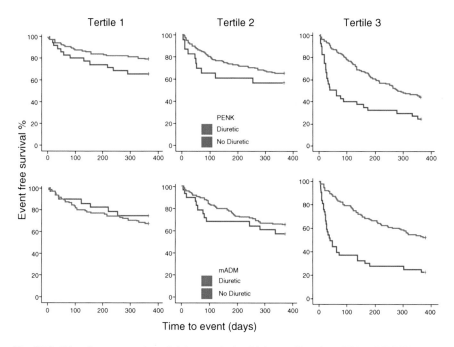

Fig. 23.3 Diuretics are more beneficial to survival at higher tertiles of mADM and PENK

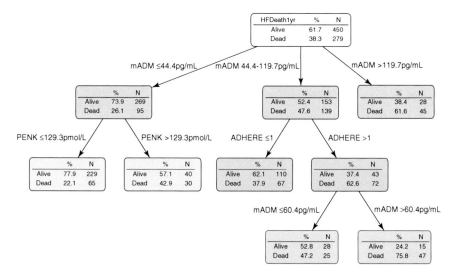

Fig. 23.4 CART diagram showing how patients could be risk stratified with mADM, PENK and the ADHERE score

neprilysin inhibitors, measurement of propeptides rather than bioactive peptides may indicate prognosis more accurately, and this has to be considered in future research.

References

1. Marino R, Struck J, Maisel AS, Magrini L, Bergmann A, Di Somma S. Plasma adrenomedullin is associated with short-term mortality and vasopressor requirement in patients admitted with sepsis. Crit Care. 2014;18:R34.
2. Ernst A, Köhrle J, Bergmann A. Proenkephalin A 119–159, a stable proenkephalin A precursor fragment identified in human circulation. Peptides. 2006;27:1835–40.
3. Ishimitsu T, Ono H, Minami J, Matsuoka H. Pathophysiologic and therapeutic implications of adrenomedullin in cardiovascular disorders. Pharmacol Ther. 2006;111:909–27.
4. Lainchbury JG, Cooper GJ, Coy DH, Jiang NY, Lewis LK, Yandle TG, Richards AM, Nicholls MG. Adrenomedullin: a hypotensive hormone in man. Clin Sci. 1997;92:467–72.
5. Nagaya N, Satoh T, Nishikimi T, Uematsu M, Furuichi S, Sakamaki F, Oya H, Kyotani S, Nakanishi N, Goto Y, Masuda Y, Miyatake K, Kangawa K. Hemodynamic, renal, and hormonal effects of adrenomedullin infusion in patients with congestive heart failure. Circulation. 2000;101:498–503.
6. Eto T, Kato J, Kitamura K. Regulation of production and secretion of adrenomedullin in the cardiovascular system. Regul Pept. 2003;112:61–9.
7. Sugo S, Minamino N, Shoji H, Kangawa K, Kitamura K, Eto T, Matsuo H. Interleukin-1, tumor necrosis factor and lipopolysaccharide additively stimulate production of adrenomedullin in vascular smooth muscle cells. Biochem Biophys Res Commun. 1995;207:25–32.
8. Maisel A, Mueller C, Nowak R, Peacock WF, Landsberg JW, Ponikowski P, Mockel M, et al. Mid-region pro-hormone markers for diagnosis and prognosis in acute dyspnea: results from the BACH (Biomarkers in Acute Heart Failure) trial. J Am Coll Cardiol. 2010;55:2062–76.
9. Neumann JT, Tzikas S, Funke-Kaiser A, Wilde S, Appelbaum S, Keller T, Ojeda-Echevarria F, Zeller T, Zwiener I, et al. Association of MR-proadrenomedullin with cardiovascular risk factors and subclinical cardiovascular disease. Atherosclerosis. 2013;228:451–9.
10. Wu AH, Tabas J, Stein J, Potocki M, Mueller C, McCord J, Richards M, et al. The effect of diabetes on the diagnostic and prognostic performance of mid-region pro-atrial natriuretic peptide and mid-region pro-adrenomedullin in patients with acute dyspnea. Biomarkers. 2012;17:490–7.
11. Funke-Kaiser A, Havulinna AS, Zeller T, Appelbaum S, Jousilahti P, Vartiainen E, et al. Predictive value of midregional pro-adrenomedullin compared to natriuretic peptides for incident cardiovascular disease and heart failure in the population-based FINRISK 1997 cohort. Ann Med. 2014;46:155–62.
12. Potocki M, Breidthardt T, Reichlin T, Morgenthaler NG, Bergmann A, Noveanu M, Schaub N, et al. Midregional pro-adrenomedullin in addition to b-type natriuretic peptides in the risk stratification of patients with acute dyspnea: an observational study. Crit Care. 2009;13:R122.
13. Maisel A, Mueller C, Nowak RM, Peacock WF, Ponikowski P, Mockel M, Hogan C, et al. Midregion prohormone adrenomedullin and prognosis in patients presenting with acute dyspnea: results from the BACH (Biomarkers in Acute Heart Failure) trial. J Am Coll Cardiol. 2011;58:1057–67.
14. Peacock WF, Nowak R, Christenson R, DiSomma S, Neath SX, Hartmann O, Mueller C, et al. Short-term mortality risk in emergency department acute heart failure. Acad Emerg Med. 2011;18:947–58.
15. Shah RV, Truong QA, Gaggin HK, Pfannkuche J, Hartmann O, Januzzi Jr JL. Mid-regional pro-atrial natriuretic peptide and pro-adrenomedullin testing for the diagnostic and prognostic evaluation of patients with acute dyspnoea. Eur Heart J. 2012;33:2197–205.
16. Cinar O, Cevik E, Acar A, Kaya C, Ardic S, Comert B, Yokusoglu M, et al. Evaluation of mid-regional pro-atrial natriuretic peptide, procalcitonin, and mid-regional pro-adrenomedullin for the diagnosis and risk stratification of dyspneic ED patients. Am J Emerg Med. 2012;30:1915–20.
17. Travaglino F, Russo V, De Berardinis B, Numeroso F, Catania P, Cervellin G, Nigra SG, Geraci F, et al. Thirty and ninety days mortality predictive value of admission and in-hospital procal-

citonin and mid-regional pro-adrenomedullin testing in patients with dyspnea. Results from the VERyfing DYspnea trial. Am J Emerg Med. 2014;32:334–41.

18. Gegenhuber A, Struck J, Dieplinger B, Poelz W, Pacher R, Morgenthaler NG, Bergmann A, et al. Comparative evaluation of B-type natriuretic peptide, mid-regional pro-A-type natriuretic peptide, mid-regional pro-adrenomedullin, and Copeptin to predict 1-year mortality in patients with acute destabilized heart failure. J Card Fail. 2007;13:42–9.

19. Lassus J, Gayat E, Mueller C, Peacock WF, Spinar J, Harjola VP, van Kimmenade R, et al. Incremental value of biomarkers to clinical variables for mortality prediction in acutely decompensated heart failure: the Multinational Observational Cohort on Acute Heart Failure (MOCA) study. Int J Cardiol. 2013;168:2186–94.

20. Neuhold S, Huelsmann M, Strunk G, Struck J, Adlbrecht C, Gouya G, Elhenicky M, Pacher R. Prognostic value of emerging neurohormones in chronic heart failure during optimization of heart failure-specific therapy. Clin Chem. 2010;56:121–6.

21. Pousset F, Masson F, Chavirovskaia O, Isnard R, Carayon A, Golmard JL, Lechat P, Thomas D, Komajda M. Plasma adrenomedullin, a new independent predictor of prognosis in patients with chronic heart failure. Eur Heart J. 2000;21:1009–14.

22. Richards AM, Doughty R, Nicholls MG, MacMahon S, Sharpe N, Murphy J, Espiner EA, et al. Plasma N-terminal pro-brain natriuretic peptide and adrenomedullin: prognostic utility and prediction of benefit from carvedilol in chronic ischemic left ventricular dysfunction. Australia-New Zealand Heart Failure Group. J Am Coll Cardiol. 2001;37:1781–7.

23. Gardner RS, Chong V, Morton I, McDonagh TA. N-terminal brain natriuretic peptide is a more powerful predictor of mortality than endothelin-1, adrenomedullin and tumour necrosis factor-alpha in patients referred for consideration of cardiac transplantation. Eur J Heart Fail. 2005;7:253–60.

24. Adlbrecht C, Hülsmann M, Strunk G, Berger R, Mörtl D, Struck J, Morgenthaler NG, Bergmann A, et al. Prognostic value of plasma midregional pro-adrenomedullin and C-terminal-pro-endothelin-1 in chronic heart failure outpatients. Eur J Heart Fail. 2009; 11:361–6.

25. von Haehling S, Filippatos GS, Papassotiriou J, Cicoira M, Jankowska EA, Doehner W, Rozentryt P, Vassanelli C, et al. Mid-regional pro-adrenomedullin as a novel predictor of mortality in patients with chronic heart failure. Eur J Heart Fail. 2010;12:484–91.

26. Bosselmann H, Egstrup M, Rossing K, Gustafsson I, Gustafsson F, Tonder N, Kistorp CN, et al. Prognostic significance of cardiovascular biomarkers and renal dysfunction in outpatients with systolic heart failure: a long term follow-up study. Int J Cardiol. 2013;170:202–7.

27. Xue Y, Taub P, Iqbal N, Fard A, Clopton P, Maisel A. Mid-region pro-adrenomedullin adds predictive value to clinical predictors and Framingham risk score for long-term mortality in stable outpatients with heart failure. Eur J Heart Fail. 2013;15:1343–9.

28. Morales MA, Maltinti M, Piacenti M, Turchi S, Giannessi D, Del Ry S. Adrenomedullin plasma levels predict left ventricular reverse remodeling after cardiac resynchronization therapy. Pacing Clin Electrophysiol. 2010;33:865–72.

29. Denning GM, Ackermann LW, Barna TJ, Armstrong JG, Stoll LL, Weintraub NL, Dickson EW. Proenkephalin expression and enkephalin release are widely observed in non-neuronal tissues. Peptides. 2008;29:83–92.

30. van den Brink OWV, Delbridge LM, Rosenfeldt FL, Penny D, Esmore DS, Quick D, Kaye DM, Pepe S. Endogenous cardiac opioids: enkephalins in adaptation and protection of the heart. Heart Lung Circ. 2003;12:178–87.

31. Bernardi P, Fontana F, Pich EM, Spampinato S, Canossa M. Plasma endogenous opioid levels in acute myocardial infarction patients, with and without pain. Eur Heart J. 1992;13:1074–9.

32. Imai N, Kashiki M, Woolf PD, Liang CS. Comparison of cardiovascular effects of mu- and delta-opioid receptor antagonists in dogs with congestive heart failure. Am J Physiol. 1994;267:H912–7.

33. Fontana F, Bernardi P, Pich EM, Capelli M, Bortoluzzi L, Spampinato S, Canossa M. Relationship between plasma atrial natriuretic factor and opioid peptide levels in healthy subjects and in patients with acute congestive heart failure. Eur Heart J. 1993;14:219–25.

34. Ng LL, Sandhu JK, Narayan H, Quinn PA, Squire IB, Davies JE, Bergmann A, Maisel A, Jones DJL. Proenkephalin and prognosis after acute myocardial infarction. J Am Coll Cardiol. 2014;63:280–9.
35. Fonarow GC, Adams Jr KF, Abraham WT, Yancy CW, Boscardin WJ, ADHERE Scientific Advisory Committee Study Group and Investigators. Risk stratification for in-hospital mortality in acutely decompensated heart failure: classification and regression tree analysis. JAMA. 2005;293:572–80.

Chapter 24
Biomarkers in Specific Disease States: Cardio-Oncology

Ugochukwu O. Egolum and Daniel J. Lenihan

Abstract Cancer related mortality has been dramatically reduced in recent decades due to more effective cancer treatments, especially chemotherapy and radiation therapy. However, the use of these treatment modalities may be limited by the risk of significant cardiac damage. The current standard for cardiac safety assessment, in order to limit cardiotoxicity, predominantly focuses on serial cardiac imaging to identify changes in left ventricular ejection fraction (LVEF). Unfortunately, this method is imperfect and frequently is a late finding. Potentially permanent cardiac damage manifesting as a significantly reduced LVEF has to occur before any important change in management is undertaken. One alternative and complimentary approach is the appropriate use of cardiac biomarkers to identify subclinical cardiac damage allowing for earlier detection and institution of cardio-protective interventions. This chapter will highlight the clinical use of cardiac biomarkers, specifically natriuretic peptides, cardiac troponins, as well as emerging biomarkers, for the detection of cardiac injury in the context of cardio-oncology.

Keywords Biomarker • Cardio-Oncology • Heart failure • Cardiac toxicity • Anthracyclines • Troponin • Natriuretic peptides

Cancer and cardiovascular diseases are by far the most common diseases resulting in mortality in the developed world [1]. The last decade has seen a profound increase cancer therapeutic options and the efficacy of those treatments [2]. Consequently, there is an ever increasing cohort of patients who are long-term survivors of childhood and adult onset cancer [3]. As this patient population ages, there is an increasing overlap with concomitant cardiovascular disease (CVD) [4–6]. It appears that CVD in survivors may be an epidemiological consequence of aging but also is

U.O. Egolum, MD • D.J. Lenihan, MD (✉)
Division of Cardiovascular Medicine, Vanderbilt University Medical Center,
Nashville, TN, USA
e-mail: daniel.lenihan@vanderbilt.edu

© Springer International Publishing Switzerland 2016   297
A.S. Maisel, A.S. Jaffe (eds.), *Cardiac Biomarkers*,
DOI 10.1007/978-3-319-42982-3_24

related to the toxicity of chemotherapy, radiation therapy or other treatments for cancer [6, 7]. Furthermore, a substantial portion of cancer patients may have pre-existing CVD which can be unmasked or exacerbated by increasingly specific che-motherapeutic agents with cardiotoxic effects. Cardiac damage may occur in a myriad of ways including arrhythmias, myocardial ischemia, hypertension, left ven-tricular (LV) dysfunction and heart failure (HF) [8–11]. Additionally, there are a host of vascular complications that may arise during and after treatment [12]. Encouragingly, there is also evidence that early detection of cardiovascular damage with initiation of cardiovascular based medical therapy can prevent and/or enhance cardiac recovery in the case of LV dysfunction but also prevention of toxicity with control of vascular complications [13–16]. The main limitation is related to detect-ing cardiovascular dysfunction at an early stage and initiating therapy before perma-nent damage occurs. The emphasis, thus, has been on cardiac imaging modalities including echocardiography with and without LV deformation (strain), multiple gated acquisition scan (MUGA) and cardiac magnetic resonance imaging (cMRI) to hopefully detect damage at an early point [17–21]. Unfortunately, the detection of a significant change in LVEF by any of these modalities is generally a late finding and usually indicates substantial underlying cardiac damage and remodeling [6, 22, 23]. The challenge at the present time is to be able to identify cardiac damage at the earliest stage prior to a reduction in LVEF and initiate therapy or modify dosing to prevent LV dysfunction. One way of achieving this goal is to utilize cardiac bio-markers to identify those at risk for developing cardiotoxicity. Overall, the advan-tage of cardiac biomarkers is that it is generally much less expensive, can be followed with ease in a serial fashion, and are less subject to interpretative variation [22]. In this chapter we will examine the data supporting the use of cardiac based biomarkers to enhance safety and cardio-protection during therapy for cancer.

B-type Natriuretic Peptide

B-type natriuretic peptide (BNP) is a neurohormone polypeptide secreted by the myocytes of the ventricles in response to increased wall stress from volume expan-sion and pressure overload and is secreted along with a 76-amino acid N-terminal pro BNP (NT-proBNP), that is biologically inactive, and eventually cleaved to the active 32 amino acid BNP [24]. The hemodynamic effects of BNP include a decrease in afterload and increase in natriuresis; thus, counteracting some of the pathophysi-ologic mechanisms responsible for the progression of HF. Robust data from the Breathing Not Properly trial (BNP trial) demonstrated that BNP was able to differ-entiate congestive heart failure (CHF) from non-CHF causes of dyspnea with good specificity and high negative predictive values. Subsequent studies also showed the utility of BNP for prognosis and risk stratification in the setting of HF [25, 26]. Additionally, NT-proBNP–guided optimal medical therapy is associated with a reduced incidence of cardiovascular death, new episodes of decompensated HF, and reduction in NT-proBNP that also correlates with LV remodeling and recovery [27]. Based on the aforementioned clinical utility, it comes as no surprise that the natri-uretic peptides, BNP/NT-proBNP, can be useful in the setting of early detection of potential cardiotoxicity due to its ability to detect subclinical disease, direct medical therapy and assist with prognostication even prior to a decline in LVEF [28, 29].

Multiple studies have looked at the utility of perturbations in BNP/NT-proBNP levels in patients with cancer undergoing treatment with chemotherapy or radia-tion (Table 24.1). In one such study, patients receiving high dose anthracyclines for breast cancer, NT-proBNP was measured at baseline and immediately follow-ing each treatment cycle [30]. There was a high degree of correlation between a rise in NT-ProBNP and a reduction in LVEF. Similar findings with natriuretic peptides were replicated in other studies primarily with the use of anthracycline-based chemotherapeutic regimens [28, 29]. The utility of BNP to assist in identi-fying those patients at risk for cardiotoxicity and LV dysfunction goes beyond the acute setting. Persistently elevated BNP is predictive of late onset adriamycin-induced cardiotoxicity and correlates with cardiac dysfunction detected over time [6, 28–30]. Furthermore, a baseline elevation of BNP can mark a patient at high risk for the development of cardiotoxicity during subsequent rounds of chemo-therapy [16].

Aside from predicting subsequent cardiotoxicity predominantly with anthracycline-based treatment, natriuretic peptide (NP) levels may indicate a potential therapeutic benefit. In one study, children with acute lymphoid leukemia (ALL) were randomized to receive doxorubicin with or without dexrazoxane (a cardioprotective free radical scavenger) and those patients given dexrazoxane tended to have reduced NT-proBNP concentrations indicating a cardioprotective effect (47 vs. 20 %, $p = 0.07$) [31]. It is especially important to have cardioprotec-tive strategies in the pediatric population that have increased long-term survival into adulthood [5, 32]. Additionally, NT-proBNP levels were lower and the LV mass was reduced in a pediatric patient population nearly 4 years after anthracy-cline treatment ($p = 0.003$) [32]. Consequently, NT-BNP/BNP levels appear to guide providers in identifying those specific patients at risk for toxicity as well as indicating what therapeutic interventions may reduce the impact of cardiac dys-function with anthracyclines.

The utility of natriuretic peptides (NP) to assist in detecting cardiac damage dur-ing cancer therapy can extend to a broader population than just those receiving known substantial cardio-toxins like anthracyclines. For instance, those patients receiving chest radiation, those at risk for development of atrial fibrillation while receiving anti-VEGF based therapy, those at risk for HF with tyrosine kinase inhibi-tors, and potentially those receiving combination therapy for multiple myeloma all may be populations in which NP may be useful [16, 33–35]. Elevated BNP levels correlate with an increased risk for radiation induced cardiomyopathy (early and late) and are directly related to the amount of radiation delivered [33]. Furthermore, NT-proBNP levels are used to stage and predict outcomes in patients with AL amy-loidosis as well as monitor response to therapy [36–38].

Table 24.1 Role of natriuretic peptides in the evaluation of chemotherapy and radiation-induced cardiotoxicity*

Reference	Population	N	Treatment	BNP type	Cutoff	BNP evaluations	Results and conclusions
Meinardi et al.	Breast cancer	39	ACs and RT	BNP	10 pmol/l	Baseline, 1 month, and 1 year after chemotherapy	BNP increased as early as 1 month after chemo; no correlation with LVEF decline
Nousiainen et al.	Non-Hodgkin lymphoma	28	CHOP	BNP	227 pmol/l	Baseline, after every cycle, and 4 weeks after last cycle	Correlation between BNP increases and parameters of diastolic function (FS and PFR)
Daugaard et al.	Various	107	ACs	BNP		Before, and at various points during treatment	BNP correlation with decreased LVEF, but baseline and BNP change could not predict LVEF decline
Perik et al.	Breast cancer	54	ACs and RT	NT-proBNP	10 pmol/l	Median 2.7 and 6.5 years after chemotherapy	BNP increased with time and was related to dose; cardiotoxic effects develop over years
Sandri et al.	Various	52	HDC	NT-proBNP	153 ng/l (M <50), 227 ng/l (M >50), 88 ng/l (F <50), 334 ng/l (F >50)	Baseline, and 0, 12, 24, 36, and 72 h after each cycle	Persistent NT-proBNP elevation at 72 h predicts later systolic and diastolic dysfunction
Germanakis et al.	Pediatric cancers	19	ACs	NT-proBNP	0.2 pmol/ml	Mean 3.9 years after chemotherapy	Correlation between NT-proBNP and LV mass decrease
Perik et al.	Breast cancer	17	ACs and T	NT-proBNP	125 ng/l	Baseline and throughout T treatment	Higher pre-treatment NT-proBNP values in those who developed HF during treatment

Author	N	Treatment	Biomarker	Cutoff	Timing	Results
Aggarwal et al.	63	ACs	BNP		Once, >1 year after treatment completion	Higher BNP in patients with late cardiac dysfunction by ECHO
Ekstein et al.	23	ACs	NT-proBNP	350 pg/ml	Before and after each AC dose	Dose-related increase in BNP from baseline seen after first AC dose
Jingu et al.	197	RT	BNP		Before, <1 month, 1–2, 3–8, 9–24, and >24 months after RT	Increased BNP over time and in those with abnormal FDG accumulation
Kouloubinis et al.	40	ACs	NT-proBNP		Before and after chemotherapy	Correlation between NT-proBNP increase and LVEF decline
Dodos et al.	100	ACs	NT-proBNP	153 or 227 ng/l for M <50 or >50; 88 or 334 ng/l for F <50 or >50	After first dose, last dose, and 1, 6, and 12 months after last dose	No significant increase in NT-proBNP with treatment; cannot replace serial ECHO for monitoring of AC-induced cardiotoxicity
Kozak et al.	30	ChemoRT	NT-proBNP		Baseline, after 2 weeks of RT, and after RT end	No change in NT-proBNP during treatment
Cil et al.	33	ACs	NT-proBNP	110 pg/ml	Before and after chemotherapy	Despite association, pre-chemo NT-proBNP did not predict for later LVEF
ElGhandour et al.	40	CHOP	BNP		Before first cycle and after sixth cycle of chemotherapy	Correlation between BNP values after chemotherapy and LVEF

(continued)

Table 24.1 (continued)

Reference	Population	N	Treatment	BNP type	Cutoff	BNP evaluations	Results and conclusions
Mavinkurve-Groothuis et al.	Pediatric cancers	122	ACs	NTproBNP	10 pmol/l (M), 18 pmol/l (F), age-adjusted in children	Once, with imaging	NT-proBNP levels related to cumulative AC dose
Nellessen et al.	Lung and breast CA	23	RT	NT-proBNP	100 pg/ml	Before RT, every week during RT for 4–6 weeks	Log-transformed NT-proBNP increased during treatment
Fallah-Rad et al.	Breast cancer	42	ACs and T	NT-proBNP		Before chemotherapy, before T, and 3, 6, 9, and 12 months after start of T	No change in NT-proBNP values over time
Feola et al.	Breast cancer	53	ACs	NT-proBNP	5 pg/ml	Baseline, after 1 month, 1 and 2 years	NT-proBNP increased acutely with treatment, and in patients with systolic dysfunction
Goel et al.	Breast cancer	36	ACs and T	NT-proBNP	110 pg/ml (age <75), 589 pg/ml (age >75)	Baseline, before and 24 h after T	No change in NT-proBNP with trastuzumab
Romano et al.	Breast cancer	92	ACs	NT-proBNP	153 pg/ml (age <50), 222 pg/ml (age >50)	Every 2 weeks during treatment, then at 3, 6, and 12 months	Interval change in NT-proBNP predicated for LV impairment at 3, 6, and 12 months
Sawaya et al.	Breast cancer	43	ACs and T	NT-proBNP	125 pg/ml	Baseline, 3 and 6 months after chemotherapy	No relation between NT-proBNP levels before and after treatment and LVEF change
D'Errico et al.	Breast cancer	60	ChemoRT	NT-proBNP	125 pg/ml	Before and after RT	Correlation between NT-proBNR V3G$_y$ for the heart, D15$_{cm}$2/Dmean and D$_{15cm}$3/D50%

Author	Cancer	N	Treatment	Biomarker	Cutoff	Timing	Findings
Lipshultz et al.	ALL	156	ACs	NT-proBNP	150 pg/ml (age <1), 100 pg/ml (age >1)	Before, and daily during induction, and after treatment	Correlation between NT-proBNP and change in LV thickness-to-dimension ratio 4 years later
Mladosievicova et al.	Childhood leukemias	69	ACs	NT-proBNP	105 pg/ml (F), 75 pg/ml (M)	Median 11 years after treatment	Increased NT-proBNP with exposure to ACs
Onitilo et al.	Breast cancer	54	Taxanes and T	BNP	200 pg/ml	Baseline and every 3 weeks during treatment	No correlation between elevated BNP values and cardiotoxicity
Prongprot et al.	pediatric cancers	30	ACs	NT-proBNP	Age-adjusted (100)	Once, with imaging	Correlation between NT-proBNP values and FS and LVEF
Sawaya et al.	Breast cancer	81	ACs and T	NT-proBNP	125 pg/ml	Before, every 3 months during and after T treatment	NT-proBNP did not change with treatment
Sherief et al.	Acute leukemias	50	ACs	NT-proBNP	Age-adjusted (107)	Once, with imaging	NT-proBNP linked to AC dose and abnormal tissue Doppler imaging parameters
Kittiwarawut et al.	Breast cancer	52	ACs	NT-proBNP	45 pg/ml	Baseline and end of fourth cycle	Correlation between NT-proBNP and FS
Ky et al.	Breast cancer	78	ACs and T	NT-proBNP		Baseline, 3 and 6 months after start of chemotherapy	No relationship between NT-proBNP values and cardiotoxicity

*From Tian S et al. [6], with permission

BNP brain natriuretic peptide, *NT* N-terminal, *AC* anthracycline, *RT* radiation therapy, *HDC* high-dose chemotherapy, *T* trastuzumab, *LVEF* left ventricular ejection fraction, *HE* heart failure, *ALL* acute lymphoblastic leukemia, *FS* fractional shortening, *PFR* peak filling rate

It should be noted that NP, although broadly useful and predictive, must be interpreted within the entire clinical context at the moment of sampling for any given patient. For example, a rapid increase in BNP/NT-proBNP in a patient undergoing chemotherapy easily could be related to a concomitant process, such acute kidney injury or volume overload, without evidence of cardiac dysfunction or toxicity. In this context, the clinician is encouraged to make a careful assessment of the volume status of the patient and attempt to define the presence of other prominent co-morbidity such as sepsis [39].

Troponin

Troponin I (TnI) and troponin T (TnT) are both cardiac specific proteins that form an integral part of the cardiac contractile unit [16, 22]. As biomarkers they are highly specific and sensitive for cardiac damage and are widely used in the diagnosis/treatment of acute coronary syndromes as currently supported by major guideline documents [40]. Elevations in troponin correlate with cardiac myocyte damage/death, however, it does not distinguish the mechanism of injury. As such, cardiac troponin has found utility in the screening of asymptomatic patients for cardiotoxicity during and after treatment [41–43]. A summary of the major clinical trials examining the utility of troponin in cardio-oncology is provided in Table 24.2 [6].

One of the larger studies to examine this topic enrolled 703 patients with various advanced malignances who were receiving high dose chemotherapy [41]. TnI was checked at initiation of therapy, and 1 month after. Cardiac function was measured and documented with echocardiography at baseline, and 1, 2, 6, and 12 months post therapy. Thirty percent of the patients had early TnI elevation, and a third of subsequently showed elevated TnI at 1 month. Reductions in ejection fraction were predicted by both early ($r = 0.78$, $p < 0.001$) and persistent elevation at 1 month ($r = 0.92$, $p < 0.001$). Not only did elevated troponin predict decline in EF, persistent elevation was able to predict the development of symptomatic HF which suggests that troponin elevation closely correlates with the cardiotoxic effects of the chemotherapeutic agents [44]. Having a positive troponin at any time predicted future cardiovascular events with a positive predictive value of 84 % and negative predictive value of 99 %. There is a suggestion that troponin I elevation may be able to predict cardiac dysfunction with other cardio-toxic therapy, such as trastuzumab, but the data has not been as consistent as initially reported [16, 45, 46]. Additionally, troponin T has shown utility in the care of patients with *light chain amyloidosis* [37, 38, 47]. Troponin levels are predictive of outcomes and decreases correlate with response to therapy and can be used to monitor disease activity in the post therapy patient with amyloidosis.

The utility of troponin to detect cardiac damage in patients who survived prior treatment of childhood cancer is a hopeful goal but has not been well established to date [48–50]. However, a study in patients with ALL treated with anthracyclines and dexrazoxane had a reduced incidence of elevated troponin underscoring the protec-

Table 24.2 Role of cardiac troponins in the evaluation of chemotherapy and radiation-induced cardiotoxicity*

Reference	Population	N	Treatment	Tn type	Cutoff	Troponin evaluations	Results and Conclusions
Hugh-Davies et al.	Breast cancer	50	ACs and RT	T	0.1 ng/ml	Pre- and post-treatment	No change in TnT after 45–46 Gy delivered to the whole breast
Lipshultz et al.	ALL	15	ACs	T	0.03 ng/ml	Baseline, and 1–3 days after each cycle	Correlation between TnT and LV end-diastolic dimension and wall thickness
Herman et al.	Animal study	37	ACs	T		Before, and 1 week after chemotherapy	TnT and histological myocardial changes in both related to cumulative doxorubicin dose
Cardinale et al.	Various	204	HDC	I	0.5 ng/ml	Before, and 0, 12, 24, 36, and 72 h after every cycle	Elevated TnI during treatment predicted for LVEF decline
Cardinale et al.	Breast cancer	211	HDC and RT	I	0.5 ng/ml	Before, and 0, 12, 24, 36, and 72 h after every cycle	Correlation between max TnI, number of positive assays, and max LVEF reduction
Auner et al.	Hematologic malignancies	78	ACs	T	0.03 ng/ml	Within 48 h of treatment start, then every 48 h during treatment	Correlation between TnT increase and median LVEF decline
Sandri et al.	Various	179	HDC		0.08 ng/ml	Before, and 0, 12, 24, 36, and 72 h after every cycle	TnI increase predicted subsequent LVEF decline
Cardinale et al.	Various	703	HDC	I	0.08 ng/ml	Before, and 0, 12, 24, 36, and 72 h after every cycle, and 1 month after treatment	Persistent TnI positivity predicted for subsequent LVEF decline
Kismet et al.	Pediatric solid cancers	24	ACs	T	0.01 ng/ml	With imaging, > 1 month after chemo	No relationship between TnT and echocardiographic abnormalities
Lipshultz et al.	ALL	76	ACs	T	0.01 ng/ml	Throughout chemotherapy	TnT persistently increased suring treatment, and predicted for cardioprotective response
Kilickap et at	Various	41	ACs	T	0.01 ng/ml	Baseline, after first and last cycle	Correlation between TnT increase and diastolic dysfunction (E/A ratio)
Perik et al.	Breast cancer	17	ACs and T	I	0.1 g/1	Before, and throughout T	No TnI elevations in 15/16 patients

(continued)

Table 24.2 (continued)

Reference	Population	N	Treatment	Tn type	Cutoff	Troponin evaluations	Results and Conclusions
Dodos et al.	Various	100	ACs	T	0.1 ng/ml	After first dose, last does, and 1, 6, 12 months after last dose	No TnT elevations detected
Kozak et al. (72)	Lung and esophageal CA	30	ChemoRT	T		Baseline, 2 weeks after start of treatment and after	TnT undetectable in 20/30 patients
Cilt et al.	Breast cancer	33	ACs	I		Before and after chemotherapy	No correlation between TnI and LVEF decline
Mavinkurve-Groothuis et al.	Various pediatric	122	ACs	T	0.01 ng/ml	Once, with imaging	No patients with elevated TnT levels
Cardinale et al.	Breast cancer	251	ACs and T	I	0.08 ng/ml	Before T, every 3 months during treatment, 1 year after start, every 6 months	Elevated TnI values are an indepaendent predictor of cardiotoccity, and LVEF recovery
Nellessen et al.	Lung and breast CA	23	RT	I	0.03 ng/ml	Before RT, every week during RT for 4–6 weeks	Log-transformed TnI increased during treatment
Fallah-Rad et al.	Breast cancer	42	ACs and T	T		Before chemotherapy, before T, and 3, 6, 9, and 12 months after start of T	No change in TNT values over time
Feola et al.	Breast cancer	53	ACs	I	0.03 ng/ml	Baseline, after 1 month, 1 and 2 years	TnI concentrations elevated at 1 month, then returned to normal
Goel et al.	Breast cancer	36	ACs and T	I	0.20 ng/ml	Baseline, before and 24 h after T	No elevated TnI values throughout
Morris et al.	Breast cancer	95	ACs and T	I	0.04– 0.06 ng/ml	Every 2 weeks during treatment, then at 6, 9, and 18 months	Elevated TnI values preceded maximal LVEF decline, but no relationship with max LVEF decline
Romano et al.	Breast cancer	92	ACs		5 or 0.08 ng/ml (age <50 or >50)	Every 2 weeks during treatment, then at 3, 6, and 12 months	No correlation between TnI change and subsequent LV impairment

(continued)

Sawaya et al.	Breast cancer	43	ACs and T	I	0.015 ng/ml	Baseline, 3 and 6 months after chemotherapy	Elevated TnI at 3 months predicted for cardiotoxicity within 6 months
D'Errico et al.	Breast cancer	60	ChemoRT	I	0.07 ng/ml	Before and after RT	No elevated TnI concentrations
Garrone et al.	Breast cancer	50	ACs	I	0.03 ng/ml	Baseline, 5, 16, and 28 months after	TnI kinetics correlated with LVEF decline
Lipshultz et al.	ALL	156	ACs		0.01 ng/ml	Before, and daily during induction, and after treatment	Lower incidence of detectable TnT during treatment with dexrazoxane
Onitilo et al.	Breast cancer	54	Taxanes and T	I	0.1 ng/ml	Baseline, and every 3 weeks during treatment	TnI undetectable throughout
Sawaya et al.	Breast cancer	81	ACs and T	I	30 pg/ml	Before, every 3 months during, and after T treatment	Elevated TnI values at end of treatment predictive of subsequent cardiotocitiy
Sherief et al.	Acute leukemias	50	ACs	T	0.01 ng/ml	Once, with imaging	No elevated TnT values
Erven et al.	Breast cancer	72	RT	I	0.13 ng/ml	Before and after RT	Higher TnI values in l-sided breast patients
Ky et al.	Breast cancer	78	ACs and T	I	121.8 ng/ml	Baseline, 3 and 6 months after start of chemotherapy	Interval change in TnI predicted cardiotoxicity

*From Tian et al. [6], with permission

Tn troponin, *AC* anthracycline, *RT* radiation therapy, *HDC* high-dose chemotherapy, T trastuzumab, *LVEE* left ventricular ejection fraction, *ALL* acute lympho-blastic leukemia

tive effect during active treatment [31]. In another study elevated troponin corre-lated with lower LV mass at 4 years post treatment [44]. Although early troponin elevation during therapy was predictive of cardiac dysfunction, post therapy tropo-nin did not correlate with risk of late onset cardiotoxicity [48].

Despite the utility of troponin as outlined above, there appears to be mixed data as it relates to the utility of troponin levels for predicting radiation induced cardio-myopathy [51, 52].

Emerging Biomarkers

There has been a desire to identify an effective biomarker to detect cardiac injury during cancer treatment and therefore other markers have been investigated.

Myeloperoxidase (MPO)

MPO is a proatherogenic enzyme produced by neutrophils that is indicative off oxidative stress and lipid peroxidation. Its prognostic role in acute coronary syn-drome and heart failure has been suggested [46, 53–55]. In the context of cancer chemotherapy, a panel of biomarkers including NT-proBNP, growth differentiation factor (GDF)-15, placenta growth factor (PlGF), c reactive protein (crp), soluble fms-like tyrosine kinase receptor (sFlt)-1, and galectin (gal)-3 in breast cancer patients receiving antracyclines and herceptin were examined [46]. In patients with 90th percentile MPO interval change from baseline the probability of cardiotoxicity at 15 months was 34.2%, and the risk of future cardiac toxicity increased with each standard deviation increase in MPO concentration (HR 1.34, $p = 0.048$). Although, the most useful biomarker tested was high sensitivity troponin I, MPO was also modestly useful in detection of cardiac damage.

C-reactive Protein (CRP)

CRP is an acute phase reactant produced in response to inflammation [56, 57]. Although its role in CAD and HF is well documented, the utility of CRP in the cardio-oncology patient population has mixed results [58, 59]. High-sensitivity CRP (hsCRP) concentrations ≥ 3 mg/l predicted impaired LVEF with 92.9% sensitivity and 45.7% specificity (PPV, 40.6%; NPV, 94.1%) in a cohort of breast cancer patients. HsCRP elevations occurred >70 days before echocardiographic changes were seen. As such, hsCRP maybe able to risk stratify patients and delineate who needs more stringent follow up [58]. Another study, in a survivorship cohort, found higher CRP values regardless of exposure to cardiotoxic treatment but poor correlation with LV mass, wall thickness, and dimension [50]. This suggests that hs-CRP may be a surrogate for overall inflammation or tumor burden in addition to drug effects.

Total Antioxidant Status (TAOS)

Total antioxidant status is a sum total of antioxidants in the blood and could potentially be used to monitor for cardiac toxicity in anthracycline based therapy [49]. A study of 29 children undergoing anthracycline based therapy for acute leukemia showed statistically significant decrease in TAOS which correlated with higher total doses of anthracyclines and subsequent reduction in LVEF.

Nitric Oxide (NO)

NO is generated by NO synthase from L-arginine in numerous cell types and is a key regulator of cardiomyocyte contractility [60]. Dysregulated NO synthesis is implicated in the pathophysiology of doxorubicin-induced cardiotoxicity [6, 60]. One study demonstrated significantly higher plasma levels of total nitrite, a stable product of NO, in children that received doxorubicin and in those with abnormal LVEF as compared to healthy controls and an increased NO may be an indicator of subclinical cardiotoxicity.

In addition to the markers discussed above, future directions include heart-type fatty acid-binding protein, cytochrome C, glycogen phosphorylase isoenzyme BB and circulating microRNAs deserve mention as potential targets.

Conclusion

With a dramatic improvement in the overall survival and outcomes of patients with cancer, cardiac damage or exacerbation of underlying cardiac disease by cancer therapy has become a critically important issue for cancer survivors and clinicians. Screening for cardiotoxicity, as per current guidelines, focuses predominantly on serial noninvasive imaging. This is costly, subject to variation in reader interpretation, and often detects changes when cardiac remodeling has already taken place. Cardiac biomarkers have emerged as an inexpensive means to serially follow patients and to potentially detect early subclinical cardiac toxicity. Biomarkers can delinate low versus high risk patients allowing for intensive screening in the later group. As such, biomarkers, can potentially reduce costs associated with unnecessary serial screening. Early, detection of subclinical cardiotoxic effects, facilitate changes in the chemotherapy regimen and/or the initiation of cardioprotective medical regimen (eg. Beta blocker) to prevent permanent cardiac remodeling.

In summary, biomarkers offer significant advantages in the detection, treatment and prognostication of cardiotoxicity. Multiple cardiac biomarkers have been studied and shown utility in this setting. However, as we look to the future with ever increasing array of available chemotherapy agents, further prospective randomized trials need to be conducted with the incorporation of cardiac biomarkers to improve our understanding of their optimal role. Eventually, cardiac biomarkers maybe implemented in every day practice and serve to replace or complement cardiac imaging.

Here we will present a patient recently seen at our medical center and illustrate how we applied biomarkers to their medical care.

Case

A 65 y/o Caucasian male, WL, with medical history of hypertension and dyslipidemia was referred to our heart failure clinic from an outside general cardiology clinic for evaluation of difficult to manage heart failure with preserved ejection fraction (HFpEF). Despite diuretic therapy, he continued to have orthopnea, edema and dyspnea with minimal activity. His echocardiogram showed mild concentric LVH, normal ejection fraction, grade II diastolic dysfunction and no significant valvular pathology. His electrocardiogram showed low voltage and a pseudoinfarct pattern raising suspicion for infiltrative cardiomyopathy. Laboratory evaluation showed a monoclonal protein spike and a bone marrow biopsy was notable for 15% clonal plasma cells and no amyloid. A cMRI demonstrated global subendocardial delayed enhancement consistent with amyloidosis. A cardiac catheterization was negative for significant coronary disease with biopsy positive for congo red staining- confirming a diagnosis of AL cardiac amyloidosis. His diuretic regimen was adjusted and with careful attention to salt/fluid intake his HFpEF symptoms improved.

He was referred to the Oncology clinic for further evaluation. At that point his troponin I was 0.12 ng/ml (<0.03 ng/ml), BNP 569 pg/ml (<100 pg/ml) and serum lamda light chain 27.19 mg/dl (0.57-2.63 mg/dl). At this point he was started on induction therapy with 6 cycles of bortezomib and dexamethasone. During induction therapy he developed worsening heart failure symptoms and a repeat echocardiogram showed ejection fraction of 35%. His troponin I and BNP increased to 0.21 ng/ml and 1006 pg/ml respectively. His cardiac dysfunction was presumed secondary to bortezomib. Based on prior reported studies this is generally reversible [52]. We adjusted his medical regimen with the addition of carvedilol, spironolactone and uptitration of his diuretic regimen. We continued and completed induction therapy. After approximately 6 months his LVEF was back to normal. Additionally, troponin I and BNP decreased to 0.13 ng/ml and 340 pg/ml respectively, signally cardiac recovery and reduction in disease activity. He subsequently underwent consolidation therapy with reduced dose melphalan and stem cell transplantation. During post-transplant follow up, troponin I normalized, BNP decreased to

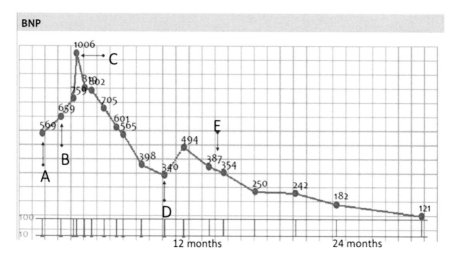

Fig. 24.1 The time course of BNP elevation (pg/ml) during the diagnosis and successful treatment of a patient with AL amyloidosis. (*A*) diagnosis, (*B*) bortezomib + dexamethasone, (*C*) LVEF drop to 35 %, (*D*) LVEF recovery/stem cell transplant, (*E*) heart failure symptoms improved

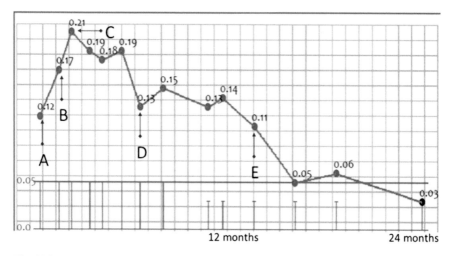

Fig. 24.2 The time course of Troponin I elevation (ng/ml) during the diagnosis and successful treatment of a patient with AL amyloidosis. (*A*) diagnosis, (*B*) chemotherapy + dexamethasone, (*C*) LVEF drop to 35 %, (*D*) LVEF recovery/stem cell transplant, (*E*) heart failure symptoms improved

120 pg/ml and serum lambda light chain decreased to the normal range <1.66 mg/dl. Overall, the biomarker activity was consistent with no amyloid disease activity and no ongoing cardiac damage. We will continue to follow him closely checking BNP and troponin levels periodically (Figs. 24.1, 24.2, and 24.3).

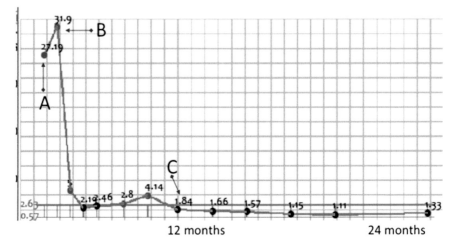

Fig. 24.3 The time course of lambda light chain levels (mg/dl) during the diagnosis and successful treatment of a patient with AL amyloidosis. (*A*) diagnosis, (*B*) chemotherapy + dexamethasone, (*C*) heart failure symptoms improved

References

1. Sanz J, Moreno PR, Fuster V. The year in atherothrombosis. J Am Coll Cardiol. 2007; 49:1740–9.
2. Hensley ML, Hagerty KL, Kewalramani T, et al. American Society of Clinical Oncology 2008 clinical practice guideline update: use of chemotherapy and radiation therapy protectants. J Clin Oncol. 2009;27:127–45.
3. Oeffinger KC, Mertens AC, Sklar CA, et al. Chronic health conditions in adult survivors of childhood cancer. N Engl J Med. 2006;355:1572–82.
4. McCabe MS, Bhatia S, Oeffinger KC, et al. American Society of Clinical Oncology statement: achieving high-quality cancer survivorship care. J Clin Oncol. 2013;31:631–40.
5. Armstrong GT, Oeffinger KC, Chen Y, et al. Modifiable risk factors and major cardiac events among adult survivors of childhood cancer. J Clin Oncol. 2013;31:3673–80.
6. Tian S, Hirshfield KM, Jabbour SK, et al. Serum biomarkers for the detection of cardiac toxicity after chemotherapy and radiation therapy in breast cancer patients. Front Oncol. 2014;4:277.
7. Armstrong GT, Kawashima T, Leisenring W, et al. Aging and risk of severe, disabling, life-threatening, and fatal events in the childhood cancer survivor study. J Clin Oncol. 2014;32:1218–27.
8. Ewer MS, Suter TM, Lenihan DJ, et al. Cardiovascular events among 1090 cancer patients treated with sunitinib, interferon, or placebo: a comprehensive adjudicated database analysis demonstrating clinically meaningful reversibility of cardiac events. Eur J Cancer (Oxford, England: 1990). 2014;50:2162–70.
9. Cheng H, Force T. Molecular mechanisms of cardiovascular toxicity of targeted cancer therapeutics. Circ Res. 2010;106:21–34.
10. Chu TF, Rupnick MA, Kerkela R, et al. Cardiotoxicity associated with tyrosine kinase inhibitor sunitinib. Lancet. 2007;370:2011–9.
11. Lotrionte M, Biondi-Zoccai G, Abbate A, et al. Review and meta-analysis of incidence and clinical predictors of anthracycline cardiotoxicity. Am J Cardiol. 2013;112:1980–4.

12. Li W, Croce K, Steensma DP, McDermott DF, Ben-Yehuda O, Moslehi J. Vascular and meta-bolic implications of novel targeted cancer therapies: focus on kinase inhibitors. J Am Coll Cardiol. 2015;66:1160–78.
13. Cardinale D, Colombo A, Sandri MT, et al. Prevention of high-dose chemotherapy-induced cardiotoxicity in high-risk patients by angiotensin-converting enzyme inhibition. Circulation. 2006;114:2474–81.
14. Kalay N, Basar E, Ozdogru I, et al. Protective effects of carvedilol against anthracycline-induced cardiomyopathy. J Am Coll Cardiol. 2006;48:2258–62.
15. Bosch X, Rovira M, Sitges M, et al. Enalapril and carvedilol for preventing chemotherapy-induced left ventricular systolic dysfunction in patients with malignant hemopathies: the OVERCOME trial (preventiOn of left Ventricular dysfunction with Enalapril and caRvedilol in patients submitted to intensive ChemOtherapy for the treatment of Malignant hEmopathies). J Am Coll Cardiol. 2013;61:2355–62.
16. Stevens PL, Lenihan DJ. Cardiotoxicity due to Chemotherapy: the Role of Biomarkers. Curr Cardiol Rep. 2015;17:603.
17. Lotrionte M, Cavarretta E, Abbate A, et al. Temporal changes in standard and tissue Doppler imaging echocardiographic parameters after anthracycline chemotherapy in women with breast cancer. Am J Cardiol. 2013;112:1005–12.
18. Schwartz RG, McKenzie WB, Alexander J, et al. Congestive heart failure and left ventricular dysfunction complicating doxorubicin therapy. Seven-year experience using serial radionu-clide angiocardiography. Am J Med. 1987;82:1109–18.
19. Thavendiranathan P, Poulin F, Lim KD, Plana JC, Woo A, Marwick TH. Use of myocardial strain imaging by echocardiography for the early detection of cardiotoxicity in patients during and after cancer chemotherapy: a systematic review. J Am Coll Cardiol. 2014;63:2751–68.
20. Plana JC, Galderisi M, Barac A, et al. Expert consensus for multimodality imaging evaluation of adult patients during and after cancer therapy: a report from the American Society of Echocardiography and the European Association of Cardiovascular Imaging. J Am Soc Echocardiogr Off Publ Am Soc Echocardiogr. 2014;27:911–39.
21. Nousiainen T, Vanninen E, Jantunen E, et al. Concomitant impairment of left ventricular sys-tolic and diastolic function during doxorubicin therapy: a prospective radionuclide ventriculo-graphic and echocardiographic study. Leuk Lymphoma. 2002;43:1807–11.
22. Christenson ES, James T, Agrawal V, Park BH. Use of biomarkers for the assessment of chemotherapy-induced cardiac toxicity. Clin Biochem. 2015;48:223–35.
23. Ewer MS, Lenihan DJ. Left ventricular ejection fraction and cardiotoxicity: is our ear really to the ground? J Clin Oncol. 2008;26:1201–3.
24. Selvais PL, Donckier JE, Robert A, et al. Cardiac natriuretic peptides for diagnosis and risk stratification in heart failure: influences of left ventricular dysfunction and coronary artery disease on cardiac hormonal activation. Eur J Clin Invest. 1998;28:636–42.
25. McCullough PA, Nowak RM, McCord J, et al. B-type natriuretic peptide and clinical judgment in emergency diagnosis of heart failure: analysis from Breathing Not Properly (BNP) Multinational Study. Circulation. 2002;106:416–22.
26. Maisel AS, Krishnaswamy P, Nowak RM, et al. Rapid measurement of B-type natriuretic pep-tide in the emergency diagnosis of heart failure. N Engl J Med. 2002;347:161–7.
27. Januzzi JL, Troughton R. Are serial BNP measurements useful in heart failure management? Serial natriuretic peptide measurements are useful in heart failure management. Circulation. 2013;127:500–7; discussion 8.
28. Nousiainen T, Vanninen E, Jantunen E, et al. Natriuretic peptides during the development of doxorubicin-induced left ventricular diastolic dysfunction. J Intern Med. 2002;251:228–34.
29. Feola M, Garrone O, Occelli M, et al. Cardiotoxicity after anthracycline chemotherapy in breast carcinoma: effects on left ventricular ejection fraction, troponin I and brain natriuretic peptide. Int J Cardiol. 2011;148:194–8.
30. Kouloubinis A, Kaklamanis L, Ziras N, et al. ProANP and NT-proBNP levels to prospectively assess cardiac function in breast cancer patients treated with cardiotoxic chemotherapy. Int J Cardiol. 2007;122:195–201.

31. Lipshultz SE, Miller TL, Scully RE, et al. Changes in cardiac biomarkers during doxorubicin treatment of pediatric patients with high-risk acute lymphoblastic leukemia: associations with long-term echocardiographic outcomes. J Clin Oncol. 2012;30:1042–9.

32. Germanakis I, Kalmanti M, Parthenakis F, et al. Correlation of plasma N-terminal pro-brain natriuretic peptide levels with left ventricle mass in children treated with anthracyclines. Int J Cardiol. 2006;108:212–5.

33. Jingu K, Nemoto K, Kaneta T, et al. Temporal change in brain natriuretic Peptide after radiotherapy for thoracic esophageal cancer. Int J Radiat Oncol Biol Phys. 2007;69:1417–23.

34. Maitland ML, Bakris GL, Black HR, et al. Initial assessment, surveillance, and management of blood pressure in patients receiving vascular endothelial growth factor signaling pathway inhibitors. J Natl Cancer Inst. 2010;102:596–604.

35. Grandin EW, Ky B, Cornell RF, Carver J, Lenihan DJ. Patterns of cardiac toxicity associated with irreversible proteasome inhibition in the treatment of multiple myeloma. J Card Fail. 2015;21:138–44.

36. Dispenzieri A, Gertz MA, Kyle RA, et al. Serum cardiac troponins and N-terminal pro-brain natriuretic peptide: a staging system for primary systemic amyloidosis. J Clin Oncol. 2004;22:3751–7.

37. Dispenzieri A, Gertz MA, Kyle RA, et al. Prognostication of survival using cardiac troponins and N-terminal pro-brain natriuretic peptide in patients with primary systemic amyloidosis undergoing peripheral blood stem cell transplantation. Blood. 2004;104:1881–7.

38. Kumar S, Dispenzieri A, Lacy MQ, et al. Revised prognostic staging system for light chain amyloidosis incorporating cardiac biomarkers and serum free light chain measurements. J Clin Oncol. 2012;30:989–95.

39. Burjonroppa SC, Tong AT, Xiao LC, Johnson MM, Yusuf SW, Lenihan DJ. Cancer patients with markedly elevated B-type natriuretic peptide may not have volume overload. Am J Clin Oncol. 2007;30:287–93.

40. O'Gara PT, Kushner FG, Ascheim DD, et al. 2013 ACCF/AHA guideline for the management of ST-elevation myocardial infarction: a report of the American College of Cardiology Foundation/American Heart Association Task Force on Practice Guidelines. Circulation. 2013;127:e362–425.

41. Cardinale D, Sandri MT, Colombo A, et al. Prognostic value of troponin I in cardiac risk stratification of cancer patients undergoing high-dose chemotherapy. Circulation. 2004;109:2749–54.

42. Cardinale D, Colombo A, Torrisi R, et al. Trastuzumab-induced cardiotoxicity: clinical and prognostic implications of troponin I evaluation. J Clin Oncol. 2010;28:3910–6.

43. Cardinale D, Sandri MT. Role of biomarkers in chemotherapy-induced cardiotoxicity. Prog Cardiovasc Dis. 2010;53:121–9.

44. Lipshultz SE, Rifai N, Sallan SE, et al. Predictive value of cardiac troponin T in pediatric patients at risk for myocardial injury. Circulation. 1997;96:2641–8.

45. Ky B, Carver JR. Biomarker approach to the detection and cardioprotective strategies during anthracycline chemotherapy. Heart Fail Clin. 2011;7:323–31.

46. Ky B, Putt M, Sawaya H, et al. Early increases in multiple biomarkers predict subsequent cardiotoxicity in patients with breast cancer treated with doxorubicin, taxanes, and trastuzumab. J Am Coll Cardiol. 2014;63:809–16.

47. Gertz MA. Immunoglobulin light chain amyloidosis: 2014 update on diagnosis, prognosis, and treatment. Am J Hematol. 2014;89:1132–40.

48. Pongprot Y, Sittiwangkul R, Charoenkwan P, Silvilairat S. Use of cardiac markers for monitoring of doxorubixin-induced cardiotoxicity in children with cancer. J Pediatr Hematol Oncol. 2012;34:589–95.

49. Erkus B, Demirtas S, Yarpuzlu AA, Can M, Genc Y, Karaca L. Early prediction of anthracycline induced cardiotoxicity. Acta Paediatr. 2007;96:506–9.

50. Lipshultz SE, Landy DC, Lopez-Mitnik G, et al. Cardiovascular status of childhood cancer survivors exposed and unexposed to cardiotoxic therapy. J Clin Oncol. 2012;30:1050–7.

51. Kozak KR, Hong TS, Sluss PM, et al. Cardiac blood biomarkers in patients receiving thoracic (chemo)radiation. Lung Cancer. 2008;62:351–5.
52. Nellessen U, Zingel M, Hecker H, Bahnsen J, Borschke D. Effects of radiation therapy on myocardial cell integrity and pump function: which role for cardiac biomarkers? Chemotherapy. 2010;56:147–52.
53. Tang WH, Tong W, Troughton RW, et al. Prognostic value and echocardiographic determinants of plasma myeloperoxidase levels in chronic heart failure. J Am Coll Cardiol. 2007;49:2364–70.
54. Baldus S, Heeschen C, Meinertz T, et al. Myeloperoxidase serum levels predict risk in patients with acute coronary syndromes. Circulation. 2003;108:1440–5.
55. Reichlin T, Socrates T, Egli P, et al. Use of myeloperoxidase for risk stratification in acute heart failure. Clin Chem. 2010;56:944–51.
56. Arruda-Olson AM, Enriquez-Sarano M, Bursi F, et al. Left ventricular function and C-reactive protein levels in acute myocardial infarction. Am J Cardiol. 2010;105:917–21.
57. Windram JD, Loh PH, Rigby AS, Hanning I, Clark AL, Cleland JG. Relationship of high-sensitivity C-reactive protein to prognosis and other prognostic markers in outpatients with heart failure. Am Heart J. 2007;153:1048–55.
58. Onitilo AA, Engel JM, Stankowski RV, Liang H, Berg RL, Doi SA. High-sensitivity C-reactive protein (hs-CRP) as a biomarker for trastuzumab-induced cardiotoxicity in HER2-positive early-stage breast cancer: a pilot study. Breast Cancer Res Treat. 2012;134:291–8.
59. Morris PG, Chen C, Steingart R, et al. Troponin I and C-reactive protein are commonly detected in patients with breast cancer treated with dose-dense chemotherapy incorporating trastuzumab and lapatinib. Clin cancer Res Off J Am Assoc Cancer Res. 2011;17:3490–9.
60. Guler E, Baspinar O, Cekmen M, Kilinc M, Balat A. Nitric oxide: a new biomarker of Doxorubicin toxicity in children? Pediatr Hematol Oncol. 2011;28:395–402.

Chapter 25
Biomarkers of Sarcopenia and Mitochondrial Dysfunction

Boris Arbit, Elizabeth Lee, and Pam R. Taub

Abstract Research over the last 20 years has led to a new understanding of the central role of mitochondrial function in the physiology of aging and the pathogenesis of cardiovascular diseases. Sarcopenia, the gradual loss of skeletal muscle mass, is the most vivid result of the progressive, global decline in mitochondrial DNA and energy production. This deterioration in cellular bioenergetics is implicated in many diseases such as heart failure and diabetes. It carries a significant economic burden, and portends decreased functional capacity and increased mortality. This chapter reviews recent research on emerging biomarkers to better diagnose mitochondrial dysfunction and sarcopenia.

Keywords Mitochondria • Sarcopenia • Biomarkers • Follistatin • Myostatin • Cardiolipin • Citrate synthase

Cellular bioenergetics, in which mitochondria play a key role, are integral to all physiological processes and result in energy production in the form of adenosine triphosphate (ATP). In nucleated cells, ATP creation is controlled by the mitochondria, which facilitates the metabolism of nutrients via oxidative respiration. At the inner mitochondrial membrane, there is a series of oxidation/reduction reactions that occur with stepwise electron transfer between five complexes and two carriers. The energy released by each of these electron transfer steps is used to pump protons from the mitochondrial matrix into the inter-membrane space, generating an electrochemical gradient across the inner mitochondrial membrane. The return of protons into the mitochondrial matrix through complex V releases the energy that drives the phosphorylation of adenosine diphosphate (ADP) to ATP. This entire process is dependent upon the integrity of the structure of the mitochondria. When the structural integrity is compromised, the mitochondrial dysfunction that follows may play a central role in the pathogenesis of cardiovascular diseases, such as ischemia

B. Arbit, MD • E. Lee, B.S. • P.R. Taub, MD, FACC (✉)
Division of Cardiovascular Medicine, Department of Medicine, University of California, San Diego, CA, USA
e-mail: ptaub@ucsd.edu

© Springer International Publishing Switzerland 2016   317
A.S. Maisel, A.S. Jaffe (eds.), *Cardiac Biomarkers*,
DOI 10.1007/978-3-319-42982-3_25

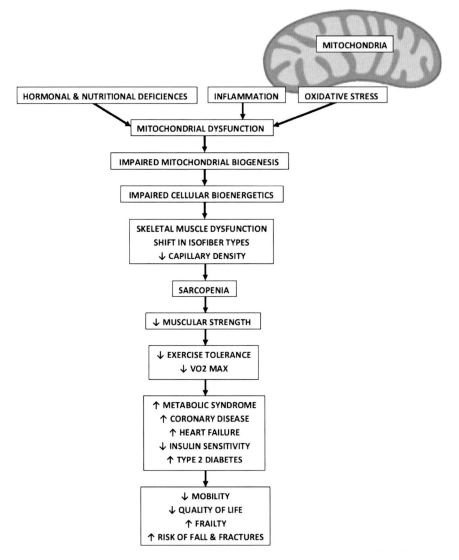

Fig. 25.1 Interaction of mitochondrial dysfunction and sarcopenia leading to decreased functional capacity

and reperfusion injury [1], atherosclerosis [2], heart failure (HF) [3], and insulin resistance (Fig. 25.1) [4].

A way to evaluate the overall performance of the mitochondria is to look at the patient's cardiorespiratory fitness. Cardiorespiratory fitness, assessed though aerobic exercise testing, is one of the most important health metrics in virtually all patient populations [5]. The level of cardiorespiratory fitness in a given individual is dependent upon the interactions between cardiovascular, pulmonary, and skeletal muscle (SkM) systems. Maximal oxygen uptake ($\dot{V}O_2$max) is a metric that best evaluates

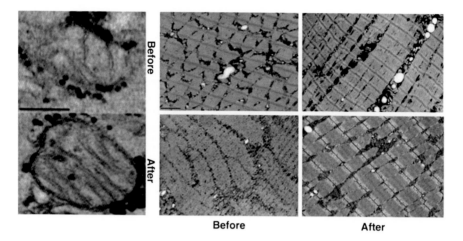

Before   **After**

Fig. 25.2 Improvement in mitochondrial cristae parallels improvement in skeletal muscle structures

aerobic endurance by measuring the maximal oxygen transport from the environment to the mitochondria. A poor $\dot{V}O_2$max is a robust, independent predictor of cardiovascular and all-cause mortality, and provides powerful risk stratification [6].

The factors that limit the $\dot{V}O_2$max are still being debated. For example, some authors have concluded that cardiac output—the capacity of the circulatory system to transport oxygen to muscle mitochondria—is a limiting factor [7]. However, there are others who argue that the skeletal muscle, which is richly endowed with mitochondria, is the limiting factor in determining $\dot{V}O_2$max. The likely answer is that both central (cardiac) and peripheral (skeletal muscle) factors contribute to exercise capacity. Studies of elderly patients have shown at the cellular, tissue, and whole-body level that SkM mitochondrial capacity and efficiency are associated with preferred walking speed, and further $\dot{V}O_2$max varied in proportion to muscle respiratory capacity [8]. Studies from our group have suggested that reversal of detrimental alterations in sarcomeric microstructure (associated with diabetes and congestive heart failure (CHF)) and restoration of cristae density may lead to improvement of $\dot{V}O_2$max (Fig. 25.2) [9, 10].

Maintaining structural and functional integrity of skeletal muscle mitochondria is important for sustained health. Disturbance in mitochondrial content and function can directly impact skeletal muscle function and consequently functional status, overall health, and quality of life.

Sarcopenia

Sarcopenia is a syndrome characterized by a progressive global loss of skeletal muscle mass and strength [11]. Baumgartner et al. proposed a method for identifying sarcopenia based on measures of lean mass obtained by dual-energy X-ray absorptiometry, defining it as skeletal muscle mass (kilograms/height(meters) [2]) less than two standard deviations below the mean of a young reference group [12]. To further refine the identification of sarcopenia, the Foundation for the National Institutes of Health Sarcopenia Project, took into account the prevalence of muscle weakness, recommending a set of sex-specific, empirically-derived cut-points for low absolute grip strength and low appendicular lean mass standardized to body mass index [13].

Sarcopenia is actually very common in the elderly population, occurring in approximately 5% of subjects at 65 years of age, and as high as 50% in subjects over 80 years old. With aging, 1–2% of muscle mass is lost per year after the age of 50. Because this is such a common ailment, sarcopenia has been a great burden on healthcare, costing between 18 and 30 billion dollars per year [14]. This burden is attributed to falls, fractures, hospitalizations, and mortality, due to the overall frailty of these patients.

Frailty, a characteristic of sarcopenia that leads to decreased health and poor quality of life, is still not well understood. There is limited knowledge about cellular pathways mediating muscle atrophy. So far, it is thought that alterations in mitochondrial function are considered a major factor underlying sarcopenia and muscle atrophy [15]. There has also been widespread speculation that the mitochondrial dysfunction arising from oxidative damage to mitochondrial DNA (mtDNA) is the central mechanism driving the aging process [16].

Several factors play a key role in mediating mitochondrial damage: the physical proximity of the electron transport chain (ETC) to the mtDNA (making it prone to oxidative damage) [17], the absence of protective histones and an efficient repair system [18], and the lack of mitochondrial introns (which makes each mutation more significant in terms of gene integrity and protein function). Aging appears to spur this process. In 146 healthy men and women aged 18–89 years, Short et al. demonstrated that mtDNA, mRNA, and mitochondrial ATP production declined with advancing age [19]. Decreased mtDNA content was correlated with decreased mitochondrial ATP production rate, which in turn, was associated with significantly lower $\dot{V}O_2$max (P <0.01). The study also showed that the amount of mitochondrial proteins (e.g., NADH dehydrogenase, pyruvate dehydrogenase alpha 1, ubiquitous mitochondrial creatine kinase, citrate synthase) was reduced in older muscles, whereas levels of DNA oxidation were increased. Bua et al. found that the number of fibers in the human vastus lateralis harboring ETC abnormalities increases from 6% at 49 years of age to 31% at 92 years of age [20].

Mitochondria in Heart Failure

Abnormalities in mitochondrial bioenergetics are a characteristic feature of several diseases of heart muscle, including systolic and diastolic HF [21]. Typically, ATP production of the normal heart exceeds any other tissue, amounting to up to 6 kg per day, a number that is many times its own weight. When ATP transfer (as phosphocreatine) and utilization becomes impaired so that insufficient high-energy phosphate bonds are transported from the mitochondria to the myofibrils, the contractile function of the muscle becomes limited [22]. Myocardial ATP levels usually remain normal until the advanced stages of HF, when they decrease by 30–40 %. In HF, myocardial phosphocreatine to ATP ratio is reduced, and has been shown to correlate with the New York Heart Association (NYHA) classes [23].

During diastole, ATP hydrolysis is required for myosin to detach from actin, calcium to dissociate from Troponin-C, and calcium to be sequestered by the sarcoplasmic reticulum. The ratio of the products of ATP hydrolysis (ADP and inorganic phosphate) to ATP must remain high in order to maintain a normal diastolic function. It is estimated that relaxation of the myocardium requires up to 15 % of the total energy cost of the cardiac cycle.

In HF, having insufficient ATP levels results in both diminished heart and skeletal muscle performance, leading to fatigue. In the skeletal muscle, there are alterations that contribute to the pathophysiology of HF such as atrophy, shift in isofiber types, decreased capillary density, oxidative capacity, and strength. At the subcellular level, there is a loss in mitochondrial volume and cristae surface density (site of ATP production). Additionally, studies have shown that patients with HF have a decreased ratio of mitochondria to myofibrils, with impaired function of the mitochondria [24]. Fortunately, the mitochondrial aberrancies of end-stage HF can be reversed. In a study of 20 patients from the Columbia Presbyterian Medical Center, Lee at al. showed an improvement of cardiomyocyte mitochondrial function in patients after long-term therapy with left ventricular assist devices [25]. The underlying pathophysiological mechanism of HF was shown to be caused by free fatty acid accumulation and calcium overload, both of which affect membrane potential. One of the central findings of this study was that mechanical unloading has a beneficial effect on cardiac metabolism in the failing myocardium.

On a systemic scale, an imbalance between catabolic and anabolic signals in CHF leads to tissue wasting and ultimately cachexia. It is defined as weight loss of $\geq 5\%$ in ≤ 12 months in the presence of an underlying illness, when accompanied by 3 out of 5 the symptomatic and biochemical criteria [26]. Cachexia is a serious complication of CHF that worsens clinical symptoms and is a strong independent risk factor for mortality. Patients with HF and cachexia had a mortality rate of 50 % at 18 months of follow-up, compared with 17 % in non-cachectic CHF patients [27].

Biomarkers of Sarcopenia

Precise assessment of skeletal muscle mass and its alterations is difficult. Currently, assessment of sarcopenia is limited to the quantification of muscle mass by magnetic resonance imaging, computed tomography, or dual energy x-ray absorptiometry scan and functional tests to quantify muscle function. It would be more cost-effective to identify reliable biomarkers that can be measured in blood to guide diagnosis and therapy in routine clinical practice and in clinical trials. There are few biomarkers for both sarcopenia and mitochondrial function that are being investigated.

Myostatin, also termed as growth/differentiation factor-8 (GDF-8) is a member of the TGF-β superfamily that is predominantly expressed in SkM. The most potent negative regulator of SkM growth, myostatins need to be inhibited for muscle growth and development to occur. This is demonstrated when systemic administration of myostatin led to skeletal muscle wasting in mice [28]. Furthermore, studies in chronic HF have shown that patients in advanced stages of HF express significantly higher concentrations of myostatin in Skm (which may explain cachexia seen in HF) [29, 30]. However, 12 patients with late stage CHF (NYHA IIIb) were able to reverse these changes through 12 weeks of exercise training, supporting the concept of exercise as an important treatment tool in chronic HF [29, 31].

On the other hand, follistatin is a secreted glycoprotein that has been recognized as a high affinity binding and neutralizing protein for several members of the TGF-β superfamily including myostatin. Follistatin antagonizes myostatin activity by binding to it and interfering with the binding of myostatin to its receptor. This interaction is seen in resistance training, where myostatin levels decrease and those of follistatin increase, leading to an increase in muscle mass. For example, administration of follistatin to Mstn−/− mice caused muscle mass to increase more than when myostatin was depleted [32, 33]. In animal trials, intramuscular and systemic administration of gene therapy vectors expressing follistatin led to increased muscle fiber hypertrophy and strength [34, 35]. Also, Brandt et al. examined 76 patients with type 2 diabetes and 92 control subjects, and showed that skeletal muscle myostatin mRNA is elevated in patients with type 2 diabetes [36]. It was associated with impaired insulin sensitivity, increased triglycerides, low-grade chronic inflammation, obesity, and a poor fitness level [36]. Follistatin also regulates other targets besides myostatin.

Many studies show that aging muscle can respond favorably following endurance training by increasing the levels of key regulators such as peroxisome proliferator-activated receptor gamma coactivator 1-alpha (PGC-1α), a master regulator of mitochondrial biogenesis. It appears that in senescent SkM, the upregulation of PGC-1α is impaired in response to endurance training and thus, may partly explain the loss of function. Interestingly, PGC-1α also seems to be involved in protecting SkM from denervation or starvation induced atrophy as seen in experiments involving PGC-1α-overexpressing transgenic mice. Thus, it serves as a vital link between mitochondrial and skeletal muscle function.

An older, well-established biomarker, serum creatinine, has been suggested to serve as a reliable muscle mass biomarker, if appropriate adjustment for kidney function and dietary meat intake is undertaken [37].

Biomarkers of Mitochondrial Function

A biomarker of mitochondrial function, citrate synthase (CS) is one of the key regulatory enzymes in the energy-generating metabolic pathway that catalyzes the condensation of oxaloacetate and acetyl coenzyme A to form citrate in the tricarboxylic acid cycle. It has been extensively used as a metabolic marker in assessing oxidative and respiratory capacity. Leek et al. showed that CS activities increased (in vastus lateralis) in response to acute exercise in six sedentary males. Another group further refined this finding by showing different responses of skeletal and cardiac muscles in CS enzymatic activity but similar responses in CS gene expression at 1 and 48 h after the last session of endurance training in 16 rats [38].

Another biomarker, cardiolipin (CL), is a major membrane phospholipid in the mitochondria and is essential for cellular energy metabolism mediated through mitochondrial oxidative phosphorylation. It has been suggested that CL plays a role in the generation of an electrochemical potential for substrate transport and ATP synthesis. CL that has undergone oxidation (oxCL) promotes delocalization and release of cytochrome c, causing its release from the mitochondria and the activation of cell death programs. Antibodies against CL cause both venous and arterial thrombosis, and are known to be of major importance in systemic lupus erythematosus, cardiovascular disease and venous thrombosis [39]. This mechanism involving cardiolipin highlights how cellular processes in mitochondria ultimately are involved in the pathogenesis of disease. Prevention of the aging-related changes in mitochondrial membrane composition, through a possible attenuation of cardiolipin oxidation was studied in yeast by Goldberg et al. [40]. The group concluded that longevity in chronologically aging yeast is programmed by the level of metabolic capacity and organelle organization they developed, in a diet-specific fashion. In 27 diabetic subjects (ages 37–70), compared to 32 non-diabetic, age-matched controls, greater mitochondrial membrane polarization and lower mitochondrial mass/cardiolipin content was measured [41].

Recently, platelet mitochondrial DNA (mtDNA) function has come to the forefront as a potential new marker of cardiovascular disease. Platelets play an important role in cardiovascular disease, in the pathogenesis of atherosclerosis and in the development of acute thrombotic events. Large amounts of ATP are required to power platelet activation, adhesion, and aggregation. Since platelets do not have a nucleus, their only DNA is mitochondrial. Thus, the understanding of mitochondrial gene expression may be critical to understanding role of platelets in cardiovascular disease. A novel experiment by Baccarelli and Byun showed significantly higher platelet mtDNA methylation in ten patients with hypertension and/or atherosclerosis aged 44–83 years old compared to 17 healthy individuals aged 22–71 years old [42]. There are also other mechanisms in mitochondrial platelet function. An increase in mitochondrial calcium levels mediates mitochondrial redox imbalance, membrane protein thiol cross-linking, and the activation of mitochondrial permeability transition pore opening. Following strong activation, increased cytosolic and mitochondrial calcium levels result in a mitochondrial membrane potential collapse. A pilot study of mitochondrial respiratory function and proteomic changes comparing platelets extracted from insulin sensitive ($n=8$) and type 2 diabetic subjects ($n=7$) showed that this collapse leads to increased mitochondrial ROS levels and platelet apoptosis [43].

Therapies Targeting Mitochondria

Over the past few years, there has been a growing body of research that looked at specific therapies aimed at improving mitochondrial function. A promising agent is a flavanol, (-)-epicatechin, which is found in cocoa. Studies with dark chocolate have shown improved insulin sensitivity and reductions in the incidence cardiovascular diseases including HF. Nogueira et al. have demonstrated that a flavanol present in cacao, (-)-epicatechin, stimulates mitochondrial biogenesis (increased volume, cristae density and protein content for oxidative phosphorylation complexes and organelle membrane) in skeletal and cardiac muscle of mice leading to improved exercise performance [44]. Subsequent research has shown that Epi-rich cocoa treatment improves SkM mitochondrial structure and in an orchestrated manner increases molecular markers of mitochondrial biogenesis resulting in enhanced cristae density [44]. For the first time, initial safety, tolerability, and pharmacokinetics of pure (-)-epicatechin in healthy human subjects have been reported. Biomarkers including platelet mitochondria complexes I, IV and citrate synthase activities demonstrated a significant increases of approximately 92, 62 and 8 %, with treatment. Average day 5 follistatin area under the curve (AUC) levels were around 2.5 fold higher vs. average day 1 AUC levels [45]. This study illustrated how biomarkers of mitochondrial function and sarcopenia (follistatin) can be used to assess the beneficial effects of (-)-epicatechin (Fig. 25.2).

Common antibiotics are establishing a new niche as modulators of mitochondrial function. Members of the tetracyclines family of antibiotics can exert cardioprotective effects by blocking mitochondrial permeability transition pore opening. Minocycline and doxycycline have been shown to inhibit mitochondrial Ca^{2+} uptake via the inhibition of the mitochondrial calcium uniporter [46]. In a rat model, following 45 min of occlusion of the left anterior descending coronary artery, synergistic inhibition of mitochondrial swelling by the combination of (-)-epicatechin and doxycycline were observed. Co-treatment with (-)-epicatechin and doxycycline led to a reduction inpalcium-induced swelling of isolated myocardial mitochondria, and a reduced infarct area of nearly 50 %, 48 h after ischemia reperfusion injury. This effect was sustained for 3 weeks [47]. Cyclosporine also inhibits the opening of mitochondrial permeability transition pores. It has also been shown to attenuate myocardial reperfusion injury in 58 patients who presented with acute ST-elevation myocardial infarction [1].

A deficit of certain hormones has been linked to myocardial dysfunction. Testosterone deficiency is a risk factor for cardiovascular diseases and coronary artery disease. Recent studies suggest a beneficial effect of physiological testosterone replacement therapy on lipid profiles and ischemic insults of the heart. A study showed that cardiac mitochondria taken from the ischemic myocardium in orchiectomized rats consequently had increased mitochondrial ROS production [48]. Testosterone replacement in this model mitigated cardiac mitochondrial dysfunction in the ischemic myocardium (improved left ventricular pressure, decreased infarct size, and reduced fatal cardiac arrhythmias) [48].

Thyroid hormone (TH) is another hormone whose deficiency has been shown to result in mitochondrial dysfunction. Supplementation of TH may offer a novel option for cardiac diseases [49]. 3,5,3'-triiodothyronine (T3), the biologically active form of thyroid hormone, significantly declines after myocardial infarction. TH has a mitochondria-targeted antioxidant protective effect following myocardial infarction [50]. In cultured cardiomyocytes, T3 treatment after MI decreased oxidative stress-induced apoptosis and increased the expression of factors involved in mitochondrial DNA transcription and biogenesis, such as hypoxic inducible factor-1α, mitochondrial transcription factor A and peroxisome proliferator activated receptor γ coactivator-1α, in the LV peri-infarct zone. Early restoration of TH halved the infarct scar size and prevented progression towards HF [51]. Low TH is common in patients with cardiac diseases, with an incidence of up to 30% in HF patients. In a recent placebo-controlled, double-blind study of 50 patients with clinically stable NYHA functional class I–III systolic HF and hypothyroidism, patients assigned to replacement therapy had increased 6-min walk distance, decreased serum N-terminal pro-brain natriuretic peptide level, and a significant increase in the left ventricular ejection fraction.

The skeletal muscle comprises up to 60% of the total body weight. Over the last 10–15 years we have gained new insight into how cellular bioenergetics and mitochondrial dysfunction come to play a central role in the pathogenesis of sarcopenia and cardiovascular diseases. Biomarkers that assess mitochondrial integrity and function are still in the early stages of development. Parallel to this, therapeutic options which are specifically targeted at the mitochondria are emerging.

References

1. Piot C, Croisille P, Staat P, et al. Effect of cyclosporine on reperfusion injury in acute myocardial infarction. N Engl J Med. 2008;359:473–81.
2. Madamanchi NR, Runge MS. Mitochondrial dysfunction in atherosclerosis. Circ Res. 2007;100:460–73.
3. Sebastiani M, Giordano C, Nediani C, et al. Induction of mitochondrial biogenesis is a maladaptive mechanism in mitochondrial cardiomyopathies. J Am Coll Cardiol. 2007;50:1362–9.
4. Kim JA, Wei Y, Sowers JR. Role of mitochondrial dysfunction in insulin resistance. Circ Res. 2008;102:401–14.
5. Arena R, Myers J, Guazzi M. The future of aerobic exercise testing in clinical practice: is it the ultimate vital sign? Future Cardiol. 2010;6:325–42.
6. Kavanagh T, Mertens DJ, Hamm LF, et al. Prediction of long-term prognosis in 12 169 men referred for cardiac rehabilitation. Circulation. 2002;106:666–71.
7. Boushel R, Saltin B. Ex vivo measures of muscle mitochondrial capacity reveal quantitative limits of oxygen delivery by the circulation during exercise. Int J Biochem Cell Biol. 2013;45:68–75.
8. Coen PM, Jubrias SA, Distefano G, et al. Skeletal muscle mitochondrial energetics are associated with maximal aerobic capacity and walking speed in older adults. J Gerontol A Biol Sci Med Sci. 2013;68:447–55.
9. Taub PR, Ramirez-Sanchez I, Ciaraldi TP, et al. Alterations in skeletal muscle indicators of mitochondrial structure and biogenesis in patients with type 2 diabetes and heart failure: effects of epicatechin rich cocoa. Clin Transl Sci. 2012;5:43–7.

10. Taub PR, Ramirez-Sanchez I, Ciaraldi TP, et al. Perturbations in skeletal muscle sarcomere structure in patients with heart failure and type 2 diabetes: restorative effects of (-)-epicatechin-rich cocoa. Clin Sci. 2013;125:383–9.

11. Cruz-Jentoft AJ, Baeyens JP, Bauer JM, et al. Sarcopenia: European consensus on definition and diagnosis: Report of the European Working Group on Sarcopenia in Older People. Age Ageing. 2010;39:412–23.

12. Baumgartner RN, Koehler KM, Gallagher D, et al. Epidemiology of sarcopenia among the elderly in New Mexico. Am J Epidemiol. 1998;147:755–63.

13. McLean RR, Kiel DP. Developing consensus criteria for sarcopenia: an update. J Bone Miner Res Off J Am Soc Bone Miner Res. 2015;30:588–92.

14. Janssen I, Shepard DS, Katzmarzyk PT, Roubenoff R. The healthcare costs of sarcopenia in the United States. J Am Geriatr Soc. 2004;52:80–5.

15. Calvani R, Joseph AM, Adhihetty PJ, et al. Mitochondrial pathways in sarcopenia of aging and disuse muscle atrophy. Biol Chem. 2013;394:393–414.

16. Miquel J, Economos AC, Fleming J, Johnson Jr JE. Mitochondrial role in cell aging. Exp Gerontol. 1980;15:575–91.

17. Herrero A, Barja G. 8-oxo-deoxyguanosine levels in heart and brain mitochondrial and nuclear DNA of two mammals and three birds in relation to their different rates of aging. Aging. 1999;11:294–300.

18. Furda AM, Bess AS, Meyer JN, Van Houten B. Analysis of DNA damage and repair in nuclear and mitochondrial DNA of animal cells using quantitative PCR. Methods Mol Biol. 2012;920:111–32.

19. Short KR, Bigelow ML, Kahl J, et al. Decline in skeletal muscle mitochondrial function with aging in humans. Proc Natl Acad Sci U S A. 2005;102:5618–23.

20. Bua E, Johnson J, Herbst A, et al. Mitochondrial DNA-deletion mutations accumulate intracellularly to detrimental levels in aged human skeletal muscle fibers. Am J Hum Genet. 2006;79:469–80.

21. Doehner W, Frenneaux M, Anker SD. Metabolic impairment in heart failure: the myocardial and systemic perspective. J Am Coll Cardiol. 2014;64:1388–400.

22. Neubauer S. The failing heart–an engine out of fuel. N Engl J Med. 2007;356:1140–51.

23. Neubauer S, Krahe T, Schindler R, et al. 31P magnetic resonance spectroscopy in dilated cardiomyopathy and coronary artery disease. Altered cardiac high-energy phosphate metabolism in heart failure. Circulation. 1992;86:1810–8.

24. Ingwall JS, Atkinson DE, Clarke K, Fetters JK. Energetic correlates of cardiac failure: changes in the creatine kinase system in the failing myocardium. Eur Heart J. 1990;11(Suppl B): 108–15.

25. Lee SH, Doliba N, Osbakken M, Oz M, Mancini D. Improvement of myocardial mitochondrial function after hemodynamic support with left ventricular assist devices in patients with heart failure. J Thorac Cardiovasc Surg. 1998;116:344–9.

26. Evans WJ, Morley JE, Argiles J, et al. Cachexia: a new definition. Clin Nutr. 2008;27:793–9.

27. Anker SD, Ponikowski P, Varney S, et al. Wasting as independent risk factor for mortality in chronic heart failure. Lancet. 1997;349:1050–3.

28. Zimmers TA, Davies MV, Koniaris LG, et al. Induction of cachexia in mice by systemically administered myostatin. Science. 2002;296:1486–8.

29. Lenk K, Erbs S, Hollriegel R, et al. Exercise training leads to a reduction of elevated myostatin levels in patients with chronic heart failure. Eur J Prev Cardiol. 2012;19:404–11.

30. Baan JA, Varga ZV, Leszek P, et al. Myostatin and IGF-I signaling in end-stage human heart failure: a qRT-PCR study. J Transl Med. 2015;13:1.

31. Souza RW, Piedade WP, Soares LC, et al. Aerobic exercise training prevents heart failure-induced skeletal muscle atrophy by anti-catabolic, but not anabolic actions. PLoS One. 2014;9, e110020.

32. Lee SJ. Quadrupling muscle mass in mice by targeting TGF-beta signaling pathways. PLoS One. 2007;2, e789.

33. Gilson H, Schakman O, Kalista S, Lause P, Tsuchida K, Thissen JP. Follistatin induces muscle hypertrophy through satellite cell proliferation and inhibition of both myostatin and activin. Am J Physiol Endocrinol Metab. 2009;297:E157–64.

34. Foley JW, Bercury SD, Finn P, Cheng SH, Scheule RK, Ziegler RJ. Evaluation of systemic follistatin as an adjuvant to stimulate muscle repair and improve motor function in Pompe mice. Mol Ther J Am Soc Gene Ther. 2010;18:1584–91.

35. Haidet AM, Rizo L, Handy C, et al. Long-term enhancement of skeletal muscle mass and strength by single gene administration of myostatin inhibitors. Proc Natl Acad Sci U S A. 2008;105:4318–22.

36. Brandt C, Nielsen AR, Fischer CP, Hansen J, Pedersen BK, Plomgaard P. Plasma and muscle myostatin in relation to type 2 diabetes. PLoS One. 2012;7, e37236.

37. Patel SS, Molnar MZ, Tayek JA, et al. Serum creatinine as a marker of muscle mass in chronic kidney disease: results of a cross-sectional study and review of literature. J Cachex Sarcopenia Muscle. 2013;4:19–29.

38. Siu PM, Donley DA, Bryner RW, Alway SE. Citrate synthase expression and enzyme activity after endurance training in cardiac and skeletal muscles. J Appl Physiol. 2003;94:555–60.

39. Wan M, Hua X, Su J, et al. Oxidized but not native cardiolipin has pro-inflammatory effects, which are inhibited by Annexin A5. Atherosclerosis. 2014;235:592–8.

40. Goldberg AA, Bourque SD, Kyryakov P, et al. Effect of calorie restriction on the metabolic history of chronologically aging yeast. Exp Gerontol. 2009;44:555–71.

41. Widlansky ME, Wang J, Shenouda SM, et al. Altered mitochondrial membrane potential, mass, and morphology in the mononuclear cells of humans with type 2 diabetes. Transl Res J Lab Clin Med. 2010;156:15–25.

42. Baccarelli AA, Byun HM. Platelet mitochondrial DNA methylation: a potential new marker of cardiovascular disease. Clin Epigenetics. 2015;7:44.

43. Avila C, Huang RJ, Stevens MV, et al. Platelet mitochondrial dysfunction is evident in type 2 diabetes in association with modifications of mitochondrial anti-oxidant stress proteins. Exp Clin Endocrinol Diabetes Off J German Soc Endocrinol German Diabetes Assoc. 2012;120: 248–51.

44. Nogueira L, Ramirez-Sanchez I, Perkins GA, et al. (-)-Epicatechin enhances fatigue resistance and oxidative capacity in mouse muscle. J Physiol. 2011;589:4615–31.

45. Barnett CF, Moreno-Ulloa A, Shiva S, et al. Pharmacokinetic, partial pharmacodynamic and initial safety analysis of (-)-epicatechin in healthy volunteers. Food Funct. 2015;6:824–33.

46. Schwartz J, Holmuhamedov E, Zhang X, Lovelace GL, Smith CD, Lemasters JJ. Minocycline and doxycycline, but not other tetracycline-derived compounds, protect liver cells from chemical hypoxia and ischemia/reperfusion injury by inhibition of the mitochondrial calcium uniporter. Toxicol Appl Pharmacol. 2013;273:172–9.

47. Ortiz-Vilchis P, Yamazaki KG, Rubio-Gayosso I, et al. Co-administration of the flavanol (-)-epicatechin with doxycycline synergistically reduces infarct size in a model of ischemia reperfusion injury by inhibition of mitochondrial swelling. Eur J Pharmacol. 2014;744:76–82.

48. Pongkan W, Chattipakorn SC, Chattipakorn N. Chronic testosterone replacement exerts cardioprotection against cardiac ischemia-reperfusion injury by attenuating mitochondrial dysfunction in testosterone-deprived rats. PLoS One. 2015;10, e0122503.

49. Forini F, Nicolini G, Iervasi G. Mitochondria as key targets of cardioprotection in cardiac ischemic disease: role of thyroid hormone triiodothyronine. Int J Mol Sci. 2015;16:6312–36.

50. de Castro AL, Tavares AV, Campos C, et al. Cardioprotective effects of thyroid hormones in a rat model of myocardial infarction are associated with oxidative stress reduction. Mol Cell Endocrinol. 2014;391:22–9.

51. Forini F, Lionetti V, Ardehali H, et al. Early long-term L-T3 replacement rescues mitochondria and prevents ischemic cardiac remodelling in rats. J Cell Mol Med. 2011;15:514–24.

Chapter 26
Biomarkers in Arrhythmias, Sudden Death, and Device Therapy

David E. Krummen and Lori B. Daniels

Abstract Biomarkers are emerging clinical tools which may provide rapid and objective quantification of distinct pathophysiologic mechanisms which contribute to atrial and ventricular arrhythmias, and may identify patients at risk for adverse response to implantable device therapy. The purpose of this chapter is to discuss our present understanding of cardiac biomarkers in these settings, with an emphasis on emerging data on diverse pathogenic processes associated with arrhythmias. Based upon the rapid growth in the number and understanding of biomarkers, there is tremendous potential to assist in the risk stratification and care of patients with cardiac arrhythmias. While presently limited in practice, the incorporation of biomarkers into routine clinical use may be dependent upon future trials of biomarker panels, or biomarkers in combination with functional or imaging studies, to achieve an acceptable clinical accuracy.

Keywords Biomarkers • Atrial fibrillation • Sudden cardiac death • Cardiac resynchronization therapy • B-type natriuretic peptide • C-reactive protein • Fibrosis • Stroke

Prediction is very difficult, especially about the future. –Neils Bohr

In clinical medicine, prediction of patients at greater risk for atrial and ventricular arrhythmias, and for adverse response to cardiac device therapy is difficult. In this role, laboratory biomarkers have tremendous potential to more objectively identify such patients who may benefit from more intensive follow-up or therapy. The purpose

D.E. Krummen, MD (✉)
Division of Cardiovascular Medicine, University of California San Diego,
San Diego, CA, USA

Division of Cardiovascular Medicine, VA San Diego Healthcare System,
San Diego, CA, USA
e-mail: dkrummen@ucsd.edu

L.B. Daniels, MD, MAS
Division of Cardiovascular Medicine, University of California San Diego,
San Diego, CA, USA

© Springer International Publishing Switzerland 2016   329
A.S. Maisel, A.S. Jaffe (eds.), *Cardiac Biomarkers*,
DOI 10.1007/978-3-319-42982-3_26

of this chapter is to discuss the potential role of biomarkers in the clinical care of patients with atrial and ventricular arrhythmias and those undergoing device implantation. Case vignettes from the authors' clinics are included to illustrate such concepts in practice. Due to the broad scope of this chapter, we will focus on major trials in biomarkers and cardiac arrhythmias, with additional emphasis on emerging biomarkers which address novel pathophysiologic processes. While much of the work in this field is not yet incorporated into routine clinical practice, this chapter is intended to provide an outlook intro the areas we believe are most promising for either future clinical use or informing us about underlying pathophysiologic mechanisms.

Biomarkers and Atrial Fibrillation

Atrial fibrillation is an arrhythmia characterized by rapid and apparently chaotic activation of the atria with irregular and often rapid activation of the ventricles. It is the most common arrhythmia presenting for clinical care [1]. Atrial fibrillation is associated with a spectrum of symptoms including palpitations, tachycardia, fatigue, chest pain, and shortness of breath. In addition, it is associated with significant morbidity due to stroke and heart failure, and with increased mortality [2]. Unfortunately, many patients present with stroke or heart failure as the first symptom of the arrhythmia. It would be clinically useful to identify patients at significant risk of atrial fibrillation and to allow earlier diagnosis (and thus earlier treatment) via more intense monitoring. Those at risk could also be targeted for aggressive preventive measures.

Atrial Fibrillation Pathogenesis

Recent research has shed important insight into the pathogenesis of atrial fibrillation. Blood-based biomarkers are suitable for evaluating a subset of these. Biomarkers presently allow evaluation of ventricular [3] and atrial stretch [4], atrial fibrosis [5], and other categories noted in Table 26.1. However, they have a limited role in evaluating other central mechanisms of atrial fibrillation such as pulmonary vein ectopy or atrial electrical remodeling, which are better evaluated during electrophysiology study [6]. Similarly, delayed enhancement magnetic resonance imaging (MRI) is better suited than biomarkers to evaluate atrial structural remodeling and to directly localize and quantify atrial fibrosis [7]. Evaluation of alterations in ion channel gene expression is presently limited to the research laboratory.

Categories of Biomarkers in AF

As shown in Table 26.1, biomarkers related to atrial fibrillation can be broadly categorized by mechanism: injury/inflammation, oxidative stress, mechanical stretch, myocardial remodeling/fibrosis, thrombosis, and renal insufficiency.

Table 26.1 Partial list of biomarkers in atrial fibrillation

Categories	Biomarkers
Injury/inflammation	CRP, IL-6, IL-1β, IL-8, TNF-α, TGF-β, IFN-γ, sCD40L, hsTn, GDF-15, SAA
Oxidative stress	ROS, NADPH oxidase activity, F2-isoprostanes, DROM
Renin-angiotensin-aldosterone system and other neurohormones	Angiotensin II receptors, ACE levels, Copeptin, MRpro-ADM
Mechanical stress	BNP, NT-proBNP, MR-proANP
Myocardial remodeling	PICP, PIIICP, MMPs, Homocysteine, GAL-3, sST2
Thrombosis	sP-sel, fibrinogen, vWf, platelet factor 4, thromboglobulin
Renal insufficiency	Cystatin C, albumin, creatinine
Other	MAP kinases, bradykinin

ACE angiotensin converting enzyme, *BNP* B-type natriuretic peptide, *CRP* C-reactive protein, *GDF* growth differentiation factor, *hsTn* highly sensitive cardiac troponin, *IL* interleukin, *MMP* matrix metalloprotein, *MR-proADM* midregional pro-adrenomedullin, *MR-proANP* midregional pro-atrial natriuretic peptide, *NT-proBNP* N-terminal pro-BNP, *vWF* von Willebrand Factor

Highlighted Studies of Biomarkers in Atrial Fibrillation

An important study correlating atrial fibrillation incidence with biomarker levels in a community cohort was reported by Schnabel and colleagues [8]. The authors studied 3120 participants from the Framingham Offspring Study and evaluated the association between ten biomarkers and incident atrial fibrillation over a median 9.7 years of follow-up. Of the markers studied, B-type natriuretic peptide (BNP) and C-reactive protein (CRP) were found to be the strongest predictors of incident atrial fibrillation. A biomarker score was derived by incorporating BNP and CRP concentrations into a risk score comprised of clinical variables. Higher tertiles of the biomarker score were highly predictive of atrial fibrillation incidence in both men and women. Additionally, BNP, but not CRP, improved atrial fibrillation risk prediction beyond that provided by well-established clinical risk factors.

A current, clinical need in cardiac electrophysiology regards the identification of patients at high risk for atrial fibrillation recurrence after ablation. Hussein and colleagues addressed this issue in a recent study, and found that elevated BNP levels are associated with post-procedural atrial fibrillation recurrence [9]. In this study, they followed 726 patients undergoing first-time ablation for lone atrial fibrillation. At baseline, BNP concentrations were associated with the burden of atrial fibrillation. In addition, patients in the highest quintile of BNP (>126 pg/ml) had nearly a six-fold increased risk of atrial fibrillation recurrence over 26 months of follow-up compared to those in the lowest quintile, after adjusting for multiple covariates.

Recent Work in Atrial Fibrillation and Atrial Fibrosis Biomarkers

Biomarkers of atrial fibrosis have also been shown to identify individuals at higher risk for atrial fibrillation. In their study of 3306 participants from the Framingham Offspring Cohort, Ho and colleagues recently reported that higher circulating concentrations of galectin-3 were associated with an increased risk of developing atrial fibrillation over a median follow-up of 10 years [10]. Future work is required to determine whether galectin-3 itself plays a role in atrial fibrillation substrate progression.

The composition of the extracellular matrix is regulated by matrix metalloproteinases (MMPs) and their tissue inhibitors (TIMP). Elevated serum MMP and low TIMP levels have been shown to predict incident atrial fibrillation [11] and atrial fibrillation recurrence after ablation [12]. Going forward, it may be possible to predict atrial fibrosis with one or more biomarkers, which could someday either supplant or complement the information gleaned from delayed enhancement MRI [7]. Notably, biomarkers have important advantages over MRI such as lower cost, availability at centers without MRI capability, and objectivity. Disadvantages include the lack of spatial information regarding fibrosis distribution which may be useful in ablation planning.

Stroke Risk in Atrial Fibrillation

In addition to the risk of arrhythmias themselves, biomarkers can help identify individuals at increased risk for stroke. Hijazi and colleagues analyzed data from the ARISTOTLE trial of apixaban in atrial fibrillation stroke prevention [13]. They found that N-terminal pro-BNP (NT-proBNP) levels are often elevated in atrial fibrillation, and are independently associated with an increased risk of stroke and mortality. Future studies are required to evaluate the exciting possibility that biomarkers may identify a subgroup of patients who may substantially benefit from anticoagulation despite a low clinical risk score for stroke.

Clinical Vignette: Patient with AF Seeking Ablation

Presentation

A 75 year-old woman with hypertension and chronic obstructive pulmonary disease (COPD) presents to clinic with atrial fibrillation, which has been present for 3 months. She has noted increased shortness of breath and heart palpitations. Her presenting electrocardiogram (ECG) is shown in Fig. 26.1. Her initial echocardiogram shows a left ventricular ejection fraction (EF) of 42 %. She and her family inquire about atrial fibrillation ablation versus medical management.

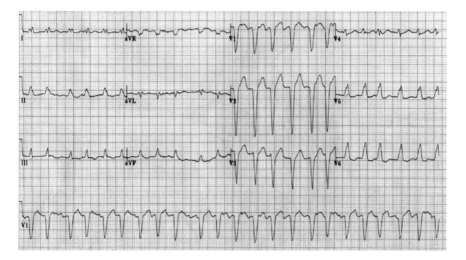

Fig. 26.1 Presenting electrocardiogram showing atrial fibrillation with rapid ventricular response (rate 135 beats per minute)

Clinical Approach

The patient is initiated on rate control medications and warfarin anticoagulation. After 3 months, her heart rate is 82 beats per minute, and she is now relatively asymptomatic, with mild dyspnea on moderate exertion. Physical examination shows euvolemia. Repeat echocardiography reveals that her EF has improved to 52%, with mild diastolic dysfunction, and her left atrial diameter is 46 mm. Her BNP concentration is 132 pg/ml.

Clinical Decision-making

The decision of whether to proceed with atrial fibrillation ablation is complex, incorporating a number of patient-specific factors including symptoms and the estimated probability of ablation success. Prior studies have shown that increased left atrial volume [14], atrial fibrillation cycle length ≤142 msec [15], BNP >126 pg/ml [9], and a high burden of atrial fibrosis [7] predict poor ablation outcome. The patient has mild dyspnea on exertion, but it is unclear whether this is due to COPD or the arrhythmia. Her left atrial 2-dimensional size by echocardiogram is enlarged, but volume quantification by CT more accurately predicts atrial fibrillation recurrence following ablation than does echocardiographic measurement [16]. Because of her elevated BNP and mild symptoms, we felt comfortable proceeding with a rate control strategy, rather than an ablation. She is now asymptomatic from atrial fibrillation with good exercise tolerance after 2 years of follow-up. Importantly, while recent studies have shown BNP to predict stroke risk [13, 17], it has not been incorporated into guidelines for anticoagulation in atrial fibrillation. She was started on warfarin due to a CHA2DS2-VASc score of 4 (age (2 points), hypertension (1 point), and female gender (1 point)).

Discussion

In this case, biomarkers helped inform the decision to pursue rate control versus rhythm control in a patient with marginal symptoms. While this decision was not entirely based upon biomarker levels, the elevated BNP provided an objective determination that she would have a lower probability of ablation success, and helped her to decide to pursue rate control.

Atrial Fibrillation Biomarkers Summary

In summary, multiple studies have shown an association between various biomarkers and risk of atrial fibrillation incidence, recurrence following ablation, and stroke. Despite this, biomarkers are not presently widely used for this purpose outside of the research setting. This is due in large part to the suboptimal performance of markers when used on an individual patient level. Additionally, studies have shown that factors such as body mass [18] and the presence of atrial fibrillation [19] impact the diagnostic cutpoints and performance of biomarkers. Alternative modalities are also available to evaluate atrial fibrillation risk, including CT and late-enhancement MRI (showing the burden of atrial fibrosis), and ECG data such as P wave duration. In the future, combining multiple biomarkers that reflect distinct pathologic processes, or combining biomarkers with imaging or functional data from ECG, may provide the increased predictive accuracy necessary to bring biomarkers to clinical practice.

Biomarkers in Ventricular Arrhythmias and Sudden Cardiac Death

There are over 700,000 sudden cardiac deaths per year in the United States and Europe, predominantly due to ventricular tachycardia and ventricular fibrillation [20]. Unfortunately, the majority of events occur in low-risk populations not predicted by a left ventricular EF less than 35 % [21], the central criterion used to determine eligibility for a primary-prevention implantable cardioverter defibrillator (ICD).

Table 26.2 Partial list of biomarkers with an association with risk of ventricular arrhythmias

Categories	Biomarkers
Inflammation	CRP, IL-6, IL-8, sCD40L
Myocardial stress	BNP, NT-proBNP
Myocyte damage	TnI, TnT
Remodeling	PICP, PIIICP, MMP, TIMP
Metabolic	Trans-18:1 oleic acid, trans-18:2 oleic acid, MMP
Renal	Cystatin-C
MicroRNAs	miRNA-1, miRNA-133
Fibrosis	Osteopontin, Galectin-3, ST2

Pathogenesis of Ventricular Arrhythmias and Biomarkers

Table 26.2 lists multiple biomarkers of various pathological processes involved in the pathogenesis of ventricular arrhythmias. As in atrial fibrillation, biomarkers address a subset of known contributing factors, such as inflammation, myocardial stress, remodeling, and fibrosis; other diagnostic modalities are currently required to assess alternative pathologic processes. These processes (and the diagnostic tests used to assess for them) include: abnormal calcium handling (T-wave alternans [22]), conduction abnormalities (signal-averaged ECG [23]), ventricular ectopy (Holter monitoring [24]), scar distribution (delayed enhancement MRI [25]), genetic abnormalities (ECG, genetic testing), pro-arrhythmic substrate alterations (electro-physiology study [26]) and ischemia (echocardiographic or nuclear stress testing). Thus, laboratory biomarkers can presently provide only a limited assessment of sudden cardiac death risk.

Highlighted Studies of Biomarkers in Ventricular Arrhythmias

Berger and colleagues were among the first to show that elevated BNP concentrations predict risk of sudden cardiac death (SCD) among patients with chronic heart failure [27]. In this study of 452 patients with a left ventricular EF of 35 % or less, those with a BNP of 130 pg/mL or higher had only an 81 % rate of sudden-death free survival at 3 years, compared to a rate of 99 % among those with BNP below that cutpoint. Subsequently, a prospective study by Tapanainen et al. of 521 patients with acute myocardial infarction found that after a mean follow-up of 43 months, only BNP and low EF were significant predictors of sudden cardiac death, with elevated BNP ≥23 pg/ml being the most powerful predictor (hazard ration 4.4) [28].

More recently, Francia et al. assessed whether plasma osteopontin and galectin-3 predicted the risk of sustained ventricular tachycardia/ventricular fibrillation in a small cohort of 75 heart failure patients with ICDs [29]. They found that osteopontin >74 ng/ml and galectin-3 > 17 ng/ml were associated with lower arrhythmia-free survival in this high-risk cohort even after adjusting for clinical factors including EF. Larger studies are required to determine whether these biomarkers improve the prediction of sudden cardiac death when used in conjunction with conventional risk factors.

Combinations of Biomarkers and SCD

In an interesting substudy of the MUSIC trial of ambulatory heart failure patients, Pascual-Figal and colleagues evaluated 36 cases of SCD and 63 control patients matched for age, sex, and left ventricular EF [30]. They found that soluble ST-2 and NT-proBNP both predicted patients at risk for sudden death. Notably these two biomarkers provided independent and complementary information, and patients with elevated levels of both biomarkers were at substantial risk (~70%) of SCD.

SCD in the General Population

Empana and colleagues evaluated 9771 asymptomatic European men from the PRIME study, a multicenter prospective cohort designed to identify risk factors for coronary heart disease, and measured high sensitivity CRP, fibrinogen, and IL-6 concentrations [31]. Of these, IL-6 > 0.48 pg/ml was an independent predictor of sudden death, with a hazard ratio of 3.06 compared with subjects with the lowest tertile of IL-6 ($\leq$0.06 pg/ml). Neither of the other two markers were significant predictors of SCD. Future work is required to determine if IL-6 is involved in mechanisms which contribute to arrhythmia risk, and if this can be translated into a clinically actionable tool.

Biomarkers of Renal Insufficiency

Recently, renal biomarkers have also been evaluated for their ability to improve sudden cardiac death risk prediction. Cystatin C, a marker of kidney dysfunction, was found by Deo and colleagues to be independently associated with sudden cardiac death risk [32] in an analysis of 4465 elderly participants from the Cardiovascular Health Study without prevalent cardiovascular disease at baseline. Notably cystatin C, but not estimates of renal function based upon creatinine levels, remained independently predictive of sudden death after adjusting for traditional risk factors. The authors suggest that the association between cystatin C and SCD is mediated by kidney dysfunction, which may alter the electrophysiological properties of the myocardium and increase the risk for SCD even in individuals with only mild renal impairment and with no clinical evidence of cardiovascular disease.

Summary of Biomarkers and Ventricular Arrhythmias/SCD

In summary, several biomarkers have shown an association with increased risk of ventricular arrhythmias and SCD. As with atrial fibrillation, they are not widely used clinically at this time, however studies of combinations of biomarkers have been promising. Alternatively, biomarkers in combination with other modalities such as T wave alternans, electrophysiology study, signal-averaged ECG (similar to preliminary work by Yamada and colleagues [33]), or scar imaging via CT or MRI may provide the required positive predictive value and negative predictive values that can ultimately lead to widespread clinical acceptance.

Biomarkers to Predict Adverse Response to Device Therapy

Implantable devices such as pacemakers are commonly used in the treatment of symptomatic bradycardia. Beyond simple pacemakers, patients with congestive heart failure, low EF, and conduction system disease, particularly left bundle branch block, may require cardiac resynchronization therapy (CRT), which involves pacing both the left and right ventricles to improve ventricular efficiency [34]. It would be clinically useful to predict patients at risk for poor response to device therapy, to allow closer monitoring, more aggressive medical therapy, and earlier referral for advanced heart failure interventions such as left ventricular assist device or transplantation.

Pathogenesis of Heart Failure Associated with Device Therapy

As shown in Table 26.3, biomarkers are suited to evaluate a number of pathophysiologic processes associated with device therapy-induced development of heart failure. Other factors include electrical dyssynchrony (assessed by ECG [35]), mechanical strain (assessed by speckle tracking on echocardiography [36]), scar distribution (assessed by sestamibi perfusion imaging and other modalities [37]), and lead positioning (assessed by chest radiography [38]).

Table 26.3 Partial list of biomarkers in device therapy and CRT

Categories	Biomarkers
Inflammation	CRP, IL-6
Myocardial stress	BNP, NT-pro BNP, ANP
Myocyte damage	TnI, TnT
Remodeling	PICP, PIIICP, MMP-9, TIMP-1
Fibrosis	Galectin-3
Renal	Cystatin-C
Other	GDF-15, Annexin A5, OPN

Adverse Response to Pacemaker Therapy

A certain proportion of patients undergoing pacemaker implantation will experience adverse left ventricular remodeling and heart failure, likely due at least in part to dyssynchrony induced by extensive pacing of the right ventricle. Chwyczko and colleagues randomized 31 patients with pacemakers implanted to treat sinus node dysfunction to either standard therapy, or to an algorithm designed to reduce the amount of right ventricular pacing [39]. Comparing exercise tolerance, left ventricular EF, and BNP concentrations between the two study arms, they found that plasma BNP concentrations rose were higher in the group with more right ventricular pacing, and were correlated with worsening exercise tolerance and heart failure symptoms. Future studies are required to determine if routine BNP testing improves upon physical examination, symptoms, and routine management in the identification of patients with pacemaker-mediated cardiomyopathy.

Non-responders to CRT

Despite significant advances in our understanding of optimal implantation techniques, approximately 30% of patients will have a suboptimal response to CRT [40, 41]. Because of the significant risks and costs associated with this therapy, it would be advantageous to identify patients at risk for nonresponse to better inform patient selection. Furthermore, identification of patients with suboptimal response early after implant may prompt consideration of more advanced heart failure therapies such as left ventricular assist device or cardiac transplantation.

Highlighted Studies in Biomarkers and CRT

Pitzalis and colleagues studied the prognostic value of BNP in the management of patients receiving CRT [42]. They found that patients with elevated BNP levels 1 month following CRT implantation had significantly worse prognosis. Specifically, a BNP level >91.5 pg/ml had 89% sensitivity and 59% specificity for HF progression after 12 months. The authors concluded that such patients should be considered for more intensive medical management and referral for advanced heart failure therapies.

More recently, Marfella and colleagues evaluated mRNA expression and response to CRT [43]. In 81 heart failure patients who were eligible for CRT, they screened 84 microRNA (miRNA) candidates and found that increased expression of five mRNAs ($p < 0.01$ for all) predicted favorable response to CRT. The authors concluded that miRNA profiling can provide objective evaluation of disease severity and therapeutic response to CRT in patients with heart failure. Furthermore, they proposed that screening for genetic polymorphisms in miRNA–mRNA regulatory pathways may enable physicians to tailor personalized therapies for such patients in the future.

Clinical Vignette: Patient with Heart Failure and Left Bundle Branch Block

Presentation

A 46 year-old man with nonischemic cardiomyopathy, EF 25%, NYHA class III heart failure symptoms, and left bundle branch block presented to clinic for management. He had been treated with optimal medical therapy including maximum doses of beta blocker and ACE inhibiter for more than 9 months, and underwent successful CRT implantation with favorable left ventricular lead positioning in the mid-lateral left ventricle (Fig. 26.2, red arrow). Three months later, he presents with fatigue, dry cough, and progressive dyspnea on exertion. He gives a history of sick contacts, and believes he has caught the same cold that his wife had last week. Physical examination is difficult due to the patient's obese body habitus, and jugular venous pressure cannot be accurately determined. Lung and heart sounds are distant. He is tachycardic with a regular rhythm but frequent premature beats, and no audible S3. The extremities are slightly cool to palpation with trace pedal edema. Laboratory evaluation is notable for an elevated white blood cell count without a left shift, and a BNP of 528 pg/ml. Chest X-ray shows likely interstitial edema versus atypical pneumonia.

Clinical Approach

Although the history could suggest either a respiratory or a cardiovascular etiology for the patient's current decompensation, physical examination, chest X-ray, and the BNP level are most consistent with fluid overload. Device interrogation shows normal CRT function, but a relatively low percentage of biventricular pacing (85%, compared with a goal of 98% or greater [44]), due to frequent ectopy. The patient is admitted for CHF management.

Clinical Decision Making

Over the next few months, a number of interventions are attempted to improve the patient's heart failure and response to CRT. First, ablation of the premature ventricular complex source is successfully performed, which increases the percent of biventricular pacing to 96%. The patient experiences a slight improvement in symptoms, but subsequently has a repeat heart failure exacerbation. He is then sent for a

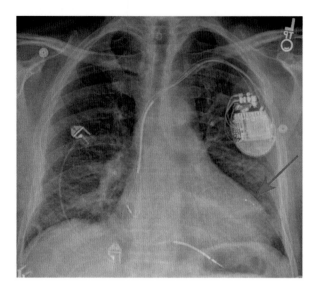

Fig. 26.2 Chest X-ray showing CRT device with favorable LV lead positioning (*red arrow*)

cardiac resynchronization echocardiogram, in which CRT pacing timings are adjusted to potentially optimize individual response to CRT [45]. No significant benefit is noted, and shortly thereafter the patient again presents with fluid overload, elevated BNP (1102 pg/dl), and decreased LV function (EF 18 %), and requires intravenous inotropic support. He is ultimately referred for left-ventricular assist device implantation, and is presently listed for transplantation.

Discussion

With respect to biomarkers, the initial elevated BNP was helpful in distinguishing a heart failure exacerbation from an upper respiratory infection, though it could be argued that physical examination and chest X-ray may have been sufficient. In reality, and especially in obese patients such as this one, physical signs can be challenging. The elevated BNP also identified this patient as likely to be a poor responder to CRT therapy, prompting consideration of further interventions such as more aggressive medical therapy, ventricular ectopy ablation, resynchronization echocardiography, and eventually referral for a left ventricular assist device. In this case, although the biomarkers may have contributed to diagnosis and risk assessment, a number of other clinically relevant factors were also taken into consideration when generating the patient's action plan. As such, this case illustrates a central barrier to routine recommendation of biomarker use in assessment of response to device therapy – lack of data showing additional benefit above and beyond standard practice.

Summary of Biomarkers and Device Therapy

In summary, biomarkers have been shown to help predict which patients are at increased risk of nonresponse to both standard pacemakers and CRT. Interesting new work shows that evaluation of miRNAs which regulate the expression of genes governing adaptive and maladaptive cardiac remodeling may provide clinical insight into the outcomes of such patients, and may eventually lead to personalized therapy. However, routine clinical use of biomarkers, including miRNAs, to drive decisions about device therapy remains elusive; future work is required to illustrate the optimal strategy to incorporate such tests into practice.

Conclusions

As noted in the opening quotation by Neils Bohr, predicting future events is difficult. Recent advances in our understanding and use of cardiac biomarkers may facilitate this process, and allow more accurate prediction of patients at risk for atrial and ventricular arrhythmias, and identification of individuals at risk for adverse response to device therapy. Additional trials are required to show the clinical utility of routine use of biomarkers in such clinical settings.

References

1. Chugh SS, Blackshear JL, Shen WK, Hammill SC, Gersh BJ. Epidemiology and natural history of atrial fibrillation: clinical implications. J Am Coll Cardiol. 2001;37:371–8.
2. Stewart S, Hart CL, Hole DJ, McMurray JJ. A population-based study of the long-term risks associated with atrial fibrillation: 20-year follow-up of the Renfrew/Paisley study. Am J Med. 2002;113:359–64.
3. Beck-da-Silva L, de Bold A, Fraser M, Williams K, Haddad H. Brain natriuretic peptide predicts successful cardioversion in patients with atrial fibrillation and maintenance of sinus rhythm. Can J Cardiol. 2004;20:1245–8.
4. Wozakowska-Kaplon B, Opolski G, Kosior D, Janion M. An increase in plasma atrial natriuretic peptide concentration during exercise predicts a successful cardioversion and maintenance of sinus rhythm in patients with chronic atrial fibrillation. Pacing Clin Electrophysiol. 2000;23:1876–9.
5. Rosenberg MA, Maziarz M, Tan AY, et al. Circulating fibrosis biomarkers and risk of atrial fibrillation: The Cardiovascular Health Study (CHS). Am Heart J. 2014;167:723–8. e2.
6. Krummen DE, Bayer JD, Ho J, et al. Mechanisms of human atrial fibrillation initiation: clinical and computational studies of repolarization restitution and activation latency. Circ Arrhythm Electrophysiol. 2012;5:1149–59.
7. Marrouche NF, Wilber D, Hindricks G, et al. Association of atrial tissue fibrosis identified by delayed enhancement MRI and atrial fibrillation catheter ablation: the DECAAF study. JAMA. 2014;311:498–506.

8. Schnabel RB, Larson MG, Yamamoto JF, et al. Relations of biomarkers of distinct pathophysiological pathways and atrial fibrillation incidence in the community. Circulation. 2010;121:200–7.

9. Hussein AA, Saliba WI, Martin DO, et al. Plasma B-type natriuretic peptide levels and recurrent arrhythmia after successful ablation of lone atrial fibrillation. Circulation. 2011; 123:2077–82.

10. Ho JE, Yin X, Levy D, et al. Galectin 3 and incident atrial fibrillation in the community. Am Heart J. 2014;167:729–34. e1.

11. Kalogeropoulos AS, Tsiodras S, Rigopoulos AG, et al. Novel association patterns of cardiac remodeling markers in patients with essential hypertension and atrial fibrillation. BMC Cardiovasc Disord. 2011;11:77.

12. Okumura Y, Watanabe I, Nakai T, et al. Impact of biomarkers of inflammation and extracellular matrix turnover on the outcome of atrial fibrillation ablation: importance of matrix metalloproteinase-2 as a predictor of atrial fibrillation recurrence. J Cardiovasc Electrophysiol. 2011;22:987–93.

13. Hijazi Z, Wallentin L, Siegbahn A, et al. N-terminal pro-B-type natriuretic peptide for risk assessment in patients with atrial fibrillation: insights from the ARISTOTLE Trial (Apixaban for the Prevention of Stroke in Subjects With Atrial Fibrillation). J Am Coll Cardiol. 2013;61:2274–84.

14. Costa FM, Ferreira AM, Oliveira S, et al. Left atrial volume is more important than the type of atrial fibrillation in predicting the long-term success of catheter ablation. Int J Cardiol. 2015;184C:56–61.

15. Matsuo S, Lellouche N, Wright M, et al. Clinical predictors of termination and clinical outcome of catheter ablation for persistent atrial fibrillation. J Am Coll Cardiol. 2009;54:788–95.

16. Parikh SS, Jons C, McNitt S, Daubert JP, Schwarz KQ, Hall B. Predictive capability of left atrial size measured by CT, TEE, and TTE for recurrence of atrial fibrillation following radiofrequency catheter ablation. Pacing Clin Electrophysiol PACE. 2010;33:532–40.

17. Hijazi Z, Oldgren J, Andersson U, et al. Cardiac biomarkers are associated with an increased risk of stroke and death in patients with atrial fibrillation: a Randomized Evaluation of Long-term Anticoagulation Therapy (RE-LY) substudy. Circulation. 2012;125:1605–16.

18. Daniels LB, Clopton P, Bhalla V, et al. How obesity affects the cut-points for B-type natriuretic peptide in the diagnosis of acute heart failure. Results from the Breathing Not Properly Multinational Study. Am Heart J. 2006;151:999–1005.

19. Richards M, Di Somma S, Mueller C, et al. Atrial fibrillation impairs the diagnostic performance of cardiac natriuretic peptides in dyspneic patients: results from the BACH Study (Biomarkers in ACute Heart Failure). JACC Heart failure. 2013;1:192–9.

20. Atwood C, Eisenberg MS, Herlitz J, Rea TD. Incidence of EMS-treated out-of-hospital cardiac arrest in Europe. Resuscitation. 2005;67:75–80.

21. Stecker EC, Vickers C, Waltz J, et al. Population-based analysis of sudden cardiac death with and without left ventricular systolic dysfunction: two-year findings from the Oregon Sudden Unexpected Death Study. J Am Coll Cardiol. 2006;47:1161–6.

22. Rosenbaum DS, Jackson LE, Smith JM, Garan H, Ruskin JN, Cohen RJ. Electrical alternans and vulnerability to ventricular arrhythmias. N Engl J Med. 1994;330:235–41.

23. Gomes JA, Mehra R, Barreca P, el-Sherif N, Hariman R, Holtzman R. Quantitative analysis of the high-frequency components of the signal-averaged QRS complex in patients with acute myocardial infarction: a prospective study. Circulation. 1985;72:105–11.

24. Yarlagadda RK, Iwai S, Stein KM, et al. Reversal of cardiomyopathy in patients with repetitive monomorphic ventricular ectopy originating from the right ventricular outflow tract. Circulation. 2005;112:1092–7.

25. Nazarian S, Bluemke DA, Lardo AC, et al. Magnetic resonance assessment of the substrate for inducible ventricular tachycardia in nonischemic cardiomyopathy. Circulation. 2005; 112:2821–5.

26. Krummen DE, Hayase J, Vampola SP, et al. Suppressing ventricular fibrillation by targeted rotor ablation: proof-of-concept from the canine laboratory to the first human case. J Cardiovasc Electrophysiol. 2015;26:1117–26.

27. Berger R, Huelsman M, Strecker K, et al. B-type natriuretic peptide predicts sudden death in patients with chronic heart failure. Circulation. 2002;105:2392–7.
28. Tapanainen JM, Lindgren KS, Makikallio TH, Vuolteenaho O, Leppaluoto J, Huikuri HV. Natriuretic peptides as predictors of non-sudden and sudden cardiac death after acute myocardial infarction in the beta-blocking era. J Am Coll Cardiol. 2004;43:757–63.
29. Francia P, Adduci C, Semprini L, et al. Osteopontin and galectin-3 predict the risk of ventricular tachycardia and fibrillation in heart failure patients with implantable defibrillators. J Cardiovasc Electrophysiol. 2014;25(6):609–16.
30. Pascual-Figal DA, Ordonez-Llanos J, Tornel PL, et al. Soluble ST2 for predicting sudden cardiac death in patients with chronic heart failure and left ventricular systolic dysfunction. J Am Coll Cardiol. 2009;54:2174–9.
31. Empana JP, Jouven X, Canoui-Poitrine F, et al. C-reactive protein, interleukin 6, fibrinogen and risk of sudden death in European middle-aged men: the PRIME study. Arterioscler Thromb Vasc Biol. 2010;30:2047–52.
32. Deo R, Sotoodehnia N, Katz R, et al. Cystatin C and sudden cardiac death risk in the elderly. Circ Cardiovasc Qual Outcomes. 2010;3:159–64.
33. Yamada T, Fukunami M, Shimonagata T, et al. Prediction of paroxysmal atrial fibrillation in patients with congestive heart failure: a prospective study. J Am Coll Cardiol. 2000;35:405–13.
34. Tracy CM, Epstein AE, Darbar D, et al. 2012 ACCF/AHA/HRS focused update of the 2008 guidelines for device-based therapy of cardiac rhythm abnormalities: a report of the American College of Cardiology Foundation/American Heart Association Task Force on Practice Guidelines. J Am Coll Cardiol. 2012;60:1297–313.
35. Moss AJ, Hall WJ, Cannom DS, et al. Cardiac-resynchronization therapy for the prevention of heart-failure events. N Engl J Med. 2009;361:1329–38.
36. Suffoletto MS, Dohi K, Cannesson M, Saba S, Gorcsan 3rd J. Novel speckle-tracking radial strain from routine black-and-white echocardiographic images to quantify dyssynchrony and predict response to cardiac resynchronization therapy. Circulation. 2006;113:960–8.
37. Xu YZ, Cha YM, Feng D, et al. Impact of myocardial scarring on outcomes of cardiac resynchronization therapy: extent or location? J Nucl Med Off Publication Soc Nucl Med. 2012;53:47–54.
38. Thebault C, Donal E, Meunier C, et al. Sites of left and right ventricular lead implantation and response to cardiac resynchronization therapy observations from the REVERSE trial. Eur Heart J. 2012;33:2662–71.
39. Chwyczko T, Dabrowski R, Maciag A, et al. Potential prevention of pacing-induced heart failure using simple pacemaker programming algorithm. Ann Noninvasive Electrocardiol Off J Int Soc Holter Noninvasive Electrocardiol, Inc. 2013;18:369–78.
40. Bristow MR, Saxon LA, Boehmer J, et al. Cardiac-resynchronization therapy with or without an implantable defibrillator in advanced chronic heart failure. N Engl J Med. 2004;350:2140–50.
41. Cleland JG, Daubert JC, Erdmann E, et al. The effect of cardiac resynchronization on morbidity and mortality in heart failure. N Engl J Med. 2005;352:1539–49.
42. Pitzalis MV, Iacoviello M, Di Serio F, et al. Prognostic value of brain natriuretic peptide in the management of patients receiving cardiac resynchronization therapy. Eur J Heart Fail. 2006;8:509–14.
43. Marfella R, Di Filippo C, Potenza N, et al. Circulating microRNA changes in heart failure patients treated with cardiac resynchronization therapy: responders vs non-responders. Eur J Heart Fail. 2013;15:1277–88.
44. Hayes DL, Boehmer JP, Day JD, et al. Cardiac resynchronization therapy and the relationship of percent biventricular pacing to symptoms and survival. Heart Rhythm Off J Heart Rhythm Soc. 2011;8:1469–75.
45. Thomas DE, Yousef ZR, Fraser AG. A critical comparison of echocardiographic measurements used for optimizing cardiac resynchronization therapy: stroke distance is best. Eur J Heart Fail. 2009;11:779–88.

Chapter 27
Biomarkers in Cardio-Renal Dysfunction

Nicholas Phreaner, Alex Pearce, and Alan S. Maisel

Abstract In cardiorenal syndrome (CRS), cardiac and renal dysfunction coexist, creating a complex clinical picture. This commonly encountered scenario is associated with increased morbidity and mortality. Cardiorenal biomarkers are emerging as a tool to help define CRS pathophysiology and direct patient care. Emerging novel biomarkers such as neutrophil gelatinase-associated lipocalin (NGAL), cystatin C (CysC), kidney injury molecule-1 (KIM-1), and proenkephalin (pro-ENK) can help identify renal impairment earlier, further delineate etiology and potentially guide treatment in the future. In this chapter, we will discuss cardio-renal syndrome, definitions of renal injury, the limitations of creatinine as a biomarker, and new biomarkers for cardio-renal dysfunction.

Keywords Cardio-renal syndrome • Acute kidney injury • Creatinine • Neutrophil gelatinase-associated lipocalin (NGAL) • Cystatin C (CysC) • Proenkephalin (pro-ENK) • Kidney injury molecule-1 (KIM-1) • Heart Failure • Cardiorenal biomarkers

Case Report

A 63-year-old man presents to the emergency department with acute dyspnea. He has a history of hypertension, hyperlipidemia and heart failure with preserved ejection fraction. He has mild chronic kidney disease (CKD) stage II and his baseline creatinine is 1.2 mg/dL. The patient has normal temperature and blood pressure. His heart rate is 94 beats per minute, respiratory rate is 18 breaths per minute and he is sating 89 % on room air. His exam is significant for warm extremities, elevated

N. Phreaner, MD (✉) • A. Pearce, MD
Department of Medicine, Division of Cardiovascular Medicine,
University of California, San Diego, San Diego, CA, USA
e-mail: nphreaner@ucsd.edu

A.S. Maisel, MD, FACC
Department of Medicine, Division of Cardiovascular Medicine, University of California San Diego, San Diego, CA, USA

Department of Medicine, Coronary Care Unit and Heart Failure Program, Veterans Affairs San Diego Healthcare System, San Diego, CA, USA

© Springer International Publishing Switzerland 2016   345
A.S. Maisel, A.S. Jaffe (eds.), *Cardiac Biomarkers*,
DOI 10.1007/978-3-319-42982-3_27

Table 27.1 Case report selected history, medication list and laboratory results

Past medical history			Hypertension		
			Hyperlipidemia		
			Heart failure with preserved ejection fraction		
Prior to admission medications			Atorvastatin 20 mg daily		
			Lisinopril 10 mg daily		
Discharge medications			Atorvastatin 20 mg daily		
			Furosemide 20 mg oral twice daily		
Clinic medications			Atorvastatin 20 mg daily		
			Furosemide 40 mg twice daily		
			Lisinopril 5 mg daily		
Test (Reference range)	Baseline	Admission	24 h	Discharge	Clinic
Creatinine (0.7–1.4 mg/dL)	1.2	1.8	1.9	1.5	1.3
BNP (<100 pg/mL)	212	837	–	358	415

jugular venous distention and bilateral crackles at the bases of his lungs. His initial laboratory results show a creatinine of 1.8 mg/dL and B-type natriuretic peptide (BNP) of 837 ng/mL (Table 27.1). The patient is admitted to the hospital for acute decompensated heart failure (ADHF) and acute kidney injury (AKI).

On hospital day one, the patient is treated with intravenous diuretics and his outpatient angiotensin converting enzyme (ACE) inhibitor is held. The patient has 3.5 l of urine output over 24 h and has symptomatic improvement in dyspnea and decreased supplemental oxygen requirements. An echocardiogram shows an ejection fraction of 48 % (previously 62 %). A low dose beta-blocker is initiated and the patient tolerates this medication well.

On hospital day two, the patient's creatinine is noted to be elevated above his admission value and his diuretic dose is reduced by half. Over the course of hospitalization, the patient is slowly decongested with intravenous diuretics and is transitioned to oral loop diuretics prior to discharge. Due to improvement in respiratory status and return to the patient's dry weight, the patient is discharged on hospital day 5 with new prescriptions for a diuretic and beta-blocker. He is told to follow up with his cardiologist in clinic. Because of the AKI during the admission, his ACE inhibitor is held upon discharge.

In clinic 3 weeks after discharge, the patient's weight has increased by 3 lb and though the patient does not describe dyspnea, he reports decreased exercise tolerance. Labs are repeated and are notable for a BNP of 415 ng/mL and a creatinine of 1.3 mg/dL. His diuretic dose is increased and a low dose ACE inhibitor is initiated.

Introduction

Renal and cardiac functions are intricately connected. Physiologically, the heart and kidney work together to ensure adequate systemic perfusion. The heart is sensitive to hemodynamic changes and the kidney plays a central role in maintaining intravascular volume.

The relationship between heart failure and renal dysfunction is complex and is encompassed under the definition of cardiorenal syndrome (CRS). CRS is commonly encountered in clinical practice and is correlated with significantly increased morbidity and mortality. Studies show a significant increase in ≥1 year mortality in patients with heart failure (HF) and moderate to severe renal impairment [1]. Additionally, in patients admitted for ADHF, decreased renal function present at admission and progressive decline in renal function during hospitalization are both associated with prolonged length of stay and poor outcomes [2, 3].

The association between cardio-renal dysfunction and increased mortality makes early identification important in clinical management. Cardiorenal biomarkers are emerging as a tool to help define CRS pathophysiology and direct patient care. BNP and N-terminal pro-B-type natriuretic peptide (NT-proBNP) are well established as useful tools for the diagnosis and treatment of heart failure. Likewise, creatinine is routinely used as a marker of renal function in most settings. These traditional biomarkers, however, cannot identify the underlying cause of cardiorenal syndrome. Novel biomarkers, such as cystatin C (CysC), kidney injury molecule-1 (KIM-1), proenkephalin (pro-ENK), and neutrophil gelatinase-associated lipocalin (NGAL) are emerging as useful tools in earlier detection of renal impairment and delineating the underlying cardiorenal pathophysiology. In this chapter, we will discuss cardiorenal syndrome, definitions of renal injury, the limitations of creatinine as a biomarker, and new biomarkers for cardio-renal dysfunction.

Cardio-Renal Syndrome

The heart and the kidney are closely linked through a myriad of complex interactions. Damage of one organ, heart or kidney, can subsequently lead to dysfunction in the other. There is a cyclical relationship between cardiac and renal function. In the acute setting, poor cardiac function and reduced stroke volume leads to decreased renal perfusion. Decreased renal perfusion results in the activation of compensatory neurohormonal systems. The sympathetic nervous system and the renin-angiotensin-aldosterone system (RAAS) trigger renal arteriolar vasoconstriction and promote increased sodium retention. These mechanisms function to maintain plasma volume and preserve organ perfusion. However, increased fluid volume creates additional cardiac stress. Additionally, increased venous backflow can also lead to renal congestion and changes in renal structure and function.

Cardiorenal syndrome is subdivided into five categories (Fig. 27.1) [4]. Four categories are based on chronicity, acute versus chronic, and the organ affected first,

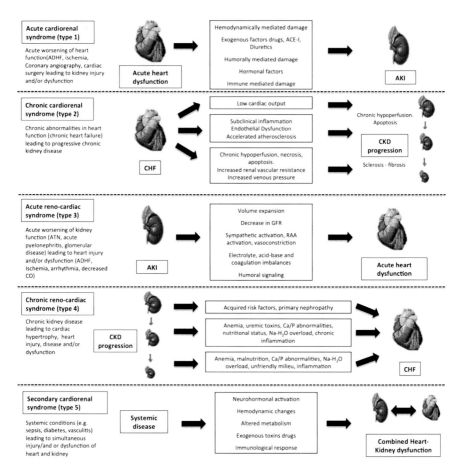

Fig. 27.1 Types and pathophysiology of cardiorenal syndrome. *AKI* Acute kidney injury, *Ca/P* Calcium/phosphorous, *CHF* Congestive heart failure, *ADHF* Acute decompensated heart failure, *CKD* Chronic kidney disease, *GFR* Glomerular filtration rate, *HF* heart failure, *RAA* Renin-angiotensin-aldosterone, *CO* Cardiac output (Adapted from Ronco et al. [27], with permission)

heart or kidney. A fifth category of cardiorenal syndrome encompasses simultaneous cardiac and renal dysfunction as a product of a systemic insult.

In CRS type 1 (Acute cardiorenal syndrome) and CRS type 2 (Chronic cardiorenal syndrome) there is primary cardiac dysfunction. In CRS type 1 acute decompensated heart failure leads to AKI. Both decreased renal perfusion as a result of decreased cardiac output and renal congestion due to increased central venous pressure lead to renal injury. CRS type 1 is extremely common. In patients with HF, AKI complicates approximately 1 in 4 hospital admissions [5].

Type 2 CRS (Chronic cardiorenal syndrome) occurs when chronic cardiac dysfunction leads to progressive kidney disease. Progressive chronic kidney disease resulting from chronic cardiac dysfunction can, in part, be attributed to long-term diminished renal perfusion, subclinical inflammation, and subsequent vascular damage. Similar to CRS type 1, renal congestion also appears to contribute to renal damage in type 2 CRS.

In CRS type 3 (Acute reno-cardiac syndrome), an abrupt decline in renal function leads to acute cardiac decompensation. Acute tubular necrosis (ATN), acute pyelonephritis, and urinary obstruction are all examples of processes that can lead to an abrupt decrease in renal function. RAAS activation to compensate for ongoing renal dysfunction enhances vasoconstriction and promotes fluid retention, increasing blood pressure and cardiac work, predisposing the heart to acute decompensation. The development of AKI in a patient with a history of heart failure also affects management. For example, when a chronic HF patient develops AKI physicians will often abruptly stop HF medications such as diuretics and ACE inhibitors to prevent additional renal injury but at the same time create a predisposition for acute cardiac decompensation.

In CRS type 4 (Chronic reno-cardiac syndrome), chronic kidney disease leads to cardiac dysfunction. There is a strong correlation between end-stage renal disease and cardiovascular disease. Chronic inflammatory changes secondary to volume overload, uremia, acidemia as well as accelerated atherosclerosis are all implicated as possible mechanisms adversely affecting the heart.

Physician perceptions of patients with both advanced renal disease and chronic cardiovascular disease are also important. Studies suggest that patients with end-stage CKD were less likely to receive medications such as aspirin, beta-blockers, or ACE inhibiters after myocardial infarction, despite evidence that mortality was similar between CKD patients and non-CKD patients receiving similar treatment regimens [6]. Although many of these medications need to be appropriately titrated for renal disease, they can still be safely administered.

Lastly, CRS type 5 (Secondary cardiorenal syndrome) encompasses concomitant renal and cardiac dysfunction as a result of a systemic disorder. Systemic diseases may include diabetes, sepsis, and vasculitis.

Creatinine and AKI

Acute Kidney Injury

Type 1 CRS, primary cardiac dysfunction leading to AKI, is the most commonly encountered type of cardiorenal syndrome. Understanding the definition of AKI is important in evaluating biomarkers for cardiorenal syndrome. There are several different classifications of AKI. The two most commonly utilized criteria are RIFLE (risk of renal dysfunction; injury to the kidney; failure of kidney function, loss of kidney function and End-stage kidney disease) and AKIN (Acute Kidney Injury Network).

In order of increasing severity, the RIFLE Criteria divide patients into five cohorts (risk, injury, failure, loss, and ESRD) [7]. Risk is defined as an increase in serum creatinine ≥1.5× baseline or a decrease in GFR ≥25 %. Injury is indicated by an increase in serum creatinine ≥2.0× baseline or decrease in GFR ≥50 %. A rise in serum creatinine ≥3.0× baseline, a decrease in GFR ≥75 %, or a serum creatinine ≥4 mg/dl with an acute rise from baseline of ≥0.5 mg/dl is classified as failure. Loss of kidney function is defined as acute renal failure (ARF) for >4 weeks. Finally, ESRD is a complete loss of kidney function >3 months.

The AKIN Criteria is similar to RIFLE with a few adjustments. The AKIN Criteria divides declining kidney function into three stages. AKIN Stage 1 defines AKI as an increase in serum creatinine ≥1.5× baseline as well as an increase ≥0.3 mg/dL from baseline within the first 48 h. Similar to the RIFLE definition of injury, AKIN Stage 2 is defined by an increase in serum creatinine ≥2× baseline. AKIN stage 3 correlates with RIFLE failure but also includes patients that require initiation of renal replacement therapy (RRT) [8]. Urine output parameters are addressed as separate criteria in both classification systems. A decrease in urine output <0.5 m/kg/h for more than 6 h defines AKI. However, urinary tract obstruction must also be excluded.

Limitations of Creatinine

There are several limitations to the classification schemes for AKI. AKI criteria are best applied to a patient with optimal volume status, which presents a challenge in the HF patient population. Additionally, both criteria heavily rely on serum creatinine, a marker that comes with its own set of limitations.

Creatinine is affected by age, gender, muscle mass, and hydration status. Creatinine only begins to rise when greater than 50 % of GFR is lost and once a steady state is reached [9]. Thus, creatinine cannot detect ongoing, dynamic changes in kidney function. Creatinine can also overestimate and underestimate GFR, depending on the clinical scenario. Creatinine is freely filtered by the glomerulus, but is also secreted at variable rates. In early kidney injury, especially during the first several days, creatinine secretion is increased, thus creatinine overestimates GFR [10]. In addition, as creatinine reaches substantially high levels, it less accurately correlates with GFR. Although creatinine is well known, extensively researched, and easily accessible, there are limitations in its role as a biomarker for renal function. These limitations have sparked interest in novel biomarkers in cardiorenal dysfunction.

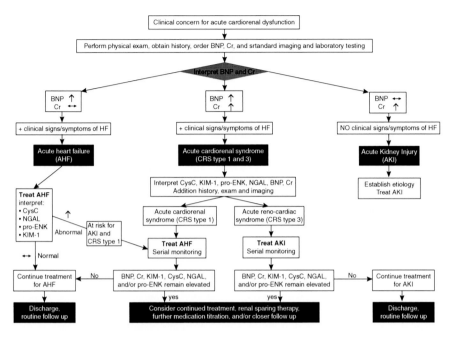

Fig. 27.2 Proposed algorithm for acute cardiorenal dysfunction. *BNP* B-type natriuretic peptide, *Cr* Creatinine, *AHF* Acute Heart Failure, *CRS* Cardio-renal syndrome, *AKI* Acute kidney injury, *CysC* Cystatin C, *NGAL* Neutrophil gelatinase-associated lipocalin, *pro-ENK* Proenkephalin, *KIM-1* Kidney injury molecule-1

Novel Biomarkers in Cardio-Renal Syndrome

The rapid diagnosis and treatment of CRS is important for improving outcomes, however, there are limitations to diagnosing CRS with history and physical exam alone. An ideal biomarker for AKI in the setting of acute or chronic heart failure would be sensitive and specific in its role of identifying the location of renal injury, establishing chronicity, etiology, prognosis and response to treatment. At this time, no single ideal biomarker exists, rather, a panel of biomarkers may soon be used to piece together a better understanding of a patient's cardio-renal status (Fig. 27.2).

Neutrophil Gelatinase-associated Lipocalin

Neutrophil gelatinase-associated lipocalin (NGAL) is a 25-kDa transport protein that is expressed by neutrophils and other epithelial cells. Although expressed in many human tissues, NGAL is significantly upregulated in the kidney in response to structural tubular damage [11]. Serial measurements of NGAL could monitor for renal injury associated with therapeutic interventions, such as diuretics used in the treatment of ADHF. NGAL can also identify ongoing renal damage earlier than creatinine. In early AKI, NGAL can be easily measured in the urine and serum 48–72 h before a rise in creatinine. The utilization of NGAL to quickly detect AKI could play a key role in the diagnosis and management of CRS type 1 and 3.

Most research on NGAL has focused on early detection of AKI. In a meta-analysis, NGAL achieved an area under the receiver-operating curve (AUC-ROC) of 0.782 in the detection of AKI in adults across all settings including cardiac surgery, critically ill patients, and after contrast infusion [12]. In addition, admission levels of serum NGAL were able to predict the development of worsening renal function in patients admitted with ADHF [13]. This was especially true in patients that presented with preserved renal function at admission, representing patients with CRS type 1. These studies depict a future role for NGAL in establishing renal dysfunction on admission and monitoring for early renal injury during hospitalization for heart failure.

In addition to detecting AKI, NGAL has prognostic utility. Elevated NGAL has been shown to have prognostic utility in patients even in the setting of normal creatinine. In a meta-analysis of critically ill patients, elevated NGAL was associated with increased risk of subsequent renal replacement therapy initiation and increased hospital mortality compared to patients with normal creatinine and normal NGAL levels [14]. In addition, plasma NGAL measured at discharge in patients admitted with ADHF was a strong prognostic indicator of 30-day outcomes. Patients that had elevations in both NGAL and BNP were at particularly high risk [15]. Within the setting of CRS, NGAL could be used to establish early subclinical renal injury and identify patients at higher risk for progressive renal dysfunction, possibly leading to therapeutic changes and improved outcomes. Although more trials are needed to establish the clinical usefulness of NGAL, it appears to add additional clinical information to more traditional biomarkers in establishing the diagnosis and prognosis of CRS.

Cystatin C

Unlike NGAL, Cystatin C (CysC) it is not a marker of tubular damage but rather a biomarker that correlates with GFR, similar to creatinine. CysC is produced by all nucleated cells, is freely filtered by the glomerulus and is not secreted by the tubules. CysC garners advantage over creatinine because it does not appear to be influenced by age, gender or muscle mass, which suggests that it could be a better predictor of GFR in certain patient populations [16]. CysC is also advantageous because it can identify AKI earlier. CysC has been shown to rise 24–48 h prior to creatinine in AKI [17].

In addition to being a stand-alone or supplemental biomarker to assess renal function, CysC has been shown to have prognostic value in heart failure and

CRS. Relatively small raises in CysC during the first 48 h of hospitalization in patients admitted with ADHF was associated with increased length of stay and was shown to be an independent predictor of 90 day mortality [18]. The independent prognostic value of CysC may be due to its superior ability to detect small changes in GFR. However, the ability of CysC to estimate GFR has recently been under scrutiny. In an analysis of 1621 middle-aged patients from the general population, CysC was not better than creatinine at estimating GFR [19].

More studies are needed to establish a definitive role for CysC as a biomarker in CRS, however current evidence would support the use of a marker of renal function such as CysC in addition to markers of renal injury in a future kidney biomarker panel.

Kidney Injury Molecule-1

Kidney injury molecule-1 (KIM-1) is a transmembrane protein that is highly expressed in undifferentiated proximal tubule epithelial cells in response to ischemic or toxic injury. Urinary KIM-1 has been shown to be elevated in patients with ischemia induced acute tubular necrosis but not in patients with CKD or other causes of AKI [20]. KIM-1 could be used to identify the etiology of kidney injury and also establish chronicity, thus differentiating type 3 and type 4 CRS.

In a study that looked at biomarker responsiveness to cessation and reinitiation of loop diuretic therapy, KIM-1 appeared to reflect subclinical renal dysfunction in response to diuretic discontinuation. In patients with chronic heart failure at presumed euvolemia, urinary KIM-1 and urinary N-acetyl-beta-D-glucosaminidase (NAG) levels were collected after discontinuation of baseline diuretic therapy and again after reinitiation of diuretics. Both urinary KIM-1 and urinary NAG levels increased significantly after diuretics were held and returned to baseline levels after diuretic reinitiation [21]. Creatinine levels remained unchanged during the study. This would suggest venous congestion plays a role in subclinical renal dysfunction and emphasizes a place in clinical practice for the use of tubular injury biomarkers, such as KIM-1, in the early detection of type 1 CRS. Early results are promising, but larger clinical studies are needed to further establish the clinical utility of KIM-1.

Proenkephalin

Enkephalins are endogenous opioids found in various organ systems that modulate many processes related to cellular and physiological stress. Proenkephalin A 119–159 (pro-ENK) is a stable precursor fragment of proenkephalin A and acts as a surrogate biomarker for enkephalins [22]. Pro-ENK is elevated in the setting of renal disease and accumulates with decreasing GFR. Recent studies suggest that Pro-ENK may also be a marker of the inflammatory processes that cause AKI. Pro-ENK has been shown to correlate closely with creatinine in cardiac surgery patients and to be elevated preoperatively in patients that go on to develop postoperative AKI [23]. In addition to predicting patients that are at risk for AKI, serial monitoring of pro-ENK throughout admission may reflect ongoing insults to the cardiorenal system, for instance factors leading to decompensation or from therapeutic interventions. In patients admitted after acute myocardial infarction, pro-ENK levels correlate with GFR, cardiac function and poor outcomes, but not with infarct size as determined by troponin elevation [24]. As a biomarker for cardiorenal syndrome, pro-ENK may prove to have utility in predicting risk and prognosis in AKI and cardiorenal syndrome although more studies are needed to fully establish the clinical utility of pro-ENK as a biomarker in cardiorenal disease.

Natriuretic Peptides

The physiologic interactions between cardiac and renal systems are intricate, and likewise, the relationship between natriuretic peptides and renal dysfunction is complex. Patients with CKD tend to have increased intravascular volume, elevated blood pressure, and increased ventricular mass, which can all lead to physiologic elevations in BNP and NT-proBNP. Though higher cutoffs have been suggested in patients with GFR <60 mL/min/1.7 m^2, natriuretic peptides retain sensitivity and specificity in the diagnosis of heart failure and are powerful predictors of prognosis in patients with CKD [25, 26]. When combined with biomarkers of renal function and injury, natriuretic peptides can add information about a patient's cardiac function and thus allow the clinician to differentiate the type of CRS and titrate therapy accordingly.

Summary

In the case report, the patient presents with elevated BNP and creatinine. The patient's clinical presentation falls within the cardio-renal syndrome, but the etiology of his decompensation is unknown on admission. Biomarkers for tubular injury, such as NGAL or KIM-1 could be used on admission to establish the etiology of renal dysfunction. Differentiating CRS type could improve outcomes by guiding the practitioner to use either renal sparing therapy or more aggressive treatment with diuretics. Biomarkers such as CysC might be used throughout admission to better approximate GFR and serial sampling of pro-ENK may help monitor ongoing insults to the cardiorenal system and predict which patients are at risk for worsening renal function. In the case, the patient's diuretic dose was decreased and ACE inhibitor held when the creatinine increased 24 h after admission. A panel of biomarkers may better differentiate between true kidney injury and improving GFR with a slowly recovering creatinine. A better understanding of renal function might have shortened the length of stay for the patient in the case. In addition, serial biomarker sampling and biomarker levels on discharge have been shown to correlate with response to treatment and with prognosis. A persistent elevation of BNP, creatinine, CysC, pro-ENK or NGAL might prompt further titration of heart failure medication prior to discharge or closer follow up after discharge. In the clinical case, measurement of biomarkers on discharge might have prompted reinitiation of ACE inhibitor, change in diuretic dose, or closer follow, thus avoiding fluid accumulation after discharge.

In conclusion, cardiac and renal function are intricately related. Use of traditional biomarkers, such as creatinine and BNP are important in defining AKI, HF and CRS, but these tests have limitations. Novel biomarkers in this field are promising and further studies should continue to define their clinical utility in cardiac and renal dysfunction.

References

1. Smith GL, Lichtman JH, Bracken MB, et al. Renal impairment and outcomes in heart failure: systematic review and meta-analysis. J Am Coll Cardiol. 2006;47(10):1987–96.
2. Forman DE, Butler J, Wang Y, et al. Incidence, predictors at admission, and impact of worsening renal function among patients hospitalized with heart failure. J Am Coll Cardiol. 2004;43(1):61–7.
3. Heywood JT, Fonarow GC, Costanzo MR, et al. High prevalence of renal dysfunction and its impact on outcome in 118,465 patients hospitalized with acute decompensated heart failure: a report from the ADHERE database. J Card Fail. 2007;13(6):422–30.
4. Ronco C, Haapio M, House AA, et al. Cardiorenal syndrome. J Am Coll Cardiol. 2008; 52(19):1527–39.
5. Damman K, Navis G, Voors AA, et al. Worsening renal function and prognosis in heart failure: systematic review and meta-analysis. J Card Fail. 2007;13(8):599–608.
6. Ljungman S, Kjekshus J, Swedberg K. Renal function in severe congestive heart failure during treatment with enalapril (the cooperative north scandinavian enalapril survival study [CONSENSUS] trial). Am J Cardiol. 1992;70(4):479–87.
7. Bellomo R, Ronco C, Kellum JA, et al. Acute renal failure–definition, outcome measures, animal models, fluid therapy and information technology needs: the second international consensus conference of the acute dialysis quality initiative (ADQI) group. Crit Care. 2004; 8(4):R204–12.
8. Mehta RL, Kellum JA, Shah SV, et al. Acute kidney injury network: report of an initiative to improve outcomes in acute kidney injury. Crit Care. 2007;11(2):R31.
9. Bellomo R. Acute renal failure. Semin Respir Crit Care Med. 2011;32(5):639–50.
10. Ferguson MA, Waikar SS. Established and emerging markers of kidney function. Clin Chem. 2012;58(4):680–9.
11. Supavekin S, Zhang W, Kucherlapati R, et al. Differential gene expression following early renal ischemia/reperfusion. Kidney Int. 2003;63(5):1714–24.
12. Haase M, Bellomo R, Devarajan P, et al. Accuracy of neutrophil gelatinase-associated lipocalin (NGAL) in diagnosis and prognosis in acute kidney injury: a systematic review and meta-analysis. Am J Kidney Dis. 2009;54(6):1012–24.
13. Aghel A, Shrestha K, Mullens W, et al. Serum neutrophil gelatinase-associated lipocalin (NGAL) in predicting worsening renal function in acute decompensated heart failure. J Card Fail. 2010;16(1):49–54.

14. Haase M, Devarajan P, Haase-Fielitz A, et al. The outcome of neutrophil gelatinase-associated lipocalin-positive subclinical acute kidney injury: a multicenter pooled analysis of prospective studies. J Am Coll Cardiol. 2011;57(17):1752–61.

15. Maisel AS, Mueller C, Fitzgerald R. Prognostic utility of plasma neutrophil gelatinase associated lipocalin in patients with acute heart failure: the NGAL EvaLuation along with B-type NaTriuretic peptide in acutely decompensated heart failure (GALLANT) trial. Eur J Heart Fail. 2011;13(8):846–51.

16. Lassus J, Harjola VP. Cystatin C: a step forward in assessing kidney function and cardiovascular risk. Heart Fail Rev. 2012;17(2):251–61.

17. Herget-Rosenthal S, Marggraf G, Husing J, et al. Early detection of acute renal failure by serum cystatin C. Kidney Int. 2004;66(3):1115–22.

18. Lassus JP, Nieminen MS, Peuhkurinen K, et al. Markers of renal function and acute kidney injury in acute heart failure: definitions and impact on outcomes of the cardiorenal syndrome. Eur Heart J. 2010;31(22):2791–8.

19. Eriksen BO, Mathisen UD, Melsom T, et al. Cystatin C is not a better estimator of GFR than plasma creatinine in the general population. Kidney Int. 2010;78(12):1305–11.

20. Han WK, Bailly V, Abichandani R, et al. Kidney injury molecule-1 (KIM-1): a novel biomarker for human renal proximal tubule injury. Kidney Int. 2002;62(1):237–44.

21. Damman K, Ng Kam Chuen MJ, MacFadyen RJ, et al. Volume status and diuretic therapy in systolic heart failure and the detection of early abnormalities in renal and tubular function. J Am Coll Cardiol. 2011;57(22):2233–41.

22. Ernst A, Köhrle J, Bergmann A. Proenkephalin A 119–159, a stable proenkephalin A precursor fragment identified in human circulation. Peptides. 2006;27(7):1835–40.

23. Shah KS, Taub P, Patel M, et al. Proenkephalin predicts acute kidney injury in cardiac surgery patients. Clin Nephrol. 2015;83(1):29–35.

24. Ng LL, Sandhu JK, Narayan H, et al. Proenkephalin and prognosis after acute myocardial infarction. J Am Coll Cardiol. 2014;63(3):280–9.

25. McCullough PA, Duc P, Omland T, et al. B-type natriuretic peptide and renal function in the diagnosis of heart failure: an analysis from the Breathing Not Properly Multinational Study. Am J Kidney Dis. 2003;41(3):571–9.

26. Anwaruddin S, Lloyd-Jones DM, Baggish A, et al. Renal function, congestive heart failure, and amino-terminal pro-brain natriuretic peptide measurement: results from the ProBNP Investigation of Dyspnea in the Emergency Department (PRIDE) Study. J Am Coll Cardiol. 2006;47(1):91–7.

27. Ronco C, McCullough P, Anker SD, et al. Cardio-renal syndromes: report from the consensus conference of the Acute Dialysis Quality Initiative. Eur Heart J. 2010;31(6):703–11.

Chapter 28
Biomarkers in Heart Failure with Preserved Ejection Fraction

Robert Colbert, Rohit Mital, and Nicholas Marston

Abstract Chronic heart failure is increasing in prevalence throughout the world and is a leading cause of morbidity and mortality in developed countries (Phan et al., Int J Cardiol 158:337–343, 2012). Clinical research has focused primarily on patients with left ventricular systolic dysfunction with reduced ejection fraction (HFrEF), but it is now understood that up to half of all patients with heart failure have preserved ejection fraction (HFpEF) (Phan et al., Int J Cardiol 158:337–343, 2012). The patients who suffer from HFpEF are usually older, have worse systemic hypertension, and are more often female compared to patients with reduced left ventricular ejection fraction. Mortality can be high for patients with HFpEF, with 70 % of all-cause mortality attributed to cardiovascular etiologies (Phan et al., Int J Cardiol 158:337–343, 2012). Multiple biomarkers have demonstrated a role in HFpEF and may be used to help aid in clinical decision-making. These include traditional markers such as naturetic peptides and troponin, as well as novel markers such as ST2 and Galectin-3.

Keywords Biomarkers in heart failure with preserved ejection fraction • Ejection fraction and biomarkers • Heart failure and preserved ejection fraction

Chronic heart failure is increasing in prevalence throughout the world and is a leading cause of morbidity and mortality in developed countries [1]. Clinical research has focused primarily on patients with left ventricular systolic dysfunction with reduced ejection fraction (HFrEF), but it is now understood that up to half of all patients with heart failure have preserved ejection fraction (HFpEF) [1]. The patients who suffer from HFpEF are usually older, have worse systemic hypertension, and

R. Colbert, BS
University of Minnesota Medical School, Minneapolis, MN, USA

R. Mital, MD
Department of Internal Medicine, University of California, San Diego, Medical Center, San Diego, CA, USA

N. Marston, MD (✉)
Department of Internal Medicine, UCSD Medical Center, San Diego, CA, USA
e-mail: nmarston@ucsd.edu

© Springer International Publishing Switzerland 2016
A.S. Maisel, A.S. Jaffe (eds.), *Cardiac Biomarkers*,
DOI 10.1007/978-3-319-42982-3_28

are more often female compared to patients with reduced left ventricular ejection fraction. Mortality can be high for patients with HFpEF, with 70% of all-cause mortality attributed to cardiovascular etiologies [1]. Multiple biomarkers have demonstrated a role in HFpEF and may be used to help aid in clinical decision-making. These include traditional markers such as naturetic peptides and troponin, as well as novel markers such as ST2 and Galectin-3. This chapter discusses each of these markers and their clinical utility in the HFpEF population.

Natriuretic Peptides

Perhaps the best described biomarkers used in acute dyspnea to diagnose heart failure are the natriuretic peptides. Of the multiple subtypes of natriuretic peptides which play a role in protection against volume overload, B-type natriuretic peptide (BNP) is a useful biomarker in heart failure because it is synthesized and released primarily from the ventricles in response to ventricular expansion and pressure overload. BNP mediates relaxation of the myocardium and regulates increases in ventricular volume through mechanisms aimed at reducing both preload and afterload via diuresis, vasodilation, and modulation of the renin-angiotensin-aldosterone system [2]. A precursor of BNP, pre-proBNP, is cleaved to proBNP and subsequently into BNP and NT-proBNP, the active and inactive components, respectively [3]. Both the BNP and NT-proBNP are now frequently used biomarkers in the evaluation of acute dyspnea.

While BNP and NT-proBNP have been shown to have high sensitivity for heart failure, recent studies have focused specifically on the role of natriuretic peptides in HFpEF. A study by Yamaguchi, et al. demonstrated that patients with HFpEF also have an elevation in BNP compared to control [4]. However, Iwanaga and colleagues showed that BNP levels may be higher in patients with depressed LV ejection fraction. More specifically, they found patients with HFpEF had median BNP levels of 105 pg/ml compared to 265 pg/ml in the HFrEF group [5]. Nonetheless, elevated BNP appears to independently predict all-cause mortality and hospitalization due to heart failure regardless of LV ejection fraction. A study by Van Veldhuisen, et al. found that LV ejection fraction alone is not associated with increased mortality, and that for a given BNP value the prognosis for patients with HFpEF was the same as for patients with HFrEF [6] (Fig. 28.1). In patients with chronic heart failure, the Val-HEFT study showed that outpatients with the highest increase in BNP levels on therapy had the highest rates of morbidity and mortality [7]. This suggests that BNP has significant value in predicting risk and prognostication for patients with HFpEF and may be useful in guiding management decisions.

Several studies have established cutoff points for BNP or NT-proBNP levels in acute dyspnea. The Breathing Not Properly Study used a cutoff value of BNP of 100 pg/ml, and reported 90% sensitivity and 76% specificity in diagnosing heart failure [8]. The PRIDE study set an NT-proBNP cutoff <300 pg/ml to rule out heart

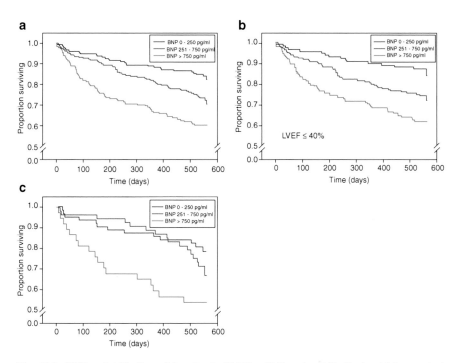

Fig. 28.1 BNP and ALL-Cause Mortality in LVEF ≤40% and >40%. Kaplan-Meier survival curves of the association between BNP and all-cause mortality in all heart failure patients (**a**),in patients with EF <40% (**b**), and in patients with LVEF >40% (**c**) (From Van Veldhuisen et al. [6], with permission.)

failure, citing a negative predictive value of 99% [9]. BNP and NT-proBNP typically correlate well to one another, although they have different absolute levels. One major difference between BNP and NT-proBNP is half-life, which is only 20 min for BNP and 1-2 h for NTproBNP. However, both assays maintain similar performance characteristics in patients with acute heart failure [3]. Of note, natriuretic levels can be falsely elevated in the elderly, females and renal dysfunction, and can be falsely low in obese patients and flash pulmonary edema [3].

Cardiac Troponins

The role of cardiac troponin is well established in acute coronary syndrome, but is also proving to have significance in heart failure. Troponins are a group of proteins involved in the modulation of muscle contraction by their effect on interaction between actin and myosin in striated muscle. The three cardiac troponins are troponin I (inhibitory), troponin C (calcium binding) and troponin T (tropomyosin binding). The cardiac troponins are encoded by a separate gene than the skeletal isoforms and vary in their structure, and thus specific assays measuring the cardiac isoforms are useful in investigation of myocardial injury [10]. Many different mechanisms may be responsible for troponin release in heart failure, including myocyte necrosis as a result of subendocardial ischemia, inflammation and oxidative stress causing cardiomyocyte damage, and altered calcium handling amongst others [11]. This detection of subclinical myocardial damage can be clinically useful in acute and chronic heart failure.

A study by Dinh, et al. showed that high sensitivity Troponin T (hsTnT) is elevated in patients with HFpEF independent of coronary artery disease, suggesting that persistent myocardial injury may play a role in the pathogenesis of HFpEF [12]. However, Santhanakrishnan and colleagues found that although HFpEF patients did have elevated hsTnT compared to control patients, hsTnT levels were higher in HFrEF patients. This may provide insight into the individual mechanisms of each of these processes and suggests HFrEF is a more myocardial specific process whereas HFpEF may be a more systemic condition [13]. Regardless of mechanism, the ADHERE study showed that the presence of positive troponin in the decompensated heart failure patient was indicative of higher risk compared to patients with negative troponin. Those with elevated troponin required more cardiac procedures, longer hospital stays, and had a higher rate of in-hospital mortality [14].

In general, the levels of troponin in heart failure patients tend to be lower and lack the acute rise and fall characteristic of acute coronary syndrome. In clinical practice, detection of heart failure based on troponin levels varies greatly depending on the assay and cutoffs utilized. In the ADHERE trial, cutoffs of TnI >0.4 ng/ml and TnT >0.01 µg/l were used and positive levels were seen in 75 % of patients with decompensated heart failure [14]. A study by the Val-HEFT investigators suggested that hsTnT may have significant value in heart failure, as TnT was positive in 92 % of patients in heart failure when a cutoff of >0.001 ng/ml was used [15]. More work will need to be done with high sensitivity troponin and heart failure to determine utility. In the meantime, it is clear that positive troponins are common in HFpEF and the degree to which they are elevated is associated with worse outcomes.

Galectin-3

Galectin-3 is a protein that belongs to the family of soluble β-galactoside-binding lectins. These proteins bind to polysaccharides, or glycans, on the surface of cells and send signals that contribute to a variety of cellular processes [16]. Galectin-3 is secreted by activated macrophages in response to aldosterone stimulation and promotes myofibroblast proliferation, leading to the deposition of excess collagen in myocytes. The end result is fibrosis and inflammation [16–18]. Animal models have demonstrated this effect in cardiac muscle, for example the overexpression of galectin-3 in rats leads to extensive cardiac fibrosis and eventually heart failure. As the levels of galectin-3 increased, so did the severity of fibrosis [19].

Human studies have evaluated galectin-3 and its performance as a surrogate marker of cardiac remodeling and fibrosis. While previous studies included all patients with heart failure, more recent studies have focused specifically on HFpEF [16–20]. Carrasco-Sánchez, et al. found that a galectin-3 level above a median of 13.8 ng/mL is an independent predictor of all-cause mortality and readmission in patients with heart failure and preserved EF [21]. In fact, the predictive value of galectin-3 was stronger in patients with preserved EF than it was in patients with reduced EF [22]. Additionally, combining plasma galectin-3 and BNP levels increased prognostic value compared to either biomarker alone [22]. An analysis of HFpEF patients in the Aldo-DHF trial found that higher galectin-3 levels at baseline were associated with worse clinical condition and an increase in galectin-3 over time was associated with an increased risk of death or hospitalization [23]. These results again held true after adjusting for naturietic peptide levels. Finally, Chen and colleagues performed a meta-analysis of nine studies that measured galectin-3 as a continuous variable and the pooled results showed that for every 1 % increase in galectin-3, the risk of all-cause mortality increased by 28 % (HR 1.28, 95 % CI 1.10–1.48) [24].

Currently, the clinically available assay categorizes heart failure patients with galectin-3 levels >17.8 ng/mL at high risk of all-cause hospitalization or mortality [23]. In the future, clinicians may be able use galectin-3 to detect the pathophysiological progression of HFpEF. The level could be used to risk stratify patients into "remodeling" (high risk) or "non-remodeling" (low risk) to help modify their treatment plans for each individual patient [17].

ST2

ST2 is a member of the interleukin-1 (IL-1) receptor family that preferentially binds IL-33. It is expressed in many tissues and cell types, and serves as a mediator of inflammation in several diseases including asthma, rheumatoid arthritis, pulmonary fibrosis, and collagen disease [25]. More recently, ST2/IL-33 system has been shown to play a role in the pathogenesis of heart failure. ST2 exists in two forms: the membrane bound ST2 ligand (ST2L) and soluble circulating ST2 (sST2). After myocardial infarction, IL-33, ST2L, and sST2 are upregulated in fibroblasts and cardiomyocytes [26]. The binding of IL-33 to ST2L is cardioprotective, as demonstrated by the reduction in hypertrophy and myocardial fibrosis that occurs when recombinant IL-33 is administered to rat cardiomyocytes [25]. However, the administration of sST2 reversed this effect, suggesting that excess levels of sST2 bind and neutralize IL-33 [17]. The cardioprotective potential of this ST2/IL-33 system has generated a lot of interest leading to many studies in the heart failure population.

In the PRIDE study, patients who were diagnosed with acute heart failure had significantly higher sST2 levels than those who were not, and these levels helped predict 1-year mortality [16, 17]. In fact, sST2 levels were at least as predictive of

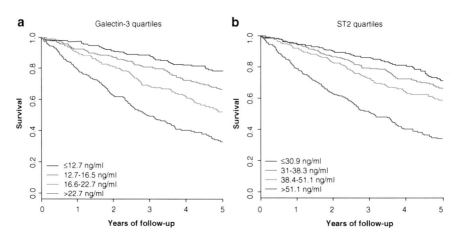

Fig. 28.2 Kaplan Meier curves according to Galectin-3 and ST2. (**a**) Survival according to Galectin-3 quartiles. (**b**) Survival according to ST2 quartiles (From Bayes-Genis et al. [31], with permission.)

death as NT-proBNP [17]. Higher levels of sST2 have also been shown to correlate with increased heart failure severity, increased ventricular filling pressures, and decreased LVEF on echocardiography [27]. sST2 has been especially promising in its ability to assess heart failure risk after acute MI. In the TIMI-14 and ENTIRE-TIMI-23 trials, high sST2 levels following an ST-elevation myocardial infarction was associated with development of heart failure and death within 30 days [17]. In another study, levels of sST2 correlated with infarct size and predicted LV functional recovery after MI [28].

Interestingly, sST2 concentrations are lower in HFpEF than in HFrEF, although the sST2 level remains an independent predictor of mortality regardless of LVEF [29]. A study of patients with severe heart failure with reduced EF revealed that percentage changes in levels of sST2 are better able to predict cardiovascular admission or worsening renal function than NT-proBNP [30]. In a comparison of sST2 and galectin-3, it appears that sST2 outperforms galectin-3 in predicting 5-year mortality in patients with chronic heart failure [31] (Fig. 28.2). This suggests that sST2 may be especially useful in the outpatient setting and may allow for improved risk stratification and tailored management in the future [32].

Conclusion

Heart failure with preserved ejection fraction is a complex disease with multiple factors contributing to cardiac dysfunction. Identifying high-risk patients early is important to allow for appropriate management and interventions [21]. The biomarkers covered in this chapter serve as tools for the clinician to diagnose and assess disease severity and progression. While more research is needed in the field, the current evidence provides a promising glimpse into how these biomarkers may be used to improve heart failure management in the future.

Case 1: Utility of HFPEF Biomarkers in the Inpatient Setting

A 69 year old man presents to the emergency department with a 5 day history of shortness of breath on exertion and lower extremity swelling. He normally performs manual labor on his ranch without any problem. However, over the past several days he has had shortness of breath with work and even when walking around his house. Two days ago, he reports being unable to lie flat in bed and woke up multiple times with shortness of breath. He also complains of being unable to fit into his shoes because of the swelling. The patient's past medical history is significant for long-standing hypertension and hyperlipidemia for which he takes losaratan, nifedipine and atorvastatin. He is a current smoker with a 30 pack year history. Vital signs on presentation are significant for blood pressure of 125/80, heart rate of 80, respiratory rate of 18, and SpO_2 of 90 % on room air. Physical examination reveals regular rate and rhythm with no audible murmur or extra heart sounds, bibasilar crackles, JVP elevated to 15 cm, and 5 mm pitting edema in the lower extremities bilaterally to the knees. Chest radiograph demonstrates cardiomegaly and increased broncho-vascular markings with bilateral pleural effusions consistent with cardiogenic pulmonary edema. BNP and BNPP are noted to be markedly elevated, with levels of 1384 pg/ml (ref range <100 pg/ml) and 14,610 pg/ml (ref range 0–899 pg/ml), respectively. Troponin T is 0.09 ng/ml (ref range <0.01 ng/ml). Echocardiogram reveals mild concentric LV hypertrophy with moderate enlargement of left atria, normal LV size and systolic function and left ventricular ejection fraction of 63 %. Mild diastolic dysfunction with impaired relaxation is noted. A diagnosis of heart failure with preserved ejection fraction is made and the patient is admitted to the hospital for further evaluation and treatment.

Case 2: Utility of HFPEF Biomarkers in the Inpatient Setting

A 76-year-old woman presents to the clinic with symptoms of dyspnea and exercise intolerance over the last 3 weeks. Normally she walks about one mile every day, but she has recently noticed increased fatigue and trouble breathing after about 3 blocks. At the end of the day, she also notices increased swelling around her ankles that does not completely resolve by morning. She denies fever, chest pain, cough, orthopnea, PND, lightheadedness, or syncope. She is widowed and lives at home by herself. Her past medical history is significant for hypertension and type II diabetes for 10 years for which she takes HCTZ and metformin. Vital signs show a blood pressure of 160/90, heart rate of 75, and normal respiratory rate and O2 saturation. Physical exam reveals normal S1 and S2 with no detectable murmurs and clear breath sounds. Her JVP is estimated at about 10 cm. Chest radiograph reveals mild cardiomegaly and trace pulmonary edema. BMP and CBC are within normal limits. NT-proBNP levels are mildly elevated at 400 pm/mL (ref range <220 pm/mL). The soluble ST2 (sST2) level is elevated at 35 ng/mL (ref range for women 7.2–33.5 ng/mL) and the galectin-3 level (Gal3) is at 16.1 ng/mL (median in patients with HF 13.8 ng/mL). Echocardiography is subsequently obtained which reveals increased thickness of the left ventricle with normal size cavity, left atrial enlargement, and a left ventricular ejection fraction of 65 %. Doppler studies show a decreased early (*E*) mitral valve flow velocity and slightly increased late (*A*) mitral valve flow velocity (*E/A* ratio of 0.4). Tissue Doppler shows abnormal left ventricular relaxation. These studies are consistent with a diagnosis of mild diastolic heart failure, or heart failure with preserved ejection fraction (HFpEF). The patient is started on lisinopril for blood pressure control, Lasix for diuresis, and instructed to follow a salt-restricted diet. Follow up is scheduled for 2 weeks later.

References

1. Phan TT, Shivu GN, et al. The pathophysiology of heart failure with preserved ejection fraction: from molecular mechanisms to exercise haemodynamics. Int J Cardiol. 2012;158:337–43.
2. Nakagawa O, Ogawa Y, Itoh H, et al. Rapid transcriptional activation and early mRNA turn-over of brain natriuretic peptide in cardiocyte hypertrophy. Evidence for brain natriuretic peptide as an "emergency" cardiac hormone against ventricular overload. J Clin Invest. 1995; 96:1280–7.
3. Daniels LB, Maisel AS. Natriuretic peptides. J Am Coll Cardiol. 2007;50:2357–68.
4. Yamaguchi H, Yoshida J, Yamamoto K, et al. Elevation of plasma brain natriuretic peptide is a hallmark of diastolic heart failure independent of ventricular hypertrophy. J Am Coll Cardiol. 2004;43:55–60.
5. Iwanaga Y, Nishi I, Furuichi S, Noguchi T, Sase K, Kihara Y, et al. B-type natriuretic peptide strongly reflects diastolic wall stress in patients with chronic heart failure: comparison between systolic and diastolic heart failure. J Am Coll Cardiol. 2006;47(4):742–8.
6. Van Veldhuisen DJ, Linssen GC, Jaarsma T, et al. B-type natriuretic peptide and prognosis in heart failure patients with preserved and reduced ejection fraction. J Am Coll Cardiol. 2013;61(14):1498–506.
7. Cohn JN, Tognoni G. A randomized trial of the angiotensin-receptor blocker valsartan in chronic heart failure. N Engl J Med. 2001;345:1667–75.
8. Maisel AS, Krishnaswamy P, Nowak RM, et al. Rapid measurement of B-type natriuretic peptide in the emergency diagnosis of heart failure. N Engl J Med. 2002;347:161–7.
9. Januzzi Jr JL, Camargo CA, Anwaruddin S, Baggish AL, Chen AA, Krauser DG, Tung R, Cameron R, Nagurney JT, Chae CU, Lloyd-Jones DM, Brown DF, Foran-Melanson S, Sluss PM, Lee-Lewandrowski E, Lewandrowski KB. The N-terminal Pro-BNP investigation of dyspnea in the emergency department (PRIDE) study. Am J Cardiol. 2005;95:948–54.
10. Coudrey L. The troponins. Arch Intern Med. 1998;158:1173–80.
11. Kociol RD, Pang PS, Gheorghiade M, et al. Troponin elevation in heart failure prevalence, mechanisms, and clinical implications. J Am Coll Cardiol. 2010;56:1071–8.
12. Dinh W, Nickl W, Futh R, et al. High sensitive troponin T and heart fatty acid binding protein: novel biomarker in heart failure with normal ejection fraction? A cross-sectional study. BMC Cardiovasc Disord. 2011;11:41.

13. Santhanakrishnan R, Chong JP, Ng TP, et al. Growth differentiation factor 15, ST2, high-sensitivity troponin T, and N-terminal pro brain natriuretic peptide in heart failure with preserved vs. reduced ejection fraction. Eur J Heart Fail. 2012;14(12):1338–47.
14. Peacock 4th WF, De Marco T, Fonarow GC, ADHERE Investigators, et al. Cardiac troponin and outcome in acute heart failure. N Engl J Med. 2008;358(20):2117–26.
15. Latini R, Masson S, Anand IS, et al. Prognostic value of very low plasma concentrations of troponin T in patients with stable chronic heart failure. Circulation. 2007;116:1242–9.
16. Shah KS, Maisel AS. Novel biomarkers in heart failure with preserved ejection fraction. Heart Fail Clin. 2014;10(3):471–9.
17. Iqbal N, Wentworth B, Choudhary R, et al. Cardiac biomarkers: new tools for heart failure management. Cardiovasc Diagn Ther. 2012;2(2):147–64. doi:10.3978/j.issn.2223-3652.2012.06.03.
18. Yang RY, Rabinovich GA, Liu FT. Galectins: structure, function and therapeutic potential. Expert Rev Mol Med. 2008;13:e17–39.
19. de Boer RA, Voors AA, Muntendam P, van Gilst WH, van Veldhuisen DJ. Galectin-3: a novel mediator of heart failure development and progression. Eur J Heart Fail. 2009;11:811–7.
20. Shah RV, Chen-Tournoux AA, Picard MH, van Kimmenade RR, Januzzi JL. Galectin-3, cardiac structure and function, and long-term mortality in patients with acutely decompensated heart failure. Eur J Heart Fail. 2010;12:826–32.
21. Carrasco-Sanchez FJ, Aramburu-Bodas O, Salamanca-Bautista P, Morales-Rull JL, Galisteo-Almeda L, Paez-Rubio MI, Arias-Jimenez JL, Aguayo-Canela M, Perez-Calvo JI. Predictive value of serum galectin-3 levels in patients with acute heart failure with preserved ejection fraction. Int J Cardiol. 2013;169:177–82.
22. de Boer RA, Lok DJ, Jaarsma T, van der Meer P, Voors AA, Hillege HL, van Veldhuisen DJ. Predictive value of plasma galectin-3 levels in heart failure with reduced and preserved ejection fraction. Ann Med. 2011;43:60–8.
23. Edelmann F, Holzendorf V, et al. Galectin-3 in patients with heart failure with preserved ejection fraction: results from the Aldo-DHF trial. Eur J Heart Fail. 2015;17(2):214–23. doi:10.1002/ejhf.203. Epub 2014 Nov 24.
24. Chen A, Hou W, et al. Prognostic value of serum galectin-3 in patients with heart failure: a meta-analysis. Int J Cardiol. 2015;182:168–70.
25. Anand IS, Rector TS, et al. Prognostic value of soluble ST2 in the valsartan heart failure trial. Circ Heart Fail. 2014;7:418–26.
26. Weinberg EO, Shimpo M, De Keulenaer GW, MacGillivray C, Tominaga S, Solomon SD, Rouleau JL, Lee RT. Expression and regulation of ST2, an interleukin-1 receptor family member, in cardiomyocytes and myocardial infarction. Circulation. 2002;106:2961–6.
27. Shah RV, Chen-Tournoux AA, Picard MH, et al. Serum levels of the interleukin-1 receptor family member ST2, cardiac structure and function, and long-term mortality in patients with acute dyspnea. Circ Heart Fail. 2009;2:311–31.
28. Weir RA, Miller AM, Murphy GE, et al. Serum soluble ST2: a potential novel mediator in left ventricular and infarct remodeling after acute myocardial infarction. J Am Coll Cardiol. 2010;55:243–50.
29. Manzano-Fernandez S, Mueller T, Pascual-Figal D, et al. Usefulness of soluble concentrations of interleukin family member ST2 as predictor of mortality in patients with acutely decompensated heart failure relative to left ventricular ejection fraction. Am J Cardiol. 2011;107(2):259–67.
30. Piper SE, Sherwood RA, et al. Serial soluble ST2 for the monitoring of pharmacologically optimized chronic stable heart failure. Int J Cardiol. 2015;178:284–91.
31. Bayes-Genis A, de Antonio M, Vila J, et al. Head-to-head comparison of 2 myocardial fibrosis biomarkers for long-term heart failure risk stratification: ST2 versus galectin-3. J Am Coll Cardiol. 2014;63(2):158–66.
32. Oghlakian GO, Sipahi I, Fang JC. Treatment of heart failure with preserved ejection fraction: have we been pursuing the wrong paradigm? Mayo Clin Proc. 2011;86(6):531–9. doi:10.4065/mcp.2010.0841.

Index

© Springer International Publishing Switzerland 2016
A.S. Maisel, A.S. Jaffe (eds.), *Cardiac Biomarkers*,
DOI 10.1007/978-3-319-42982-3

367